eat smart
stay well

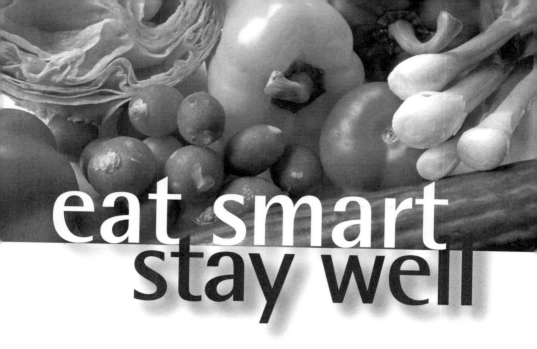

eat smart
stay well

Power foods that could save your life!

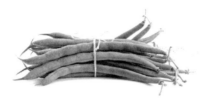

Susanna Lyle

University of Hawai'i Press
Honolulu

Text © Susanna Lyle, 2009
Typographical design © David Bateman Ltd, 2009
Photographs ShutterStock.com

Susanna Lyle asserts her right to be identified as the author of this work.

First published in 2009 by David Bateman Ltd,
30 Tarndale Grove, Albany, Auckland, New Zealand

Published in 2011 in North America by
University of Hawai'i Press
2840 Kolowalu Street
Honolulu, HI 96822
www.uhpress.hawaii.edu

Library of Congress Cataloging-in-Publication Data

Lyle, Susanna.
  Eat smart stay well : power foods that could save your life! / Susanna Lyle.
    p. cm.
  First published in 2009 by David Bateman Ltd, Auckland, New Zealand.
  Includes bibliographical references and index.
  ISBN 978-0-8248-3593-4 (pbk. : alk. paper)
  1. Nutrition. 2. Plants, Edible--Health aspects. 3. Diet in disease. I. Title.
  RA784.L96 2011
  613.2--dc22
                        2010052099

Typesetting: IslandBridge
Cover design: Sublime Design
Printed in China by Everbest Printing Co. Ltd

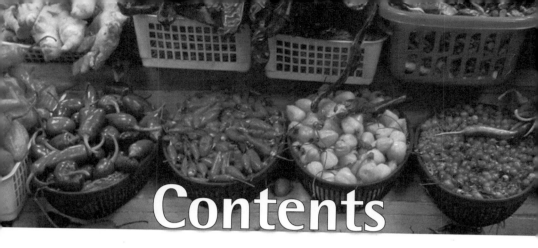

Contents

About this book

There is an ongoing surge of interest in the foods we eat and how they affect our health. Can specific foods really reduce the incidence of some of our modern-day diseases? Research is confirming this several-fold, and these findings, not surprisingly, often concur with the traditional usage of foods by our grandparents to cure a wide range of maladies.

Much exciting evidence is coming to light on the ability of many foods to reduce the development of diseases such as cancer, heart disease and diabetes. It has been estimated that 80% of heart disease, stroke, and type-2 diabetes, and 40% of cancer could be avoided through eating a healthy diet, along with regular physical activity.

Perhaps this basic and important information is coming to light now because most prior research has focused on pharmaceuticals and commercial food products: little funding has been available to study, say, the common tomato in depth. Yet, this food is one of the many that has now been shown to have wondrous health properties.

Keeping our food choices simple is an important key, as is avoiding overprocessing. In some ways, a return to the approach of our ancestors to food, but with the added knowledge from modern-day research plus access to a much wider range of ingredients, is becoming recognised as the dynamic future of food. A further recurring insight is that it is often the actual combination of a food's vitamins and compounds that determines its effectiveness. Separate these nutrients into their individual components and their efficacy is often greatly reduced; thus, regularly eating a *range* of fresh foods further enhances health and extends life span.

The most health-giving foods have been selected for inclusion within this book. Descriptions of their many benefits, the nutrients they contain, plus suggestions for their usage with other foods to optimise their overall effectiveness are included. Although 'health food' has in the past tended to be regarded as perhaps somewhat dull, I believe people's perceptions are now changing. Indeed, the majority of foods described within are bursting with flavour, and the inspiration of many of today's creative chefs, who are blending, mixing and creating delicious new combinations, is accelerating appreciation of this new food revolution.

Book layout

PART ONE: What Power Foods Can Do is the place to go if you're looking for a food for a particular health need. These foods are proven to significantly reduce the development, and sometimes even reverse the progression, of many modern-day diseases. The Top 5 food choices for specific health needs are given, as well as a range of other foods that are of benefit. There is also an 'Essential Power Foods' table that provides a guide to the main food groups recommended to achieve a complete and healthy diet.

PART TWO: Describes what it is within plant foods that are of such benefit and looks at how our understanding of the power of plant foods can be used to improve our health and wellbeing. It covers all the main food groups: proteins, carbohydrates, fibre, fats, vitamins as well as the exciting area of secondary plant compounds, such as flavanoids and polyphenolics, on which much recent research has been conducted.

PART THREE: The third and main part of this book provides information on 115 health-promoting plant foods that have been chosen for their wondrous nutritional benefits, and because they are easy to obtain (or grow). For each food, up-to-date unbiased scientific information is given, along with tasty ideas for using the foods. You will be amazed at what the humble apple, apricot and avocado can do for you — and that's just A!

For those who wish to delve deeper into these findings, there is a bibliography.

Place this book beside your recipe books so that you can confidently select which herbs, spices, fruits, nuts, vegetables and grains will help you to design a truly delicious and nutritious menu.

If you want to find out more about the health benefits of plants, you can read how to grow and enjoy over 500 food plants in Susanna's books: *Discovering Fruit & Nuts* and *Discovering Vegetables, Herbs & Spices* and visit her website: **www.growhealthy.net**

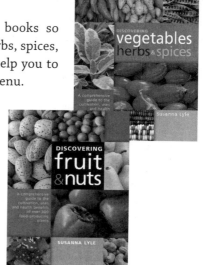

Part One:
What Power Foods Can Do

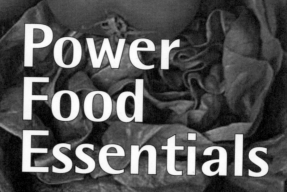

Power Food Essentials

Including representatives from the following food groups in daily meals can hugely enhance your health, enable you to live longer and reduce the risk of developing many of today's debilitating and sometimes fatal diseases.

The basic rules for cooking and eating are:

♦ choose fresh food
♦ choose food that has been altered as little as possible
♦ cook food minimally
♦ and eat plenty of plant foods.

Ensure your diet includes representatives from the following food groups.

GREEN LEAFY VEGETABLES

Key benefits
Rich in vitamin K and minerals. Brassicas are rich in isothiocyanates.

Examples
Broccoli, Brussels sprouts, chard, kale, spinach, watercress, rocket and nasturtium, horseradish, mustard and wasabi.

PURPLE AND RED BERRIES

Key benefits
Super-rich in antioxidant anthocyanins and flavonoids.

Examples
Bilberries, blackcurrant, blueberries, cherries, cranberries, elderberries, grapes, juniper berries, raspberries, sea buckthorn, strawberries, wolfberries and Goji berries.

YELLOW, ORANGE, GREEN FLESHED FRUITS AND VEGETABLES

Key benefits
Rich in carotenoids (vitamins A and C).

Examples
Apricots, carrots, guavas, kiwifruit, lemons, oranges, papaya, passion fruit, tomatoes, capsicums.

WHOLE (OR MINIMALLY PROCESSED) GRAINS

Key benefits
Wonderful fibre providers and rich in B vitamins, proteins and 'good' oils.

Examples
Amaranth, barley, beans, buckwheat, lentils, oats, peas, quinoa, rye, wheat.

NUTRITIOUS NUTS

Key benefits   Rich in 'good oils', protein, minerals and vitamin E.

Examples   Almonds, Brazil nuts, cashews, hazelnuts, peanuts, pinenuts, pistachios.

FRESH HERBS

Key benefits   Full of secondary plant compounds; both seeds and dried herbs are very rich in vitamins, minerals, protein and fibre.

Examples   Basil, cilantro, dill, lemon balm, marjoram, parsley, rosemary, sage, thyme.

CURRY

Key benefits   Exceptional levels of secondary plant compounds; also vitamins, fibre and minerals.

Examples   Cardamom, chilli, cinnamon, coriander, cumin, garlic, ginger, tamarind, turmeric.

SEEDS

Key benefits   Rich in beneficial oils, minerals, protein and fibre.

Examples   Alfalfa, linseed, pumpkin, sunflower, sesame seeds.

VITALISING VEGETABLES

Key benefits   Diverse plants that are rich in minerals, vitamins and oils.

Examples   Asparagus, avocado, beetroot, dandelion, endive, globe artichokes, horseradish, Jerusalem artichokes, olives, onions, seaweed, sweet potato.

DRIED FRUITS

Key benefits   Very rich in antioxidant secondary plant compounds and vitamins, fibre, sugar and minerals.

Examples   Apricots, currants, dates, figs, prunes, raisins.

OTHERS

Key benefits   Rich in secondary plant compounds, vitamins and minerals.

Examples   Cocoa, hops, liquorice, spirulina, tea, yeast.

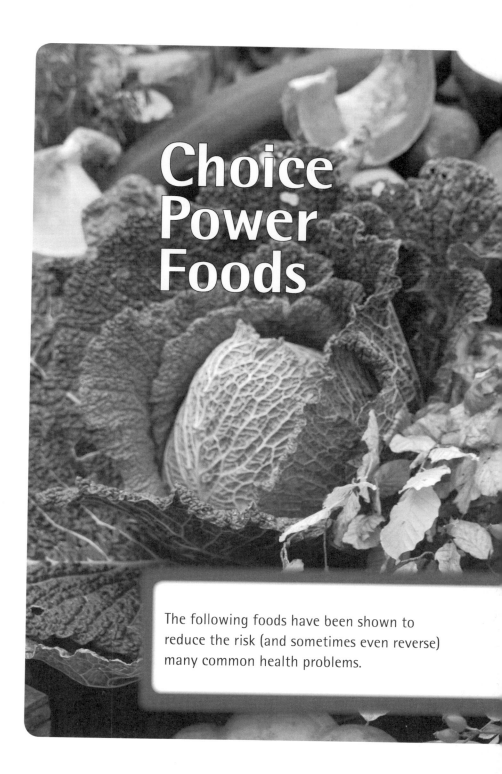

Choice Power Foods

The following foods have been shown to reduce the risk (and sometimes even reverse) many common health problems.

Allergy fighters and autoimmune-disease inhibitors

EFFECTS	Reduce susceptibility to allergies and autoimmune diseases (e.g. arthritis, osteoporosis, type-1 diabetes). Act as anti-inflammatories.
TOP 5	Avocado, bilberry, garlic, olives, pomegranate

OTHER FOOD OPTIONS	Almonds, anise, apples, barley, beetroot, blackberries, borage, buckwheat, capers, cardamom, celery, chamomile, cherries, chilli, currants, fennel, figs, ginger, grapes, hops, juniper, lemon balm, linseed, nettles, oats, onion, parsley, passion fruit, peanuts, pecans, peppercorns, pinenuts, purslane, quinoa, rosemary, safflower, sage, sea buckthorn, seaweed, spirulina, sunflower seeds, tea, tomatoes, turmeric, walnuts, watercress, wheat (whole), wolfberries and Goji berries, yeast

Blood-sugar level stabilisers

EFFECTS	Keep systems even, make energy last longer, are good for weight loss, people managing diabetes.
TOP 5	Cinnamon, oats, pinenuts, pistachios, rye

OTHER FOOD OPTIONS	Almonds, avocado, barley, Brazil nuts, buckwheat, capers, cashews, chamomile, cherries, chicory, chillies, cloves, coriander, cranberries, cumin, dandelion, elderberries, fennel, garden cress, garlic, grapes, hazelnuts, Jerusalem artichoke, kiwifruit, lemons and limes, lentils, liquorice, linseed, macadamia nuts, marjoram, mustard, peas, pecans, peppercorns, plantain, pomegranate, raspberries, rice (brown), seaweed, sesame seeds, spinach, spirulina, tamarind, tea, walnuts, wolfberries, Goji berries, yeast

Heart foods (reduce blood pressure & cholesterol)

EFFECTS	Improve heart and blood vessel health; reduce cholesterol and blood pressure. Enhance natural heart rhythm and reduce blood-clot formation.
TOP 5	Asparagus, buckwheat, cherries, pistachio nuts, rye

    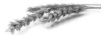

OTHER FOOD OPTIONS	Alfalfa, almonds, amaranth, apples, avocado, bananas, barley, basil, beetroots, bilberries, blackberries, blueberries, borage oil, Brazil nuts, capers, cardamom, carrots, cashews, celery, chard, chicory, Chinese greens, cinnamon, cocoa, cranberries, dandelion, dates, dill, endive, figs, garden cress, garlic, ginger, globe artichokes, grapefruit, guavas, hazelnuts, Jerusalem artichokes, kale, kiwifruit, lemons, limes, lemon balm, lentils, liquorice, linseed, macadamia nuts, marjoram, oats, onions, oranges, parsley, peas, peanuts, pecans, peppercorns, pinenuts, plantain, plums and prunes, pomegranate, raspberries, rice, rocket, rosemary, safflower, sea buckthorn, seaweed, sesame seeds, soy beans, spinach, spirulina, strawberries, sunflower seeds, sweet potatoes, tamarind, tea, tomatoes, turmeric, walnuts, wheat, wolfberries and Goji berries

Cancer deterrents

EFFECTS	Inhibit and even reverse cancer.
TOP 5 +1	Blueberries, Brussels sprouts, garden and watercress, garlic, lemons and limes, tomatoes

OTHER FOOD OPTIONS	Alfalfa, almonds, apricots, asparagus, avocado, barley, basil, beetroot, blackberries, borage, Brazil nuts, broccoli, buckwheat, carrots, celery, chamomile, chard, cherries, Chinese greens, cloves, cocoa, coriander, cranberries, cumin, currants, dandelion, dill, figs, ginger, grapefruit, grapes, guavas, hazelnuts, hops, horseradish, Jerusalem artichoke, juniper berries, kale, kiwifruit, lemon balm, liquorice, linseed, marjoram, mints, nasturtium, nettles, oats, olives, onions, oranges, parsley, peanuts, peppercorns, pistachios, plums, prunes, pomegranate, purslane, raspberries, rice, rocket, rosemary, rye, sage, sea buckthorn, seaweeds, sesame seeds, soy beans, spirulina, strawberries, sweet potatoes, tea, thyme, turmeric, walnuts, wolfberries and Goji berries

Gut foods	
EFFECTS	Ease spasms that cause indigestion, flatulence, irritable bowel and feelings of nausea.
TOP 5	Cumin, dill, ginger, lemons and limes, mint and peppermint
OTHER FOOD OPTIONS	Amaranth, anise, bananas, cardamom, cardoon, chamomile, cinnamon, dates, fennel, globe artichoke, grapefruit, guavas, hops, juniper berries, liquorice, linseed, marjoram, nettles, olives, parsley, pumpkin, purslane, tamarind, thyme, turmeric

Immune-system enhancers

EFFECTS	Enhance disease resistance and deter pathogens by acting as antibacterials, antifungals and antivirals.
TOP 5	Cumin, ginger, horseradish, rosemary, thyme

   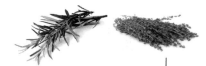

OTHER FOOD OPTIONS	Alfalfa, almonds, amaranth, anise, apricots, asparagus, avocado, basil, borage oil, Brazil nuts, broccoli, capsicums and chilli, cardamom, cashews, celery, chamomile, cinnamon, cloves, coriander, cranberries, currants, dandelion, dill, elderberries, fennel, garden cress, garlic, grapefruit, guavas, hops, juniper berries, kale, kiwifruit, lemon balm, lemons and limes, liquorice, marjoram, mints, mustard, nasturtium, nettles, nutmeg and mace, olives, onions, oranges, parsley, passion fruits, peppercorns, plums and prunes, pomegranate, pumpkin seeds, safflower, sage, sea buckthorn, sesame seeds, soy beans (soy sauce), spirulina, strawberries, sunflower seeds, tea, turmeric, watercress, wolfberries and Goji berries, yeast

Fibre foods

EFFECTS	Keep the passage of digested food regular and support healthy gut bacteria.
TOP 5	Barley, chicory, oats, plantain, rice (brown)

OTHER FOOD OPTIONS	Alfalfa, almonds, apples, asparagus, avocado, beans, Brussels sprouts, buckwheat, cardoon, dandelion, figs, Jerusalem artichokes, globe artichokes, kale, kiwifruit, lentils, oranges, peas, plums and prunes, purslane, quinoa, rye, wheat

Energy boosters	
EFFECTS	Provide quick energy sources.
TOP 5	Bananas, blackcurrants (red, white), dates, figs, prunes

OTHER FOOD OPTIONS	Apples, apricots, blackberries, beetroot, carrot, cherries, grapes (currants), guava, kiwifruit, oranges, plums, pomegranate, raspberries, strawberries, wolfberries and Goji berries

Strength builders	
EFFECTS	Build skeletal muscle.
TOP 5	Peanuts, pistachios, quinoa, soy beans, spirulina

    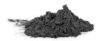

OTHER FOOD OPTIONS	Alfalfa, almonds, amaranth, beans, Brazil nuts, buckwheat, cashews, cocoa, hazelnuts, lentils, oats, peas, pecans, pinenuts, pumpkin seeds, purslane seeds, rye, safflower, seaweed (nori), sesame seeds, sunflower seeds, walnuts, wheat (whole)

Pain killers and wound healers

EFFECTS	Reduce pain, ease muscle aches, speed up skin and internal wound healing.
TOP 5	Basil, chamomile, chillies, cloves, tamarind

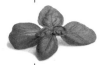

OTHER FOOD OPTIONS	Almond, cardamom, cashews, cherries, ginger, grapes, hops, horseradish, lemons, limes, marjoram, mint, nettles, nutmeg, olives, onions, oranges, parsley, passion fruit, peppercorns, pumpkin seeds, purslane, rosemary, sea buckthorn, seaweed, spinach, thyme, turmeric

Urinary tract conditioners

EFFECTS	Reduce urinary tract infections and act as diuretics.
TOP 5	Cranberries, dandelion, horseradish, juniper berries, nasturtium

   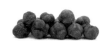

OTHER FOOD OPTIONS	Blueberries, cinnamon, grapefruit, hops, nettles, parsley, plantains, purslane, tea, watercress

Bone enhancers

EFFECTS	Build healthy bones and teeth; reduce debilitating bone diseases.
TOP 5	Kale, parsley, rocket, spinach, watercress
OTHER FOOD OPTIONS	Almonds, amaranth, apricots, asparagus, barley, broccoli, Brussels sprouts, capers, chard, chicory, Chinese greens, coriander (cilantro), dandelion, garden cress, hazelnuts, liquorice, linseed, marjoram, mustard greens, nettles, onions, peppercorns, prunes, pumpkin seeds, quinoa, rosemary, safflower, seaweed, sesame seeds, soybeans, spices (although only a little are eaten, most are very rich in calcium), thyme, walnuts

Skin and hair boosters

EFFECTS	Condition, soothe, smooth and shine. Reduce skin inflammations and infections.
TOP 5	Chamomile, lemon and lime, orange, rosemary, seaweeds

 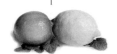

OTHER FOOD OPTIONS	Almonds, amaranth, apples, avocado, basil, borage, Brazil nuts, cardamom, cashews, cocoa, dandelion, garlic, ginger, guava, linseed, macadamia nuts, nettles, oats, olives, parsley, passion fruit, pecans, pinenuts, pomegranate, pumpkin seeds, purslane, sage, sea buckthorn, sesame seeds, sweet potatoes, tamarind, tea, thyme, watercress, wolfberries and Goji berries

Eyesight improvers

EFFECTS	Delay age-related sight problems and improve vision.
TOP 5	Apricots, bilberries, pinenuts, spinach, sweet potatoes

   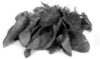

OTHER FOOD OPTIONS	Almonds, asparagus, avocado, borage, broccoli, Brussels sprouts, buckwheat, capers, carrots, chard, chicory, chilli and sweet peppers, coriander (cilantro), endive, cranberries, dandelion, garden cress, kale, kiwifruit, lentils, marjoram, mustard greens, nasturtium, nettles, oranges, parsley, passion fruit, peas, peanuts, pistachios, pumpkin, rocket, rosemary, tamarind, thyme, tomatoes, turmeric, watercress, wolfberries and Goji berries

Brain foods

EFFECTS	Improve neuronal activity, promote calm, are antidepressants and can reduce neurological disease.
TOP 5	Chamomile, hops, lemon balm, passion fruit, turmeric

OTHER FOOD OPTIONS	Almonds, beetroots, blueberries, broccoli, chard, cherries, chicory, Jerusalem artichoke, chilli, cocoa, cranberries, dates, fennel, garlic, grapes, hazelnuts, kiwifruit, lentils, liquorice, linseed, nettle, nutmeg and mace, oats, onions, parsley, peanuts, pistachios, pomegranate, purslane seeds, quinoa, rice (brown), sage, sesame seeds, spinach, spirulina, sunflower seeds, wolfberries and Goji berries, yeast

Women's foods

EFFECTS	Help manage menstrual problems, are good during pregnancy and relieve menopausal symptoms (also see Bone foods).
TOP 5 +2	Hops, liqourice, linseed, pomegranate, sage, soy beans, sesame seeds
OTHER FOOD OPTIONS	Alfalfa, amaranth, anise, asparagus, avocado, beetroots, Brazil nuts, Chinese greens, cocoa, dill, fennel, ginger, hazelnuts, lentils, marjoram, mustard, nettle, orange, parsley, passion fruit, peanuts, raspberries, rye, safflower, seaweed, spinach, sunflower seeds, thyme, wheat (whole), wolfberries and Goji berries, yeast

Men's foods

EFFECTS	Increase sperm production and health and provide other overall benefits.
TOP 5	Brazil nuts, olives, pinenuts, pumpkin seeds, tomatoes

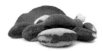

OTHER FOOD OPTIONS	Anise, barley, broccoli, cardamom, coriander, chillies, cloves, coriander, cumin, currants, figs, garlic, guava, kale, kiwifruits, marjoram, mustard, nettles, nutmeg and mace, oats, parsley, pecans, rosemary, rye, sesame seeds, spirulina, sunflower seeds, tea, thyme, wheat (whole), wolfberries and Goji berries, yeast

Tooth-strengthening foods

EFFECTS	Reduce bacterial tooth decay and keep the mouth healthy.
TOP 5	Avocado, olives, pinenuts, spirulina, wolfberries

OTHER FOOD OPTIONS	Apples, basil, cardamom, cashews, chamomile, cinnamon, cloves, cranberries, cumin, elderberries, fennel, hops, lemon balm, liquorice, nutmeg, mace, peppercorns, pomegranate, purslane, rosemary, sage, strawberries, tea, thyme

Lung cleansing foods

EFFECTS	Eases coughs, flu and other chest complaints by soothing muscle spasms.
TOP 5	Cocoa, horseradish, liquorice, nasturtium, watercress

   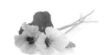

OTHER FOOD OPTIONS	Anise, chillies, cranberries, currants, elderberries, garlic, ginger, guavas, hops, juniper berries, marjoram, mints, nettle, nutmeg and mace, onions, peppercorns, rosemary, sunflower seeds, thyme

Liver, gall bladder and 'blood cleaners'

EFFECTS	Enhance liver health and act as 'blood tonics'.
TOP 5	Dandelion, globe artichoke, liquorice, sage, seaweed

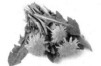   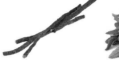 

OTHER FOOD OPTIONS	Almonds, apples, beetroot, bilberries, borage oil, capers, chard, chicory, cumin, fennel, figs, grapefruit, hops, juniper berries, nutmeg and mace, olives, oranges, parsley, pistachios, rosemary, safflower, sea buckthorn, sesame seeds, tomatoes, turmeric

Part Two:
How Power Foods Work

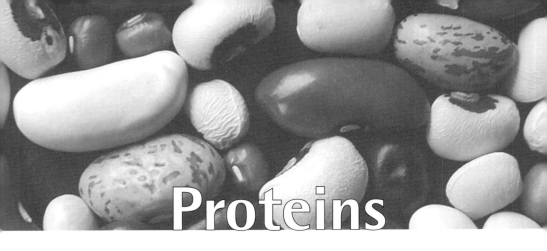

Proteins

Proteins are vital. They are needed for many processes within the body, from their inclusion within enzymes, to their use in the formation of all cells and every body fluid, except bile and urine. Proteins are often very large, complex molecules. As enzymes, these complex molecules are essential for virtually every stage of every biochemical reaction: they speed up the change of converting one compound to another. Without them, life would cease within seconds.

Proteins are made up of subunits of fairly simple molecules called amino acids. It is the arrangement of amino acids into chains and the folding and linking of these that determines the amazing complexity of the many proteins within our bodies.

Amino acids

Although hundreds of different amino acids are present in the body, only 22 are involved in protein construction. Of these, 10 are essential amino acids, meaning that they cannot be synthesised by the body and, therefore, must be supplied in the diet. They are: histidine, isoleucine, leucine, lysine, methionine, phenylalanine, threonine, tryptophan, valine and arginine. With the latter only being essential in young children.

Foods that supply all the essential amino acids are classified as being a complete protein. Many plant foods do have all the essential amino acids, e.g. amaranth, buckwheat, quinoa, spirulina, soy. Eggs are an almost perfect protein food. Dairy products and meat contain good amounts of most essential amino acids, though meat can be deficient in phenylalanine. Plant foods often do not contain good amounts of all the essential amino acids. In particular, lysine and tryptophan are often lacking. Also, wheat and rice are short of lysine, particularly if processed, but can be combined with grains such as sorghum or legumes to supply this missing amino acid.

Other staple foods deficient in amino acids are corn (lysine, tryptophan), legumes (methionine) and some nuts (lysine, sometimes methionine). Fruits and veggies have less protein and may be short of methionine. However, conversely, vegetarian diets, which are often low in methionine and lysine, have been shown to help prevent cardiovascular disease, and increased uptake of non-essential amino acids, such as arginine, alanine, glycine and serine, reduce arterial disease and retard development of some cancers. Also, greater vegetable protein and decreased meat protein intake have been shown to reduce the development of osteoporosis in a group of older women.

Essential amino acids

Arginine

Enhances the immune system and is involved in growth. Indirectly benefits the health and elasticity of blood vessels and the gut; thus, may improve blood flow, and reduce angina and blood pressure. Can exacerbate herpes. Found in abundance within sperm; deficiency leads to low sperm counts.	Seafood, fish, soy, seeds, spirulina, wholegrain cereals, brown rice, cocoa, nuts, raisins.

Histidine

Needed for maintenance of nerve cells and repair of tissues, and for pain control. Widens small blood vessels, so may lower blood pressure. Makes histamine in allergic reactions. Has been used to treat rheumatoid arthritis, allergies, ulcers and anaemia.	Meats, brown rice, wholegrain cereals and leafy vegetables.

Isoleucine

Stabilises and regulates blood sugar and energy levels. Is very important in construction of enzymes and muscles. Seems to be deficient in people suffering from some mental and physical disorders. Can be broken down for energy, particularly during prolonged exercise.	Egg, soy, spirulina, seaweed, almonds, cashews, lentils, chickpeas, rye, seeds, other legumes, dairy.

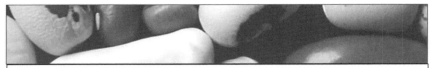

Leucine

Builds muscle and sterol compounds; forms human growth hormone. Can reduce and sometimes even stop the muscle wasting that occurs as we age. Increases endurance and enhances energy. Helps lower blood-sugar levels. Because genes that produce leucine-rich areas are damaged in Parkinson's disease, leucine has been considered as a supplement for this disease. Bodybuilders often take this as a supplement.	Egg, spirulina, dairy, fish, peas, beans, lentils, leafy vegetables, Goji and wolfberries.

Lysine

Linked with activity of B vitamins. Helps convert fatty acids into energy and lower cholesterol. Helps the body absorb and conserve calcium; aids formation of collagen, thus may be important in helping prevent osteoporosis. Often increased within the diet after sports injuries. May speed recovery and reduce recurrence of breakouts of herpes (both oral and genital) and shingles infections (though should also reduce intake of arginine-rich foods).	Fish, nuts, legumes (particularly soy), fenugreek seeds, watercress, spirulina. Lacking in corn, rice and wheat.

Methionine

Is the only essential sulphurous amino acid; its contribution of sulphur to the body is important. Has antioxidant properties and helps detoxify heavy metals. Helps prevent disorders of the hair, skin and nails. Involved in synthesis of bile salts, thus assisting breakdown of fats, but also encourages fat breakdown around the liver. Promotes excretion of oestrogen and reduces histamine levels. Deficiencies may increase birth defects; works with folate. Too much methionine increases production of homocysteine, which is strongly linked with increased heart disease.	Fish, seafood, cereals and grains (wheat, rice, corn), spirulina, seaweed, sesame. Low concentrations in legumes and some nuts.

Phenylalanine

Used in the brain to produce neurotransmitters that promote alertness and vitality; elevates mood, decreases pain, aids memory and learning. Inhibits breakdown of opiate-like substances – may help reduce chronic pain. Stimulates a hormone that suppresses appetite. Can increase blood pressure in hypotension. Used to reduce symptoms of arthritis, menstrual cramps, migraines, obesity, Parkinson's disease and schizophrenia.	Meat, fish, nuts, spirulina, seaweed, avocado, bananas, brown rice, legumes, beans, soy, leafy greens, sunflower, corn, sesame.

Threonine

Used in formation of connective tissues, bone, tooth enamel, and in production of neurotransmitters. Works with phenylalanine to elevate mood. Deficiency may be associated with irritability in children. Enhances the immune system. Involved in fat metabolism. Helps prevent build-up of fat in the liver.	Watercress, spirulina, egg, fish, whole cereals, nuts, pulses, bananas, leafy vegetables, alfalfa.

Tryptophan

Involved in neuronal activity. Crucial in the formation of serotonin, which induces sleep. Helps reduce anxiety and depression. Regulates appetite and stabilises mood. May help with hormone-related depressive symptoms. Improves immune-system functioning.	Pumpkin seeds, brown rice, cocoa, oats, bananas, dates, legumes, peanuts. Lacking in maize.

Valine

Involved in muscle metabolism and co-ordination and tissue repair. Used as an energy source by muscles. May promote mental vigour, calm emotions and be helpful in treating liver and gallbladder disease.	Sesame seeds, spirulina, legumes, soy, leafy greens, peanuts, cheese, fish, watercress, asparagus, mushrooms, whole grains, soy.

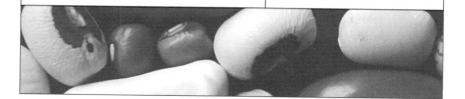

Sugars, carbohydrates and fibre

Carbohydrate is an important part of the diet: it should contribute 55% of our energy intake. It is mostly digested within the small intestine. Some carbohydrates can be broken down by enzymes within the gut into their smallest units and are absorbed, others cannot be broken down (e.g. cellulose), or are only partially broken down by gut bacteria (e.g. inulin). These 'fermented' carbohydrates may be partially absorbed, though much is excreted as insoluble fibre.

Carbohydrates are classified according to their size: one- and two-joined units are called mono- (e.g. glucose) and disaccharides (e.g. sucrose), respectively. Those with between three and nine units are termed oligosaccharides (e.g. inulin, raffinose); and those with more than ten units are polysaccharides (e.g. starch, cellulose, pectins, mucilages).

Their size and complexity determines how long they take to be digested. Sugars and simple carbohydrates are absorbed much more rapidly causing rapid increases in blood-sugar level compared with larger carbohydrates, which are digested more slowly. Apart from obesity concerns, it is thought that the rapid absorption of refined foods, such as sugar and refined carbohydrates can lead, in the longer term, to imbalanced glucose control.

The glycaemic index (GI) gives an indication of how long it takes for carbohydrates to be broken down and used by the body. Its numerical value signifies the speed at which carbohydrates and sugars increase blood-glucose levels – the higher a food's glycaemic number, the faster it is broken down and the more rapidly blood-glucose levels rise. Foods that are broken down slowly give energy over a longer period and are more beneficial than quick-energy foods, unless a quick burst of energy is required. Most vegetables, cereals and seeds have low GI numbers, whereas refined products, such as white flour and rice, which have had their outer, fibre-rich layers removed, have a high GI. Conversely, foods that contain fibre, proteins and fats slow down the absorption of carbohydrates – seeds, nuts and legumes have low GI numbers. They provide nutrients and energy over a long time period. Foods with lower scores are often rich in dietary fibre.

Glycaemic Index (GI) Numbers

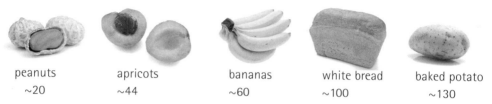

peanuts	apricots	bananas	white bread	baked potato
~20	~44	~60	~100	~130

The higher a food's GI number, the faster it is broken down into simple sugars and the more rapidly blood-glucose levels rise. Foods that are broken down slowly give energy over a longer period – in this case, a handful of raw peanuts will satisfy the body's need for energy much longer than a slice of white bread, or baked potato.

Sugars

The most common simple sugars found in foods are fructose, glucose and sucrose and maltose. They are particularly common in fruits and the sap of plants, but also in some storage roots such as sweet potatoes and beets. Because they are eaten along with other fibre and nutrients they don't cause rapid rises in blood-sugar levels.

Too much refined sugar eaten regularly can cause high blood pressure, pancreatic disorders, kidney and gallstones. Rapid increases and decreases in blood-sugar levels increase development of type-2 diabetes and can also adversely affect mental state. Hypoglycaemia (rapid onset of low blood sugar) can develop a couple of hours after eating a high-sugar meal, causing irritability, anger, anxiety, headaches, sudden tiredness and chilling of hands and feet. This can be managed by simply replacing a sugar-filled snack with one rich in nuts.

Unprocessed foods usually have a mix of at least two sugar types, whereas processed foods are often dominant in a particular sugar type: agave nectar, corn syrup and soda drinks are all rich in fructose. Balance is best, and sugars should be eaten with fibre to slow their uptake and reduce rapid insulin release.

Fructose

Monosaccharide fructose has a lower GI than glucose or sucrose, and yet is perceived as being sweeter. It is often recommended diabetics use this instead of sucrose. It does not initiate the insulin response or raise blood-glucose levels, as it is metabolised in the liver rather than throughout the body like glucose. It is added to many prepared foods, such as baked goods, making them taste sweeter, improving texture, adding a satisfying flavour and aroma. It browns easily when cooked (quicker than sucrose) and provides a longer shelf life. However, fructose consumed in excess can have negative effects. Its browning reactions have been associated with a greater risk of some types of cancer. High fructose diets may increase the risk of arthritis, kidney stones, cardiovascular disease and type-2 diabetes, and reduce the availability of copper and zinc. Apples and pears are rich in fructose and although very healthy can cause infant diarrhoea. Cloudy juice, which includes its fibre, reduces this problem.

Glucose

Monosaccharide glucose is readily absorbed by the body and is then transported within blood to all tissues, where much is used to produce energy. It is the most important sugar type metabolised to produce energy. Glucose is also a precursor to the synthesis of many compounds, including proteins and lipids. It is essential to every cell, but particularly brain cells. Foods richest in glucose include dates, honey, pomegranates, plums, figs, cherries and blueberries, but also tomatoes. In contrast, most nuts and seeds, and grains such as rice and wheat, contain virtually no glucose.

Sucrose

Disaccharide sucrose is a larger molecule than fructose or glucose, it takes a little longer to break down, and so does not taste as sweet. It is readily absorbed in the gut and transported in the blood to tissues, where much is used to produce energy. It is composed of both glucose and fructose. Apricots are rich in glucose and sucrose.

Maltose

A less common disaccharide, maltose is found in germinating seeds (e.g. barley, corn). It consists of two units of glucose, and is much less sweet than glucose or fructose.

Fibre

Fibre has been proven to have beneficial effects on digestion, reducing colorectal (colon and rectal) cancers, easing digestive disease and aiding many other processes. Ideally, we should consume ~70% of our diet as complex carbohydrates (carbohydrate and fibre). Fibre slows the absorption of sugar, reducing the peaks and troughs of insulin production (a hormone that controls blood-sugar levels and its storage), thus reducing the risk of type-2 diabetes. Greater intake of fibre also significantly inhibits development of coronary atherosclerosis and reduces its progression in those who already have this disease.

Fibre includes many plant substances, some of which can be fully digested, whereas others are only partially or not digested at all. Much depends on whether or not they are fermentable – are able to be broken down (even partially) by our gut bacteria. They are also known as viscous (soluble in water) or insoluble, with most fermentable fibre also being viscous and soluble. Plants provide all our fibre, with even fruits supplying good amounts, e.g. apples, blueberries, dates, guavas, olives, oranges, raspberries.

Unfermentable (insoluble) fibre does not significantly react with our gut bacteria, nor does it affect blood-cholesterol levels, but it does deactivate intestinal toxins, inhibit the adhesion of pathogenic bacteria to the gut wall, reduce excess permeability of the intestines and is linked to decreased risks of colon and breast cancer. Fibre-rich diets have been shown to significantly reduce the incidence of gallstones. Wheat bran and whole grains, as well as the skins of many fruits, vegetables and seeds, are rich sources of insoluble fibre.

Soluble (fermentable) and insoluble (unfermentable) fibre

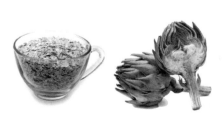 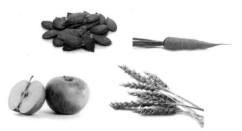

Oats and artichokes are two excellent sources of soluble fibre.

Plants provide all our fibre – whole grains and the skins of many fruit, vegetables and seeds are rich sources of this type of fibre.

Viscous (soluble) and fermentable fibre acts like a sponge, absorbing many times their own weight of water. Swollen, fibre binds around waste-food particles, aiding their passage through the gut. Helps make the passage of stools easier, constipation and haemorrhoids are relieved, and the risk of more serious diseases, such as diverticular disease and bowel cancer, are reduced. It also absorbs cholesterol. An excellent form of soluble fibre is oats. The gel formed from this fibre traps cholesterol-like substances and then eliminates them before they are absorbed into the blood stream. People who eat a high-fibre diet have lower total cholesterol levels and are less likely to develop cardiovascular disease.

Fermentable, viscous fibre helps reduce type-2 diabetes as it helps control blood-sugar levels: it slows the absorption of glucose and delays gastric emptying, thus smoothing out blood-sugar peaks and troughs after eating. The delay in gastric emptying also means that we feel fuller for longer after eating. Fermentable fibre also forms complexes with bile acids, which are manufactured by the liver from cholesterol. These complexes are treated as waste and removed from the body. The liver then uses more cholesterol to make new bile acids, thus taking more cholesterol out of the system.

Fermentable fibre is food for 'good' bacteria within the gut. They partially ferment it to form compounds (e.g. butyric acid), which are crucial to the continual renewal and health of cells within the large intestine and colon, and reduce the incidence of colorectal cancer. These compounds also inhibit enzymes that would otherwise produce cholesterol in the liver so add to the cholesterol-lowering properties of fibre. Abundant 'good' gut bacteria also reduce the number and survival of pathogenic bacteria.

Benefits of fermentable fibre

🐾 Increases populations of 'good' gut bacteria

🐾 Reduces numbers of potentially pathogenic bacteria

🐾 Helps movement of digested food through the gut

🐾 Reduces constipation

🐾 Produces beneficial compounds (e.g. butyrate) that we absorb

🐾 Increases our absorption of calcium and magnesium

🐾 Lowers blood-sugar levels and improves insulin response

- Reduces elevated serum-cholesterol and triglyceride levels

- Lowers blood pressure

- Stimulates the immune system

- Promotes the synthesis of B vitamins

- Helps reduce the development of colorectal cancer and other intestinal disorders (e.g. irritable-bowel syndrome).

Examples of fermentable, viscous fibre are oats and artichokes, whereas wheat contains more cellulose and is largely unfermentable. However, both fibre types significantly reduce (by 15–33%) the development of coronary heart disease, prevent diverticulitis (where pouches of inflamed tissue form in the colon), plus help with weight loss (high-fibre diets give a feeling of fullness without being absorbed), and reduce blood-sugar levels, serum LDLs (low-density lipids) and triglycerides.

Selected plant-fibre types

Beta-glucans	Soluble, glucose-type fibre that is viscous and fermentable. Common in many plants (e.g. oats, barley, mushrooms, yeast, spirulina).
Inulin and oligofructose	Also called fructo-oligosaccharides, is composed of complex chains of fructose. Viscous and partially fermentable by gut bacteria. Occur widely within plants from the sunflower family, chicory, artichokes, endive, lettuce, etc., and also within onions. Also known as a 'prebiotic', inulin stimulates growth of 'good' bacteria. Is undigested, so does not result in weight gain. Does not affect blood glucose or stimulate insulin secretion, so good for diabetics. Inulin and oligofructose can reduce serum-triglyceride and cholesterol levels, with significant improvements seen in a short time. However, inulin can cause flatulence and bloating.

Pectins	Mucilaginous, viscous fibre that develops thickening properties when heated. Fermentable by gut bacteria. Common in many fruits (e.g. apples, citrus rind – particularly grapefruit). Proven to lower serum-cholesterol levels, so reduces the incidence of thrombosis. May also help prevent colorectal cancer. Used to treat constipation and diarrhoea.
Psyllium	A fermentable fibre that is abundant within plantain seeds, i.e. *Plantago* species. Has huge moisture-absorbent properties and is linked with significant health benefits.
Xyloglucan	Beneficial to the digestive system and protects against damage caused by UV light. Tamarind is very rich in this fermentable fibre.

Fats

Fats can be classified as either saturated or unsaturated. Unsaturated fats are liquid at room temperature. It is now well established that saturated fats are detrimental to good health. We also know that unsaturated fats are 'good', but that they do vary in their health value: the balance between omega-3 and omega-6 fatty acids, and the type of omega-6 fat affects us differently. Some fats are essential to the diet, including vitamins A, D, E and K, but also omega-3 and omega-6 fatty acids. Many seeds and nuts are excellent sources of these. However, only about 15% of our diet should consist of fats. If eating more than this amount, ensure adequate intake of vitamin C, zinc, chromium, and selenium in particular, but also fibre, iodine, manganese, coenzyme Q10, magnesium and niacin. These help reduce the formation of blockages within arteries.

Fats fulfil many crucial structural, biochemical and physiological processes. Triglycerides form the greater part of every cell membrane within our bodies. Saturated fats have all their chemical sites filled with hydrogen ions. In contrast, unsaturated fats have only some sites filled with hydrogen, thus also contain one to several double bonds. Unsaturated fats are liquid at room temperature.

Unsaturated fats

Found primarily in seeds, nuts, seafood and fish. Classified into two main types: monounsaturated and polyunsaturated. Of the two, polyunsaturates can be more easily broken down.

Monounsaturated fats

These have only one double bond (e.g. oleic acid, palmitoleic acid): they are less liable to become rancid and oxidise compared to polyunsaturates. They are liquid at room temperature, but become semi-solid when cooled. Good sources are olives, almonds, grape seeds, avocados, peanuts, pecans, cashews, linseed, safflower, sesame, sunflower, macadamia, wholegrain wheat and oatmeal. Are easily broken down within the body. Can lower total serum-cholesterol and LDLs ('bad' cholesterol), and raise high-density lipids (HDLs, 'good' cholesterol). These fats should form a generous proportion of the fats we eat (e.g. oleic acid within olive oil). Mediterranean diets contain lots of oleic acid, which is thought responsible for the lower rates of heart disease and cancer within these countries.

Polyunsaturated fats

These have multiple double bonds, and remain soluble even at low temperatures. Combining them with protective, antioxidant-rich foods, i.e. those that contain vitamins C and E, selenium, flavonoids and zinc, extends 'shelf-life' considerably.

Most polyunsaturates can be made within the body, with the exceptions of α-linolenic acid (an omega-3 essential fatty acid) and linoleic acid (an omega-6 essential fatty acid), which must be included in the diet. They are vital to all cell membranes, conferring fluidity, flexibility, permeability and promote the activity of membrane-bound enzymes. They are required as precursors to the formation of other fatty acids, are involved with both increasing and reducing inflammation, affect our mood and behaviour, modulate cellular communication and affect DNA activity. Several large studies confirm that coronary disease occurs significantly less in those who eat a diet rich in these types of fatty acids. They also reduce inflammatory bowel disease and some kidney disorders, and may actually decrease the amount of fat stored. Deficiency in essential fatty acids results in increased susceptibility to infection and slow wound healing. Pregnant women and young children, in particular, need generous amounts of omega-3 fatty acids, as deficits can cause long-term adverse effects.

Omega-3 essential fatty acids (e.g. α-linolenic acid)

Including more omega-3 fatty acids (e.g. α-linolenic acid) in the diet can reduce coronary heart disease by more than 50% in both men and women. Stabilises heart beat, decreases risk and growth of blood clots, decreases serum triglyceride levels, improves elasticity of blood vessels and decreases inflammation. Also decreases levels of 'bad' cholesterol (LDLs, see page 46). Because elevated levels of triglycerides are common in those with type-2 diabetes, including more omega-3 oils in the diet is recommended. Omega-3 fatty acids may also protect against rheumatoid arthritis. They are linked with the retinal membranes and visual pigment (rhodopsin), so enhance visual health.

Omega-3s are integral to the formation and health of the nervous system and brain. A lack of omega-3s results in symptoms such as impaired memory and decreased learning efficiency. It is thought that a lower ratio of omega-3 to omega-6 fatty acids in brain membranes is linked to a greater incidence of depression. People with major depression often have significantly decreased omega-3 fatty acids. These people may also develop increased levels of inflammatory compounds. Arachidonic acid (an omega-6 fatty acid) is a precursor of these compounds, whereas omega-3 fatty acids inhibit their formation. Some data demonstrate that including omega-3s in the diets of psychiatric patients has decreased the symptoms of several mental disorders. There is growing evidence that this simple therapy may help alleviate depression, bipolar disorder, schizophrenia, anxiety, eating disorders, attention-deficit disorders, addiction and autism. And, without the need to use drugs that often have unpleasant side effects.

Good sources of omega-3 fatty acids

   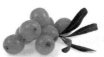

 linseed   hazelnuts   walnuts   sea buckthorn   kiwifruit

The modern Western diet is often skewed towards more omega-6s than omega-3s, i.e. a ratio of 10:1, compared to 1–3:1 in the past. Research now recommends increasing omega-3s in the diet to readjust this ratio, and that this increase be accompanied by vitamin E-rich foods (e.g. nuts and seeds). Because omega-6 arachidonic acid can cause a greater inflammatory response to injuries, allergies, infections, atherosclerosis and some cancers, more omega-3s in the diet can rebalance this ratio and reduce inflammation.

Main sources of omega-3s are oily fish and linseed (flax), but also walnuts, hazelnuts, seeds, spirulina, perilla, chia sage, hemp seed, kiwifruit, purslane, sea buckthorn, lingonberries, green vegetables and soya beans.

Good sources of omega-6 fatty acids

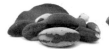

Brazil nuts   pecan nuts   pumpkin seeds   sunflower seeds   pinenuts

---

Omega-6 essential fatty acids (e.g. linoleic acid, gamma-linolenic acid (GLA), arachidonic acid)

Linoleic acid is an essential fatty acid that is sourced from plants. Consuming foods rich in linoleic acid lowers total cholesterol and reduces LDLs and triglycerides. However, they can also lower 'good' cholesterol (i.e. HDLs). Linoleic acid is important within the brain. It can be converted to arachidonic acid, which is crucial for the production of several hormones and has many functions within the body, including the inflammatory response, though its response can sometimes be excessive (see above).

GLA, in contrast, has anti-inflammatory properties, which may help treat autoimmune diseases such as multiple sclerosis, psoriasis and lupus. Has been shown to reduce rheumatoid arthritis. GLA also has tumour- and metastasis-suppressing properties, can reduce blood pressure by widening blood vessels, inhibit cholesterol production and strengthens the immune system. It is being trialled for use in HIV treatment.

Omega-6 oils are found particularly in borage and blackcurrant seed oil, but also within many nuts and seeds (e.g. safflower, sunflower, pinenuts, corn oil, soya bean oil, pecans, Brazil nuts, pumpkin, sesame).

Saturated fats

These can be divided into two types: long- and medium-chain saturated fats. They occur in many animal and dairy products, as well as tropical oils, such as coconut and palm, and are very stable.

Long- and medium-chain saturated fats are absorbed and dealt with quite differently by the body. Due to their smaller size, medium-chain fats can be absorbed directly from the small intestine and are transported directly to the liver where they can be converted to energy. In contrast, long-chain fats need to be extensively broken down and treated with enzymes and bile before they can be absorbed and transported, via the lymphatic system, to the main blood circulation, which distributes them around the body, including to fat layers and the liver. In the liver, they undergo further processing before they can be used for energy. Long-chain fatty acids also cause total serum-cholesterol level to rise, and are implicated in the development of some cancers. In contrast, medium-chain fats have even been suggested to help with weight loss, as they are not utilised by the body in the same way as long-chain fats. Medium-chain fats (e.g. lauric acid) are found in large amounts in coconut and palm oils.

Cholesterol

Cholesterol is a lipid-like, waxy substance used by the body structurally and in many metabolic processes. It is a major component of cell membranes and is used in the synthesis of steroids and bile salts. Although some cholesterol is obtained through the dietary intake of dairy products, meat, eggs and fish, much is produced by the liver, and the amount produced is determined by the type of fat that is eaten. Interestingly, because dietary cholesterol is derived from the cell membranes of animals, plants contain virtually no cholesterol. It is the amount of cholesterol that the body produces that can cause problems, and saturated fats, which occur at high levels in dairy products and fatty meats, encourage the body's production of excess cholesterol. Most seeds and nuts contain larger ratios of unsaturated fats, which do not have this effect.

Cholesterol attaches to a protein to travel around the body. The liver forms two main types of lipoprotein: low density lipoproteins (LDL) and high density lipoproteins (HDL). (There are also very low density lipoproteins.) Both are required and are essential for good health. Elevated blood-cholesterol levels need to be monitored; however, of more importance is the actual ratio between LDL/HDL: the lower it is the better.

Low-density lipoproteins: LDLs contain 60–70% cholesterol. Enables transport of cholesterol from the liver to all body cells, including smooth muscle, which is what arteries are composed of. This cholesterol, in excess, initiates the formation of deposits in arteries and, as a consequence, can result in increased risk of heart disease, though it is not the only factor to cause arterial clots.

High-density lipoproteins: HDLs contain 20–30% cholesterol. They transport cholesterol away from tissues and back to the liver, where it is recycled or eliminated. Greater amounts of HDL lower levels of cholesterol within the body and reduce the risk of heart disease.

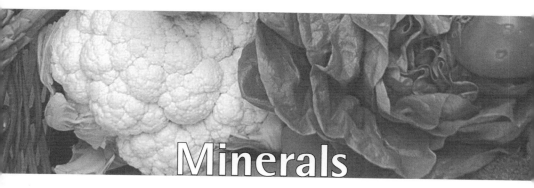

Minerals

Inorganic substances make up only 4% of the body's weight, with most found in bones, yet are crucial to biological processes. Minerals such as calcium and phosphates are needed to build bones; others, often termed micronutrients, are only required in tiny amounts and yet a deficiency can cause serious disease. Most minerals are adequately provided for in a balanced diet, exceptions and deficiencies often occurring in a region where a particular mineral is lacking in the soil (e.g. boron, zinc, selenium).

Essential minerals

Boron

Needed for healthy bones and joints. Deficiency is linked to arthritis. Affects the reproductive system and brain; a lack is linked to increased risk of prostate cancer and osteoporosis.

> raisins, soya beans, avocado, almonds, hazelnuts, kidney beans, sweet corn.

Sources

47

Calcium

Approximately 99% is found in bones and teeth. Is also used for muscle activity and nerve-impulse transmission. Important in maintaining constriction and relaxation of blood vessels (it can lower blood pressure) and for secretion of hormones such as insulin. Is strongly linked to decreasing the development of non-genetically linked colorectal cancers (i.e. by 20–25%). Increased calcium also reduces incidence of kidney stones: it may reduce oxalate build-up, one of the main causes of stones: so, eat your spinach with a yoghurt dressing. Adequate calcium during pregnancy may reduce the incidence of pre-eclampsia and, in children (in particular) may protect against lead toxicity (e.g. from exhaust gases). Needs vitamin D for absorption and usage. Required with vitamin K for blood clotting. High sodium intake increases calcium loss from the body; post-menopausal women could consider reducing sodium intake. More calcium and vitamin D in the diet and adequate exercise reduce the incidence of osteoporosis. Protein-rich diets cause more calcium to be lost from the body; studies show that vegetarians have better uptake rates. Acidic foods, such as citrus help its absorption; excess magnesium reduces its absorption. During digestion, calcium can reduce iron uptake.

Sources
dairy, beans, shellfish, kale, spinach, rhubarb, broccoli, soya beans, sesame seeds, almonds.

Copper

Antioxidant properties. Used to make melanin and in the formation of connective tissue (including capillaries) and bone. Deficiency can raise blood pressure. Important for tissue healing and for sheathing nerve cells. Involved with neurotransmitters that affect mood and metabolism. Benefits the immune system. Required with iron to synthesise red blood cells. Too much copper is toxic and inhibits absorption of vitamin C and zinc; conversely, high levels of zinc, vitamin C or fructose inhibit copper absorption.

Sources
whole grains, eggs, beans, nuts (e.g. cashews, Brazil nuts, pecans), seeds (e.g. pumpkin seeds), beets, spinach, asparagus, brown rice, papaya, chocolate, potatoes, fish.

Chromium

Needed only in small amounts yet is crucial in controlling blood-sugar levels. The greater the intake of sugar, the more chromium is required. Deficiency causes peaks and troughs in blood-sugar levels, leading to erratic mood changes, i.e. when blood-sugar levels plunge (hypoglycaemia), and possibly to development of type-2 diabetes. More of this mineral is required as we age and during pregnancy. Possible to have too much, so it is best to get chromium through foods rather than as a supplement.

> brewer's yeast and molasses, also in whole grains and kiwifruit.
>
> **Sources**

Fluorine

Found in bones and teeth. Improves tooth strength and reduces caries, though may also increase osteoporosis. Too much can make teeth brittle. Its necessity as an essential mineral is controversial.

> fish and tea; small amounts found in most foods.
>
> **Sources**

Iodine

Essential in the production of thyroid hormone, which regulates metabolism, growth rate, development and reproductive function. Intrinsic in the formation of the brain and growth in the unborn child and young children. Indirectly involved with controlling cholesterol levels. Isothiocyanates, found in brassicas and millet, can block thyroidal uptake of iodine. Isoflavones, found in soya beans, can inhibit thyroid synthesis.

> seafood, seaweeds, vegetables grown near the coast, brassicas, peanuts, cassava, soya beans.
>
> **Sources**

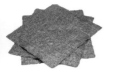

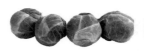

Iron

Most is found in red blood cells, which are crucial oxygen transporters. Needed for DNA synthesis; the formation of energy-carrying ATP; production and maintenance of neurotransmitters; liver detoxification; connective fibre and bone; bile acids. Too little causes anaemia and too much can cause serious disease; therefore, it is best to increase intake of iron-rich foods rather than take supplements.

Iron comes in two dietary forms: non-haeme and haeme. Each has different absorption rates. All iron in plants and ~60% from animal sources is non-haeme and is absorbed slowly, only partially and is dependent on the presence of other substances. Haeme iron (found in meat) is more rapidly and easily absorbed. Non-haeme iron absorption is improved by eating foods rich in vitamin C, other organic acids (e.g. malic, citric) and zinc. Absorption is inhibited in particular by compounds found in legumes (e.g. soya beans), phytosterols, tea, calcium-rich foods, other positively charged minerals and oxalates. Deficiency of vitamin A can increase iron deficiency, causing anaemia; therefore, it is best to treat anaemia with extra carotenoids as well as iron.

> **Sources** pumpkin seeds, oily fish, seeds, sweet potato, spinach, meats, shellfish, eggs, legumes, nuts.

Magnesium

Most is found in bone (60%), with much of the remainder found in muscle. Involved in muscle contraction, nervous-impulse transmission, normal heart rhythm, energy production, bone mineralisation and production of antioxidant enzymes. Present in ~300 enzymes and involved in fatty-acid and protein synthesis. Helps initiate reactions within and between cells. Adequate magnesium within the diet may help reduce blood pressure, improve elasticity of blood vessels and has been used to reduce the risk of heart attacks. Is likely to improve glucose metabolism and insulin sensitivity in diabetics. May help prevent pre-eclampsia in pregnancy. Extra magnesium in the diet of older people may increase bone-mineral density and decrease osteoporosis in post-menopausal women. Important in the formation of tooth enamel. Deficiency is linked to diabetes, high cholesterol, spasms of blood vessels, increased pre-menstrual tension, repetitive strain injury, cramps and depression. High intake of zinc (as supplements) and of protein can inhibit uptake of magnesium. Need a balance between calcium and magnesium uptake.

> abundant in dark green leafy vegetables, some nuts and whole grains, pumpkin seeds, legumes (particularly soya beans), taro, sweet corn, chocolate, seafoods.   **Sources**

Manganese

Required in small amounts for red blood-cell synthesis, urea formation, reproduction, growth, wound healing and insulin release. Deficiency can cause hearing loss, problems with balance. Taken with calcium, it may help prevent osteoporosis, and taken with glucosamine it may help relieve joint pain. Its uptake is linked with iron and zinc.

> wheatgerm, whole grains, green vegetables, chard, nuts, seeds, oysters, sweet potatoes, pumpkin seeds, tofu, chocolate, tea.   **Sources**

Nitrogen

Required to build amino acids and thus proteins: enzymes, DNA, RNA and many other important molecules.

> meat, dairy products, legumes, seeds, nuts (see amino-acid notes above).   **Sources**

Phosphorus

Abundant within the body, with almost equal amounts of phosphate and calcium within bones and teeth. Vital for making energy-carrying ATP. Is a key part of cell membranes and a component of many enzymes, DNA and RNA. Very important in buffering pH and gaseous exchange in blood. In many plants, phosphate occurs mostly as phytate (a phosphate/protein molecule): found particularly in the outer layers and germ of whole grains (wheat, rye, oats) and legumes (particularly broad beans). However, humans lack the 'right' enzymes to digest phytate effectively, i.e. only ~50% of potential phosphate is digested. But, an enzyme found in yeast and gut bacteria can help break it down. For this reason, yeast in bread and microbes in yoghurt makes phosphate more available than in unfermented products. So, adding yoghurt to your muesli helps release more phosphate. Phytates also bind with several minerals and reduce their bioavailability (e.g. calcium, magnesium, iron, zinc, and the vitamin niacin), but can help eliminate potentially toxic heavy metals. Phytates have been shown to act as anti-cancer agents against colon cancer, and also possibly liver, lung and breast cancers. They enhance the immune system and reduce serum-cholesterol, the incidence of kidney stones, and slow gastric emptying. Diets rich in fructose (e.g. corn syrup) and low in magnesium can increase loss of phosphate from the body and lead to deficiencies.

Sources

yoghurt is the number one provider of phosphates, with pumpkin seeds a close second. Also found within dairy, fish, meats, seeds, nuts, beans, whole grains.

Potassium

Involved in nerve-impulse transmission, muscle contraction and the pumping heart. Vital for maintaining fluid and electrolyte balance within cells. Linked with lowering blood pressure and improving bone density at all ages. Helps release energy from protein, fat and carbohydrates during metabolism. The modern diet is thought to contain about ten times more sodium compared to potassium; this ratio was reversed in our ancestors. This imbalance causes diseases such as stroke, increased blood pressure, kidney stones and osteoporosis. Fruits and vegetables are much richer in potassium than sodium. Adequate potassium and calcium are important for good bone formation and maintenance. Much can be lost through cooking.

Sources

most fruits and vegetables, particularly beans, baked potatoes, sweet potatoes, squash, pumpkin, tomatoes, leafy greens, dried apricots, honeydew melon, bananas.

Selenium

An important micronutrient and antioxidant. Is associated with sulphur-based compounds within plants. Plentiful in brassicas and plants within the onion family. Is part of several powerful antioxidant enzymes in animals. Helps repair damaged DNA, and inhibits proliferation and induces death of cancer cells (e.g. lung, liver, prostate). May also slow the progression of HIV. Selenium is essential to thyroid metabolism and, thus, normal development, growth and metabolism. Important in the immune system and improves elasticity of blood vessels, thus reducing cardiovascular disease. Works synergistically with vitamin E, another antioxidant; together, these are linked with reducing heart disease and decreasing the symptoms of asthma and arthritis. Also may enhance the efficacy of vitamin C. Selenium found in plants may have greater anticarcinogenic activity than if taken as a supplement.

very abundant in Brazil nuts, also in meat, seafood, brassicas, garlic, onion, sunflower seeds, oatmeal, mushrooms, eggs.

Sources

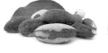

Sodium

Required for transmission of nerve-impulses, muscle contraction and for the heart pump. Is part of the pH-buffering system and helps maintain blood pressure. Intrinsically linked with water balance within the body: too much sodium causes water retention (and increased blood pressure); too little, and dehydration occurs. Helps uptake of amino acids, glucose and water from the gut. Although important, the modern diet often contains far too much. Excess sodium may be linked to increased osteoporosis, cardiovascular disease, kidney stones, gastric cancer. Excess sweating can cause a deficiency.

table salt, dairy products, meats, most processed foods.

Sources

Sulphur

After calcium and phosphorus, sulphur is the most abundant mineral found in our bodies. Can be deficient: only occurs within two amino acids: methionine and cysteine. Methionine is an essential amino acid, i.e. we cannot synthesise it, and although cysteine can be synthesised by the body, it needs a steady supply of sulphur. The other source of sulphur is from isothiocyanate and sulphur-type compounds found within the brassica and onion families. We use sulphur in several hormones (e.g. insulin) and vitamins (e.g. thiamine and biotin). Is very important within antioxidant enzymes and has antimicrobial properties. Is also important in joint health: is found in glucosamine and chondroitin. Helps regulate blood-sugar levels. Improves health of skin and hair; is said to slow greying. Many of us may be deficient in sulphur, which can lead to various problems, including increased joint disorders.

Sources   meat, eggs, dairy, beans, nuts (cashew, peanut, Brazil nuts, macadamia), brassicas and the onion family.

Zinc

Used for protein synthesis, in the structure of cell membranes, maintenance of DNA and RNA, tissue growth and development, wound healing, taste acuity, hormone production, bone mineralisation, cognitive function, foetal development, sperm production and functioning of the prostate gland. Essential to the immune system. Deficiencies cause greater susceptibility to infections. Extra zinc has been used to reduce severity of cold infections. Zinc is needed with vitamin A to produce rhodopsin, the eye pigment needed for night vision. More zinc-rich foods within the diet as people get older may boost immunity and reduce eye problems. Beneficial for skin and hair.

Sources   meat, seafoods (especially oysters), whole grains, seeds, nuts, pumpkin seeds, legumes.

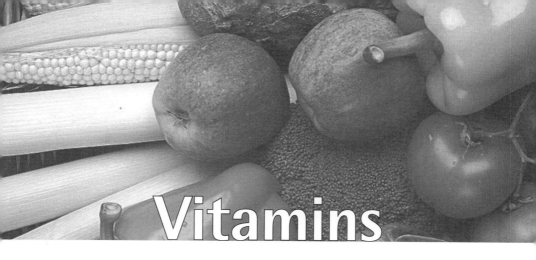

Vitamins

Vitamin A (carotenoids)

More correctly termed carotenoids, this large group of compounds give fruits and vegetables much of their vibrant orange, yellow and green colours. In plants they act as attractors of pollinators and seed dispersers, but are also powerful antioxidants and are very efficient at removing potentially damaging oxygen radicals produced in the process of photosynthesis. They also absorb certain potentially dangerous light wavelengths to protect the plant's tissues.

While α-carotene and lycopene are both carotenoids, not all carotenoids are converted to vitamin A. Provitamin compounds, e.g. α-carotene, are converted within the body to vitamin A (retinol), whereas carotenoids such as lycopene, zeaxanthin and lutein are not. Carotenoids are also classed, biochemically, as terpenes (see later).

Carotenoids are well known for improving vision: the provitamins are key in the formation of rhodopsin, needed by light-sensitive rods in the eye. A lack of these vitamins leads to poor night vision, so carrots do help us see in the dark. Carotenoids are also important for the proper formation of bones and teeth. Because they help maintain healthy epithelial cells, a lack of this vitamin leads to many digestive, urinary and respiratory infections, as well as nervous disorders and skin infections. Its maintenance of membranes helps prevent infections.

Carotenoids enhance the immune system, including the white blood cells. They also work with vitamin D and thyroid hormones to effect gene transcription and cell differentiation. Carotenoids are important within the developing embryo and also affect the production of growth hormones.

Powerful antioxidants, they have strong cancer-fighting properties. In general, carotenoids provide the greatest reduction in epithelial cancers (e.g. skin, lung, stomach, mouth, pharynx, pancreas, cervix, specific types of leukaemia), though carotene, lutein and zeaxanthin may also decrease the incidence of breast cancer in premenopausal women. They also reduce cardiovascular disease: a diet rich in carotenoids helps prevent thickening of blood vessels. Carotenoids can also successfully treat skin problems, such as acne.

There is considerable evidence that consumption of carotenoids within fruits and vegetables, rather than taken as a supplement, affords greater efficacy in the body. Also, natural sources of carotenoids are better, whereas vitamin A within supplements given in doses of just four to five times the recommended daily allowance (RDA) can be toxic. The body is unable to rid itself of excess vitamin A. Pregnant women, in particular, should avoid vitamin A supplements as in this form they can cause birth defects.

Vitamin A is fat-soluble and can be stored in the body for a long period: its storage is so effective that the body can last without additional vitamin A for a couple of years without suffering deficiency. Also, being fat-soluble, ingestion with a little oil enhances their bioavailability and uptake, as does finely chopping these foods. Eat your grated carrot and chopped tomatoes with a sprinkling of safflower oil to get their full benefits. Unlike most other vitamins and antioxidants, their value is actually increased with cooking and processing. Bile salts, iron and zinc are also needed for their digestion and absorption.

Carotenes are found abundantly within most yellow, orange and red foods, including carrots, apricots, spinach, sweet potato, cape gooseberries, papaya, greens, red peppers, oranges, melon, celery, peas.

Lycopene

Although not converted to vitamin A, this is a particularly powerful antioxidant. Recent research shows excellent health benefits from lycopene, which gives food its red colour. It seems to prevent cancers of the prostate, pancreas, stomach, breast, cervix and lung. Consumption of lycopene-rich tomatoes is inversely associated with cancer of the digestive tract. Lycopene is significantly associated with reduced prostate cancer; in several studies, risk of this cancer was reduced by between 15–55% in men who regularly ate lycopene-rich tomatoes. Lycopene may also help prevent cardiovascular disease, reduce the incidence of age-related eye disorders, and has been shown to reduce the incidence of skin cancer. It may also boost sperm concentrations. It is found particularly in tomatoes, and is hugely increased in concentrated tomato products, (e.g. sun-dried tomatoes, tomato paste). Also found in watermelons, capsicums, pink grapefruit, apricots.

Lutein and zeaxanthin

These yellow compounds absorb blue light in plants, and are the only carotenoids to occur within the lens and retina of the eye. It is thought that they protect the eye from potentially damaging short-wave blue light and, thus, are linked with preventing age-related macular degeneration and cataracts. Lutein is vital in producing a protective layer over the rods and cones at the back of eye (fovea), protecting them from UV and other oxidative damage. Eating as little as 6–10 g of these compounds a day can reduce macular degeneration by ~40% and cataracts by 20–50%. Although slowing degeneration in the elderly, they benefit the eyesight of people of all ages. These two antioxidants are found in abundance in eggs and green vegetables (kale in particular, also cress, beet greens, chicory, spinach) and within many yellow and red foods (Goji berries, oranges, corn, red peppers, marigold flowers) and kiwifruit.

Vitamin B complex

Although the B vitamins are not antioxidants, they are essential nutrients. They are all water-soluble and good quantities are found in many nuts, seeds, legumes, whole grains, leafy green vegetables, asparagus, bananas, meats and eggs, but particularly in yeast products. Being water-soluble, they are not stored for long in the body and are best eaten regularly. Also, heat destroys much thiamine, B6, pantothenic acid and folate, so only briefly cook vitamin B-rich plants if possible. Extended exposure to light and air can also decrease their efficacy, as can relatively strong acids and alkalis. Germinating seeds rich in B vitamins (e.g. rye) increases their vitamin B levels several fold, and they retain much of this value even after cooking.

All are required in many metabolic pathways and are involved in neuronal and muscular transmission, including functioning of the heart and digestive system. They are required in metabolic control, cell growth and division, production of skin and muscle, and in the immune system. B vitamins are used to convert carbohydrates and fats into energy, to produce glucose, to produce and repair DNA and RNA, and for cell signalling and differentiation. Many are linked with neuronal health and neurotransmitter production; their consumption can increase mental agility and verbal fluency, whereas a lack can cause depression, confusion, apathy, anxiety and neurodegenerative diseases, such as dementia, Alzheimer's and schizophrenia. Can reduce age-related macular degeneration. Deficiencies of the B vitamins are quite common, particularly within older people, and increased intake is recommended for this age group.

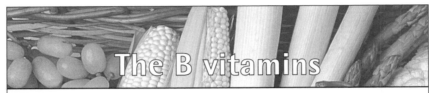

The B vitamins

Thiamine (B1, thiamin)

Needs magnesium for its metabolism. A minority have difficulty absorbing this vitamin, which leads to poor absorption of other vitamins and minerals. Tea and some seafoods, taken in large quantities, can also antagonistically affect thiamine uptake. Is destroyed by heat.	Yeast products and whole grains in particular, also oat bran, peas, legumes, seeds, nuts.

Riboflavin (B2)

Involved in metabolism of several B vitamins (folate, B6, niacin), so deficiency also affects these. It may help prevent migraines. Deficiencies can impair iron absorption. Works with vitamin A.	Wholegrain cereals, yeast products, quinoa, spirulina, milk, eggs, salmon are very good sources, but also broccoli, soya beans, asparagus, almonds, spinach.

Niacin (nicotinamide, vitamin P) (B3)

Can be derived from the amino acid tryptophan (an essential amino acid), which also needs B6 and iron, or is taken in with the diet. Is protective against cardiovascular disease: increases HDLs, reduces blood clotting, levels of LDLs and triglycerides. May reduce the incidence of mouth, throat and oesophageal cancers.	Meat, yeast products, whole grains, seeds, spirulina, peanuts, legumes.

Pantothenic acid (B5)

Derivatives of this vitamin are used in cholesterol-lowering drugs. Can increase the lifespan of mice by 20%.	Abundant within yeast products, meat, eggs, fish; also in broccoli, whole grains, sunflower seeds, legumes, mushrooms, avocado, peanuts, sweet potatoes. Gut bacteria can also produce pantothenic acid.

B6 (Pyridoxine)

Helps maintain the sodium:potassium balance. Enhances the immune system. Because it can bind to hormone cell sites such as those of oestrogen, testosterone and progesterone and reduce their activity, it is thought that it may reduce the development of some hormone-related cancers, e.g. breast. Due to its links with natural anti-depressant neurotransmitters (e.g. serotonin), it has long been considered by some as a therapy for pre-menstrual symptoms. It may help reduce morning sickness in pregnancy and is said to aid sleep and to affect dreaming. Deficiencies are relatively uncommon, though alcoholics are at more risk and possibly those on high-protein diets. May be linked with attention-deficit disorder in children. Deficiency of B6 can increase levels of homocysteine, which results in elevated risk of heart disease (see under folate, page 60). Extra B6 can improve memory, may help relieve symptoms of carpal-tunnel syndrome and give some relief in Parkinson's disease. Helps absorption of zinc, iron, B12 and protein.	Yeast products, whole grains, bananas, pistachios, beans, chickpeas, Brussels sprouts, feijoas, sorghum, brown rice, corn.

Biotin (B7)

Although required by all organisms, most is only synthesised by bacteria, yeasts, fungi and algae. Gut bacteria probably produce some absorbable biotin. It is essential for the formation of fatty acids, glucose, cell division, for replication and transcription of DNA, and many other processes. Involved in maintaining stable blood-sugar levels, and so is useful to those at risk for type-2 diabetes. Strengthens hair and nails: is most beneficial when eaten rather than applied topically. Raw egg white inhibits biotin absorption. Extra biotin is of particular importance during pregnancy.	Yeast products, peanuts, hazelnuts, almonds, avocado.

Folate (folic acid) (B9)

Important for production and maintenance of DNA, RNA and amino acids (e.g. methionine). May reduce formation of colorectal, cervical, lung, oesophageal, brain, pancreas and breast cancers. Risks of these cancers are greater with high alcohol intake, but elevated consumption of folate (>600 mcg/day) may ameliorate colorectal and breast cancer risk somewhat. A deficiency causes build up of homocysteine, which is a strong indicator of heart disease and other problems. Regular consumption of folate reduces homocysteine by 50–90%. Needed for production and maintenance of red and white blood cells. Particularly important in pregnancy when many cells are being formed; deficiency can lead to birth defects. Deficiency (with raised homocysteine levels) has been linked with increased development of dementia and Alzheimer's. However, high intakes of folic acid can mask vitamin B12 deficiency, which becomes more common in older people. Adequate B6 compliments folate usage.	Brassicas, yeast products, whole grains, spinach, avocado, asparagus, peanut, banana, barley, chickpeas, most nuts, spirulina, oranges.

Cobalamine (B12)

The only vitamin not found in fruits or vegetables. It is only made by bacteria: not plants or animals. Linked intimately with cobalt. The most common B12 deficiency is anaemia.	Very good sources are bivalves such as mussels and oysters, which siphon these microbes. Also yeast, spirulina and fermented foods such as tempeh.

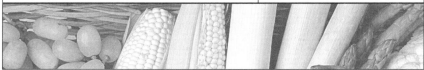

Vitamin C (ascorbic acid)

Humans cannot synthesise vitamin C; thus, it is an essential vitamin.

Vitamin C is a powerful antioxidant best known for its ability to reduce the effects of colds and flu. It has good bioavailability from food and even small amounts have great antioxidant efficacy in preventing everyday cell damage, but particularly after exposure to toxins and pollutants (e.g. smoking). It has confirmed benefits in helping eradicate cancer-causing free radicals: there is evidence of it reducing development of mouth, throat, oesophagus, stomach, colorectal, lung and breast cancers. A water-soluble vitamin, it protects the watery areas of the body, such as blood and inside cells. It also helps to recycle vitamin E, a fat-soluble antioxidant. It cannot be stored and, unlike fat-soluble vitamins (e.g. vitamin E), it needs to be consumed daily. It works much better if combined with polyphenols. Vitamin C is easily destroyed by heat when cooked or processed, and also degrades rapidly with storage or with freezing.

Vitamin C is an essential component of collagen (found within blood vessels, tendons, ligaments, bone), and helps synthesise a neurotransmitter that counteracts depression and elevates mood. It is needed for energy production, and is involved in metabolism of cholesterol into bile acids, helping to reduce blood-cholesterol levels, and also the incidence of gallstones. It protects against heart disease and stress and improves elasticity of blood vessels, so helps reduce blood pressure. It helps boost the immune system and binds with some poisons to render them harmless. Vitamin C helps increase the absorption of nutrients (e.g. iron) in the gut, and is essential for sperm production.

The recommended dosage of vitamin C is 250–400 mg a day, though some authorities only recommend ~60 mg, this being the minimum needed to stave off scurvy. As far as supplements are concerned, unlike many, it is reported that natural and supplementary ascorbic acid have equal bioavailability. However, excess consumption, i.e. regular consumption of >2000 mg/day, may cause kidney stones. Aspirin and oestrogen-based contraception pills can lower vitamin C levels within the body.

Foods that have 6–15 mg of vitamin C are regarded as a 'good' source; those with 15–30 mg are considered a 'very good' source; and those with >30 mg are 'excellent'. Sources: most fruits and vegetables, including capsicums, acerola, currants, kiwifruit, parsley, rose hips, strawberries, Goji berries, sea buckthorn.

Good sources of vitamin C

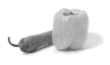   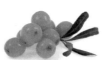

Capsicums   strawberries   parsley   sea buckthorn   kiwifruit

Vitamin E

Vitamin E is recognised as the most important lipid-soluble antioxidant in the body. It plays an important regulatory role in cell signalling and gene expression. Epidemiological studies show that high blood concentrations of vitamin E are associated with decreased risk of cardiovascular diseases and some cancers. This powerful vitamin consists of eight antioxidant compounds: of these, α-tocopherol is the main active form found in the body, though gamma-tocopherol is the main type found within most foods.

A fast-acting vitamin, it is intrinsic in maintaining integrity of cell membranes, is involved in the formation of DNA and RNA, and is needed to form red blood cells. It promotes wound healing, reduces scarring, assists normal functioning of the nervous system and is involved with vision (may reduce the incidence of cataracts). On or within the skin, it helps reduce damage done by UV light, and is a popular addition to sunscreens and anti-ageing creams. Beneficial to the liver because it neutralises some toxins. It enhances the immune system and reduces inflammatory reactions. May be of particular benefit to older people by reducing the incidence of upper-lung infections and colds, and may also protect against arthritis, diabetes, and bowel and renal disease.

Vitamin E inhibits cholesterol production in the liver, reduces serum LDL levels, relaxes blood-vessel walls, inhibits formation of blood clots and may even reverse clot formation in arteries. Regular and adequate vitamin E within the diet has been shown to reduce the incidence of heart attacks and other cardiac diseases. As an antioxidant vitamin E may reduce the incidence of prostate cancer and may benefit those with type-1 or type-2 diabetes. Ongoing studies have shown promising results for vitamin E reducing the risk of dementia caused by strokes, and improving cognitive function.

Although it can be stored in the body for longer than vitamin C, it does need to be regularly 'topped up'. Humans can only last 2–6 weeks without

---

Good sources of vitamin E

Almonds sunflower seeds amaranth seed avocado rye

an intake of vitamin E before health starts to deteriorate. Many people do not consume enough vitamin E; older people, in particular, should ensure they consume enough. It is most beneficial when taken with vitamin C.

Sources: abundant in nuts, seeds and their oils, particularly almonds, sunflowers seeds, safflower oil, palm oil, coconut, amaranth seed, soya bean oil, avocado, barley, pumpkin seeds, rice bran, wheat germ and rye.

Vitamin K

A fat-soluble vitamin, primarily important for its ability to bind calcium ions in the process of blood clotting. It works with the amino acid glutamic acid, calcium ions and several proteins to activate coagulation. A serious lack of vitamin K can cause uncontrolled bleeding; however, too much vitamin K can antagonise anticoagulant drugs such as warfarin. There is no evidence that diets rich in vitamin K increase formation of clots; conversely, a lack of vitamin K may encourage calcification of vessels, which can initiate clots.

With vitamin D, vitamin K produces compounds that prevent calcification of soft tissue and cartilage, while also ensuring normal bone growth and development. Vitamin K helps maintain strong bones; studies show that elderly people may especially benefit from extra vitamin K to reduce bone fractures and osteoporosis. A generous serving of leafy greens a day is likely to significantly improve bone health. High doses of supplementary vitamin A and E can antagonise activity of vitamin K, and long-term use of antibiotics can affect the gut bacteria that also form vitamin K. Vitamin K is poorly stored within the body, and moderate regular intake is advised.

Sources: almost all green leafy vegetables, spirulina, peas, prunes, parsley, green tea, asparagus, avocado, spring onions, fermented soya bean products and dairy.

Good sources of vitamin K

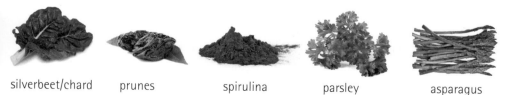

silverbeet/chard   prunes   spirulina   parsley   asparagus

Secondary plant compounds

Although often called secondary plant compounds, this multitude of compounds, a few of which are listed below, have important functions within plants and are also hugely beneficial to us.

What are antioxidants?

The colour of fruits and vegetables often reflects their nutritional value. Strongly coloured foods are packed with goodies, from dark purple and bright red berries, to large orange and yellow tropical fruits, to dark-green leafy vegetables. Antioxidant nutrients include vitamins C, E and A, coenzyme Q10, many secondary plant compounds (e.g. flavonoids), as well as the micronutrient selenium. When antioxidants are used in combination, their efficacy is often much greater than if taken individually.

Antioxidants work by reacting with destructive free radicals (charged oxygen molecules) and reactive metal cations (e.g. iron, zinc, copper, but also toxic heavy metals, such as lead, chromium, mercury) to render them harmless before they damage RNA or DNA. This prevents mutations and tumour growth. The free-radical theory of ageing (and disease promotion) is that damage gradually accumulates within our cell membranes, DNA, tissue structures and enzyme systems as we age or come into contact with toxins, and this predisposes us to many diseases. Although the body produces its own antioxidant enzymes, consuming additional antioxidant-rich foods seems almost proven to reduce this damage and tissue ageing. Antioxidants also protect and help regenerate other dietary antioxidants, such as vitamins C and E.

Plants have evolved a wide range of antioxidant compounds to protect themselves from highly reactive oxygen, produced as a by-product in photosynthesis. In addition, plants evolved other compounds as a defence against attack by insects, fungi, bacteria, herbivores, as well as from damage caused by ultraviolet (UV) radiation. Many of these compounds have now been found, often in small amounts, to have startling medicinal and dietary properties. This very large and varied group of compounds is referred to as secondary plant compounds.

Within humans, antioxidants can strengthen and increase the suppleness of smooth muscles (including arteries), reverse some of the signs of ageing, help prevent and even sometimes reduce development of some cancers, reduce heart disease (atherosclerosis), enhance the immune system, improve visual acuity, delay development of emphysema, and possibly reduce the incidence of Parkinson's and neurodegenerative diseases such as Alzheimer's.

Antioxidant-rich food can be classified into an ORAC scale (oxygen-radical-absorption capacity), with high-scoring values being the best. The table on page 66 shows ORAC values for a range of plant foods. These values are from fresh foods unless otherwise stated and are per 100 g. Note that when dried the ORAC values of fruit, such as apricots, are greatly increased.

What are secondary plant compounds?

They often have defence properties within plants, i.e. they act as a plant's immune system. They include coumarins, terpenes, isothiocyanates (from brassicas), allicin, (from garlic) and alkaloids. When injured, the plant activates compounds to deter, kill or poison the attacker, whether it be a micro-organism, insect, browsing herbivore or a human. Many of these compounds are found in the leaves, roots, unripe fruits and seed coverings of plants. In the plant, they can prevent maturation or reproduction of the pathogen. They form a physical barrier against pathogenic invasion and initiate the release of hormones (e.g. abscisic acid) that act as antibiotics, and strengthen the plant against further attack. Within us, many of these compounds have anti-cancer properties, act as antimicrobials and anti-inflammatories, enhance cardiovascular health and boost the immune system.

Plants produce other secondary compounds to attract pollinators and creatures that will eat them (i.e. ripe fruits are eaten for their flesh, but their seeds are spread inadvertently). These include the many colourful flavonoids and anthocyanins that give ripe fruits and flowers their colours. Their aromas and colours are 'designed' to lure.

Fruit/nuts/ vegetable	ORAC value	Fruit/nuts/ vegetable	ORAC value
Pecans	17,940	Rocket	1904
Elderberries (black)	14,697	Oranges	1819
Walnuts	13,541	Peach	1814
Currants, black	10,060	Beets (cooked)	1767
Hazelnuts	9645	Radishes	1736
Cranberries	9584	Macadamias	1695
Pistachio	7983	Asparagus (cooked)	1644
Goji and wolfberries	7228	Tangerine	1620
Prunes	6552	Grapefruit, pink	1548
Blueberries	6552	Spinach	1515
Artichoke, globe	6552	Brazil nuts	1419
Plums	6259	Broccoli	1362
Blackberries	5347	Grapes (red)	1260
Wine, red	5034	Lemons	1225
Raspberries	4882	Kiwifruit (gold)	1210
Almonds	4454	Olive oil, extra virgin	1150
Apple, red, with skin	4275	Apricots (fresh)	1115
Dates	3895	Onion	1034
Strawberries	3577	Capsicums, sweet, orange, raw	984
Figs	3383	Avocado	933
Cherries (sweet)	3365	Banana	879
Apricots (dried)	3234	Limes	823
Peanuts	3166	Sweet potato (cooked)	766
Raisins	3037	Pinenuts	616
Guava	2550	Peas, green	600
Pomegranate juice	2341	Celery	497
Cashews	1948	Carrots	497
Chard	1946	Pumpkin and squash (cooked)	420

Data from Nutrient Data Laboratory and Arkansas Children's Nutrition Center, 2007.

The following describes a selection of secondary plant compounds in more detail. The activities of these often explain why a particular food has the wondrous health benefits it does.

Coumarins, cinnamic acids and similar compounds

This is a large group of diverse compounds that are important plant-defence compounds, though some are also attractors. Coumarins are aromatic and are not destroyed by cooking. They are antioxidants and many can reduce development of mutagenic and carcinogenic cells and may even reduce metastasis (e.g. breast, lung, kidney, pancreas, stomach). They increase blood-vessel flow and decrease capillary permeability (should not be taken with anticoagulants), and so lower blood pressure. They have antifungal, antiviral, antibacterial and insect-deterrent properties. Many coumarins are altered by UV light; thus, they often cause adverse reactions when applied to skin that is subsequently exposed to sunlight, but they are also often used to treat skin diseases such as psoriasis, and some cancers.

Coumarins, cinnamic acids and similar compounds

Anethole and estragole

Have an anise flavour and aroma and are much sweeter than sugar. May have a protective effect on liver. Insecticidal, antiviral, antibacterial, used for respiratory infections as an expectorant and to relieve abdominal wind. As an essential oil, may have adverse effects (carcinogenic) in high quantities.	Fennel, star anise, tarragon, basil, anise, chervil, bay, marjoram.

Caffeic acid

Anticarcinogen, antioxidant, anti-inflammatory, protects against UV.	Coffee, burdock, turmeric, dandelion, artichoke, basil, thyme, oregano, apple.

Chlorogenic acid

Antioxidant and anti-diabetic. Slows glucose release after eating, and its absorption from the gut, so may reduce development of type-2 diabetes. Used in slimming foods. Is an antiviral, antibacterial, antifungal, with low toxicity. Does not lead to antimicrobial resistance (cf. antibiotics).	Coffee, strawberries, pineapple, sunflower, blueberries.

Eugenol

Antiseptic, insecticidal, antiviral, antibacterial, anaesthetic, analgesic. In high doses the pure oil may be a carcinogen. Can cause adverse skin reactions.	Bay, nutmeg, cinnamon, lemon grass, cloves.

Ferulic acid

An antioxidant. May help prevent formation and kill existing cancer cells (e.g. mouth, colon, liver, breast). With vitamins C and E it doubles protection against UV when applied to skin.	Bran, brown rice and flour, oats, many Apiaceae species (e.g. fennel, angelica, dill), coffee, artichoke, orange, pineapple, apple, peanut.

Pterostilbene

Similar to resveratrol in its efficacy; may have even greater activities. Powerful antioxidant, anti-inflammatory. Strong anti-cancer agent. Can reduce serum LDLs and triglycerides (thus reduces development of cardiovascular disease). May have neuroprotective effects. Can enhance cognitive motor skills and may inhibit progression of some types of dementia. Can lower blood sugar, so may act as an anti-diabetic.	Grapes, blueberries, bilberries, lingonberries.

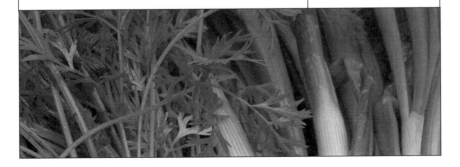

Resveratrol	
Very powerful antioxidant. Has potent anti-cancer activity. Binds to oestrogen receptors and seems to promote and antagonise oestrogen activity. It disrupts cancer-cell regulation and proliferation, initiates death of cancer cells and inhibits entry and development of cancerous cells into other tissues. There is evidence that resveratrol can inhibit the proliferation of breast, prostate, pancreatic, thyroid, stomach and colon cancers. It also inhibits enzymes that cause inflammation. Effective at reducing damage to epithelial cells (e.g. skin, lungs) and may protect against UV damage. It can reduce serum LDLs, inhibits clot formation and attachment to vessel walls, stimulates an enzyme that helps keep vessel walls supple. May reduce development of cardiovascular disease. Binds and decreases activities of some heavy metals (e.g. cadmium) and reduces toxicity produced by some pharmaceutical drugs. May have antiviral properties and increases activity of some retroviral drugs. Is also an antifungal. Mice, fish and monkeys had significantly longer lifespans when fed a high-resveratrol diet with reduced calories. May help relieve the symptoms of Alzheimer's disease.	Grapes, red wine, peanuts, blueberries, bilberries, lingonberries, cranberries.
Umbelliferone	
Can decrease plasma glucose, increase insulin, decrease serum LDLs and increase HDLs. May be good as an anti-diabetic and to inhibit cardiovascular disease. Reactive with skin, but also used in skin sunscreens.	Apiaceae species (celery, carrot, coriander, angelica), chamomile, tea, grapefruit.

Phenolics

Phenolics (and polyphenolics) are a large group of compounds that have strong health-promoting benefits. At least 5000 polyphenolics have been identified. Some protect plants from pests, disease and ultraviolet light; others are fruit and flower attractors (e.g. flavonoids, anthocyanins). Many of these compounds have synergistic activities with each other and also with vitamins. For example, phenolics eaten with vitamins A, C and E protect against cardiovascular disease, have anti-cancer properties, inhibit the development of several neurological diseases, stimulate immune function and prevent chronic disease. They also inhibit the production of inflammatory compounds, thus reducing allergic reactions.

Phenolic compounds

Ellagic acid

A powerful anticarcinogen. Significantly inhibits breast, pancreas, oesophagus, skin, colon, prostate, liver, lung and tongue cancers in rodents. It can inhibit cancer-cell division and cause the death of cancer cells. May protect 'normal' cells from the effects of chemotherapy and radiation. Also has antibacterial and antiviral properties and can reduce populations of *Helicobacter pylori* (a bacteria that can cause stomach ulcers and cancer). May reverse some toxicities within the liver and help control internal haemorrhages. Ellagic acid retains its potency after heating, freezing and other processing.	raspberries, walnuts, strawberries, cranberries, blackberries, blueberries, pomegranate, guava, grapes.

Salicylic acid

This powerful anti-inflammatory compound is found in aspirin; however, unlike aspirin, in foods it does not cause gastric problems. It is particularly rich within spices such as cumin, turmeric and paprika. As well as curing headaches, it is also taken to reduce blood pressure and inhibits the formation of clots. Significantly lowers the risk of colon cancer and possibly some forms of breast cancer. Applied to warts, it can make them disappear and helps remove dead cells and treats pore infections if applied to skin.	Cumin, turmeric, chilli, paprika, liquorice, clove, blackberries, cinnamon, peppermint, rosemary, thyme, oregano, raisins.

Rosmarinic acid

Antioxidant (stronger than vitamin E). Has anti-cancer activities. Is an anti-inflammatory. Possible use for arthritis and related autoimmune inflammatory diseases. Reduces hay fever symptoms by suppressing allergic responses and inflammation. Helps relieve mucous-membrane discomfort of the nose, throat and lungs. May reduce some types of chronic kidney diseases. Is antimicrobial and antiviral, and has been used to extend life of stored foods.	Rosemary, perilla, oregano, lemon balm, basil, thyme, sage, borage, marjoram, peppermint.

Curcumin

Efficacious in small quantities and has a wide range of medicinal benefits. Seems to slow development of Alzheimer's. Powerful antioxidant and anticarcinogen. Has antimicrobial properties. Inhibits *Helicobacter pylori,* thus reducing incidence of stomach ulcers and cancers. No toxicity to humans. Reduces inflammation from injuries and helps prevent atherosclerosis. Binds to toxic heavy metals (e.g. lead, cadmium).	Mostly in turmeric, but also mustard.

Flavonoids, anthocyanins and proanthocyanins

A large and diverse group of water-soluble often colourful compounds found in plants. They are powerful antioxidants. Epicatechins (e.g. in tea) and quercetin (e.g. in grapes, berries) are the most effective antioxidants known at this time. Proanthocyanins are also very powerful antioxidants and free-radical scavengers. They greatly enhance the activity of vitamin C in the body and have much stronger antioxidant activity than vitamins A, C and E, or selenium. They cannot be produced by the body and are only found in plants. They are important in modulating gene control, affect cell growth and division, and seem to deter development of prostate, colon, stomach, mouth, lung, breast cancers and myelogenous leukaemia. They work synergistically with vitamin E to reduce UV skin damage.

Cardiovascular disease is inversely related to consumption of many of these compounds. They lower serum LDLs ('bad' cholesterol) and triglyceride levels, while leaving HDL ('good' cholesterol) levels unchanged or elevated. They reduce absorption of cholesterol in digestion and increase bile-acid excretion. Both processes result in lowered serum-cholesterol levels. They also inhibit the formation of arterial clots, help maintain the health of capillary walls, increase cell-wall permeability, help regulate heart beat and reduce blood pressure. They can reduce atherosclerosis and stroke. They have been used to treat arterial disorders (e.g. venous insufficiency, where blood is poorly returned to the heart from the legs). They promote production of connective tissue and bone precursors, which help keep skin elastic and smooth (similar compounds are used in anti-ageing preparations).

Many of these compounds reduce inflammation, reducing development of diseases such as atherosclerosis and asthma, and they may lessen the response of allergic reactions. For example, quercetin, myricetin and kaempferol inhibit enzymes that would otherwise activate potent inflammatory compounds. These properties are being investigated to treat neurodegenerative diseases such as Parkinson's, dementia and Alzheimer's. They have been shown to reverse impaired learning and improve cognitive function. Proanthocyanins can cross the blood–brain barrier and remove and prevent lipofuscin formation in the brain and heart: lipofuscin is thought to partially initiate the ageing process.

Anthocyanins boost insulin production by up to 50%, so could help treat diabetes. They reduce blood-glucose levels and improve insulin sensitivity.

Flavonoid-like compounds can directly disrupt the function of several viruses, fungi and bacteria, e.g. HIV, herpes simplex virus, *Helicobacter pylori*. Anthocyanin-rich fruits have also long been used to improve vision, particularly night vision. A lack of these compounds can manifest itself as poor resistance to infection, bruising easily and swelling after injury.

The effectiveness of flavonoid-like compounds is greatly enhanced if taken with vitamin C, and vice versa. However, their efficacy is greatly reduced by cooking. They are readily and quickly absorbed, but also rapidly metabolised. They should be regularly included in the diet. Also, they can bind with iron to prevent its absorption, so, if taking iron supplements do not take flavonoid-rich foods within the same meal.

Sources: abundant in red wine and in most red, purple or blue fruits, particularly near the skin (e.g. bilberries, blackberries, cinnamon, plums, blueberries, cherries, cocoa, cranberries, sea buckthorn, bilberries, elderberries, pomegranates, peanuts, grapes, hawthorn, loganberries, acai berries, apples, raspberries), and some vegetables (e.g. barley, wild rice, red cabbage, red onions, sweet potato, black peppercorns, purple corn).

Flavonoids, anthocyanins and proanthocyanins

Apigenin

May inhibit development of Alzheimer's and Parkinson's. Reacts with benzodiazepine receptors in the brain to relieve anxiety and has slight sedative effects. May help with insomnia and work as an antidepressant. Anticancer for leukaemia, prostate, breast, ovarian, pancreas, skin, thyroid. May prevent invasion and development of cancer cells into other tissues	Apiaceae family (e.g. parsley, fennel, celery), chamomile, onions, basil, oranges, tea, wheat sprouts, apples, endive, ginkgo, lemon balm, beans, broccoli, olives, artichoke, cherries, cloves, coriander seeds, liquorice, linseed, grapes, leeks, barley, oregano, perilla, parsley, peppermint, tarragon.

Catechins (epicatechin, etc.)

Some of the oldest people on earth attribute their longevity to regular consumption of tea and cocoa. Very powerful antioxidants. Much stronger than vitamins C or E. Work a little like insulin (may help prevent development of type-2 diabetes), reduce heart disease and stroke by reducing serum-cholesterol and LDLs, lower blood pressure, help relax blood vessels and inhibit formation of arterial blood clots. Enhance the hormone norepinephrine, which results in relief from allergies and asthma through antihistamine-like reactions. Have shown preventive effects against skin, lung, oesophageal, breast, prostate and colon cancers. Help protect against UV damage to skin. Have proven antiviral and powerful antibiotic properties. Inhibit the replication of some bacteria (e.g. *Staphylococcus aureus*). Help reduce urinary-tract infections. Drinking green tea regularly seems to reduce body fat. Possible use for chronic fatigue syndrome.	Green and black tea, grapes, red wine, apple juice, cocoa, lentils, black-eyed peas.

Hesperidin

Best combined with rutin and vitamin C, which are abundant within citrus peel. Together they promote production of collagen, help wound healing and enhance the immune system. Can lower serum-cholesterol and blood pressure, and help keep blood vessels supple. Has been used to treat haemorrhoids and to reduce bruising. In the liver, it enhances release of stored fat and may lower the formation of fat. May help prevent bone loss. Has sedative and sleep-enhancing properties..	Citrus (especially the peel), red grapes, cherries, plums, peaches, apricots, apples, berries, green tea.

Kaempferol

Works synergistically with quercetin to reduce proliferation of cancer cells. Also reduces resistance of cancer cells to some anti-cancer drugs. Reduces cardiovascular disease.	Strawberries, gooseberries, cranberries, peas, kale, cauliflower, broccoli, leek, horseradish, grapefruit, chives, tea, apples, onions, citrus, cranberries, grapes, gingko.

Luteolin

Reduces inflammatory response of cells that can develop into Alzheimer's disease, Creutzfeldt–Jacob and multiple sclerosis. Reduces spasms within smooth muscle (e.g. gut, uterus). Has been used to treat septic shock. Gives toughness and flexibility to cartilage and tendons. May reduce age-related eye problems. Is likely to help reduce general cognitive and mental decline in ageing.	Celery, green pepper, parsley, thyme, peppermint, basil, celery, artichoke, perilla, chamomile, sage, rosemary, soya beans.

Quercetin

Works synergistically with kaempferol to reduce proliferation of cancer cells (breast, ovary, gastric colon, stomach cancers). One of the most thoroughly studied flavonoids. Reduces cardiovascular disease. Can relieve hay fever, eczema, sinusitis, asthma. Thought to inhibit release of histamines. May help relieve cystitis, chronic prostatitis and symptoms of gout. Has antiviral activity against (e.g. herpes simplex and parainfluenza type 3). May have anti-depressive properties, and helps delay progression of age-related eye problems.	Onions, tea, red grapes, cherry, apples, cranberries, raspberries, sea buckthorn, nuts, buckwheat, broccoli, prickly pear, grapefruit, green tea, tomato, lingonberries, cabbage.

Rutin

Significantly improves elasticity and health of blood vessels. Is used in several pharmaceutical preparations for venous leg ulcers, haemorrhoids. Important for maintaining health of the cardiovascular system. Can reduce inflammatory bowel disease. Has synergistic effect when taken with vitamin C, and also with hesperidin. Together, they promote production of collagen, help wound healing and enhance the immune system. Is also an antiviral. May help delay progression of age-related eye problems.	Buckwheat, apple peel, citrus fruits, red grapes, parsley, tomato, apricots, rhubarb, tea, cherries, plums, peaches, most berries.

Theaflavin

Formed from catechins and has similar properties. Has many of the above properties. Powerful cardiovascular enhancer: reduces total serum-cholesterol and LDLs, and increases HDLs. Has powerful antibacterial and antiviral properties: may inhibit replication of HIV and SARS. Can cause cell death of cancer cells, particularly prostate cancer. Reacts with androgen receptors that can initiate this type of cancer. May help reduce development of neurodegenerative disorders.	Black tea.

Terpenes

A large and important group of compounds commonly found in plants, which provide a wide range of medicinal uses. They often occur within essential oils and vary in molecular size, with smaller terpenes being aromatic (e.g. mints) and often have medicinal properties. Larger terpenes include squalene, carotenoids and steroids.

Smaller terpenes

Often have significant antimicrobial, antiseptic, antioxidant, antibacterial and anti-inflammatory properties. Are fairly rapidly metabolised, therefore ingestion of a little and often is better than large-dose intakes. Are often found in plant hairs and peel, or seed coverings. Have distinctive, pleasant aromas. A few can cause allergic skin reactions. Common within plants of the Apiaceae family (e.g. fennel, coriander, dill), and also citrus, mints, lavender, thyme, plus in many spices.

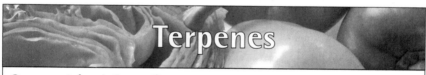

Carvacrol (and thymol)

Has a pleasant warm aroma and flavour. Anticarcinogenic and antimutagenic properties. An effective natural antibacterial (against, e.g. *Staphylococcus aureus*, *Salmonella enterica*, *Escherichia coli*). It disrupts bacterial membranes and may prevent their multiplication. Also antiviral, antifungal (e.g. the yeast *Candida*) and some protozoa (e.g. *Giardia*), and is used as an antiseptic. Used on wounds, skin infections and as a mouthwash. May help treat fungal nail infections. Has synergistic effects with similar compounds. Thymol also has most of these properties. Is widely used in dentistry for its safe antibacterial properties (against oral bacteria) and to reduce plaque. Acts as a weak tranquilliser. Has been successfully to control varroa mites that infect bees.	Oregano, marjoram, thyme, savory.

Carvone

Antimicrobial. Used in dental preparations. Eases smooth-muscle spasms. Has been used to ease indigestion and flatulence.	Caraway, dill, spearmint, peppermint, mandarin peel.

Caryophyllene

Anti-inflammatory, antibiotic, antioxidant, anticarcinogenic and an effective local anaesthetic. Antimicrobial, antifungal. Has a pleasant aromatic aroma and is used in perfumes. May have relaxing properties.	Clove, rosemary, basil, black pepper, star anise, sage, cinnamon, marjoram.

Linalool

Aromatic, spicy, pleasing. Significant insecticidal, antifungal and antibacterial properties (e.g. the yeast *Candida albicans* and bacteria *Staphylococcus aureus*, *Streptococcus* spp). Effective at controlling bacteria that cause tooth decay. Has anticarcinogenic, anti-inflammatory and local anaesthetic properties. Affects the central nervous system, acts as a mild sedative, eases spasms, reduces fevers. Often added to perfumes and soaps.	Basil, lavender, citrus rinds (e.g. bergamot), cinnamon, mint, grapevine leaves, thyme, tea, cardamom.

Limonene

Is found in >300 plants and is added to many foods. Has pine and orange aromas. Is an anticarcinogen (e.g. stomach, skin, colorectal, liver, breast, pancreas and lung cancers). Drunk with black tea, lemon peel (rich in limonene) can reduce the incidence of skin cancer by 70%. Has strong antiviral properties. Is used to dissolve cholesterol-containing gallstones. Neutralises gastric acid and eases spasms of smooth muscle, so is used to relieve heartburn, to ease gastro-oesophageal reflux and to restore normal muscular movements of the gut (peristalsis). Occasionally causes dermatitis, otherwise is non-toxic.	Citrus peel (in particular), also cherries, spearmint, dill, garlic, celery, maize, rosemary, ginger, basil.

Lupeol

Has strong ability to inhibit synthesis of the testosterone receptor and induces reactions that kill prostate cancer cells. Has been shown to be effective against cancerous pancreatic cells and in skin, head and neck cancers. Suppresses the spread of cancer cells and reduces tumour size. Is effective in only small amounts. Also an antioxidant and anti-inflammatory. May help prevent arthritis. Is an antiviral.	Aloe, figs, mangoes, calendula, capsicum, olives, grapes, melon, pumpkin, carrot, strawberries, tomatoes.

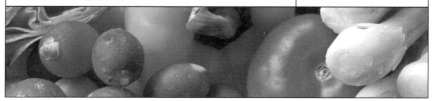

Menthol	
Applied to the skin, helps relieve pain from sprains, muscle aches, headaches and stops itching. Is often mixed with camphor (which has similar health benefits) and with capsaiscin (found in chillies). Antibacterial. Relieves sore throats when gargled. Used as a decongestant in cough preparations and to treat mouth infections. It stimulates cold-sensitive receptors in the skin and gives a cooling sensation. Used in sunburn creams. Added to several foods, perfumes and cosmetic products such as aftershave.	Peppermint, spearmint.
Zingiberene	
Helps relieve motion sickness, early morning sickness and other forms of nausea. Is an antioxidant, and has effective antimicrobial and antiviral properties. Can reduce fevers. Has antitumour and immune-enhancing effects. Can help reduce pain and anxiety. Helps reduce serum-cholesterol, and may inhibit blood clotting. Used as a fragrance and flavouring.	Turmeric, ginger, rosemary, thyme.

Larger terpenes

Saponins

Come in two main types: triterpenoid- and steroid-saponins (e.g. glycyrrhizin, found in liquorice). Some plant saponins are used as initial compounds for the production of human steroidal hormones. Historically they were widely used for their foaming characteristics in soaps, shampoo, etc. Saponins bind with cholesterol in the gut, which is then eliminated, unlocking stored cholesterol. This two-pronged action results in lowered risk for cardiovascular disease and stroke and helps with weight loss. A cholesterol-lowering drug has been synthesised from alfalfa saponins.

Several saponins enhance the immune system, particularly those within liquorice and soya beans, minimising immunologically induced liver injury. Can also help reduce stress and have sedative properties. Are able to kill or reduce the growth of many bacteria and have anti-inflammatory activity (act as anti-allergens). Saponins also have antiviral (e.g. influenza, herpes virus and possibly HIV) and antifungal activities. Some act as anticarcinogens. In some instances they can help overcome multi-drug resistance to anti-cancer drugs, thereby improving the effects of chemotherapy. However, they can reduce the absorption of carbohydrates, lipids, proteins and minerals from the gut, and larger saponins can cause disruption of cell membranes and clumping of red blood cells. But because they are very poorly absorbed from the gut, only surface gut cells are usually affected (which are readily sloughed and replaced). Heating does not significantly reduce saponin content, though fermentation does: thus products such as soya bean sauce contain very few.

Sources: alfalfa, amaranth, angelica, asparagus, aubergine, beans, beet, calendula, capsicum, fenugreek, ginkgo, ginseng, grape, hawthorn, legumes (including soya sauce), liquorice, oats, olives, onions, potatoes, quinoa, sage, spinach, sunflower, tea, tomatoes, yams.

Good sources of saponins

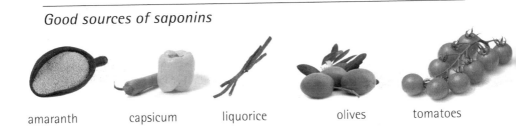

| amaranth | capsicum | liquorice | olives | tomatoes |

Phytosterols

Fat-soluble molecules which are intrinsic to plant-cell membranes. The human body cannot make them, so they need to be included in the diet. Are very similar in structure to cholesterol and, although they occur at much lower quantities in the diet, are very effective. They reduce cholesterol absorption by 50–85%, and a diet rich in phytosterols can reduce serum-cholesterol by 10% and LDLs by 13%, but leaves beneficial HDL levels unchanged. Phytosterols reduce the development of atherosclerosis and coronary heart disease.

Phytosterols may also reduce the risk of colon cancer by reducing potential carcinogenic compounds in the gut, and reduce the risk of prostate, breast, ovarian, colon and stomach cancers. They can cause death of cancer cells. They may modulate growth of oestrogen-responsive breast-cancer cells, and are of benefit to post-menopausal women. They also reduce the deleterious effects of diabetes. A diet rich in these oils is recommended to those with elevated cholesterol to complement a drug therapy. Several studies show that phytosterols can also reduce symptoms of benign prostatic hyperplasia (difficulty in urinating). They also inhibit fat storage, so are beneficial in aiding weight loss. There is even some evidence that they reduce male hair loss.

Phytosterols are necessary for an efficient immune system. They inhibit conversion of linoleic acid to inflammatory compounds and also oversee the production of hormones, such as oestrogen, testosterone and cortisol. Because these processes decline with age, it is thought that extra phytosterols within the diet may boost the endocrine system and, thus, perhaps reduce the incidence of several hormone-deficiency related diseases. Best efficacy is likely to be regular consumption, rather than occasional large intakes. Heating to a high temperature deactivates them, as does refining and hydrogenation of oils.

Sources: almonds, cashews, canola, peanuts, sesame seeds, pecans, buckwheat, saw palmetto, linseed, avocado, pumpkin seeds, sunflower seeds, pistachio, walnut, coconut, rice bran, olives, spirulina, palm oil, wheat germ, corn oils, lamb's quarters, citrus, coffee, hazelnuts, cottonseed oil, soya beans, sea buckthorn, wolfberries, ginseng, beetroot, peas, beans, tea and many vegetable oils (preferably unrefined). The bran of cereals is very rich in phytosterols, but particularly the embryo (e.g. wheat germ, rice bran).

Good sources of phytosterols

 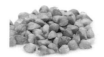 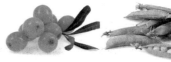

Cashews   buckwheat   hazelnuts   sea buckthorn   peas

Carotenoids

Also often known as vitamin A (see page 55). Are powerful fat-soluble antioxidants that protect membranes and other fatty areas of cells. Are generally classified as provitamins (which can be converted to vitamin A).

Provitamins include: α-carotene (e.g. carrots, pumpkins, maize, tangerine, orange); β-carotene (e.g. dark leafy greens, red, orange and yellow fruits and vegetables); and β-cryptoxanthin (e.g. papaya, tamarillo, whole wheat).

Non-provitamins include: lycopene (e.g. tomatoes, grapefruit, water-melon, guava, apricots, carrots); lutein (e.g. spinach, turnip greens, romaine lettuce, eggs, red pepper, pumpkin, mango, papaya, collards, oranges, kiwifruit, kale, peaches, squash, spinach, legumes, brassicas, prunes, sweet potatoes, honeydew melon, mustard, rhubarb, plum, avocado, pear, saffron); and zeaxanthin (e.g. wolfberries, spinach, kale, greens, maize, eggs, red peppers, pumpkin, oranges, paprika, mango, tangerine, papaya, peaches, avocado, pea, grapefruit, kiwifruit, saffron).

Good sources of carotenoid provitamins

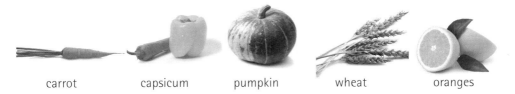

| carrot | capsicum | pumpkin | wheat | oranges |

Alkaloids

A diverse group with many being toxic, though others are highly beneficial. Some are used as recreational drugs; others are included within our everyday foods. Some are highly toxic in large amounts, but also have wondrous health benefits when given in smaller doses. Well-known examples are cocaine (from the coca plant), caffeine (from coffee), nicotine (from tobacco), morphine (from opium poppies), quinine (from Cinchona trees), theobromine (from cocoa beans), capsaiscin (from chilli), mescaline, amphetamine, ephedrine, dopamine, piperine (from black pepper), scopolamine (the main ingredient within many motion sickness pills), strychnine and quinine. Many have a bitter taste.

Caffeine

A very popular alkaloid. In plants it acts as a pesticide; in people it stimulates the central nervous system, respiration and blood circulation, increases circulation and oxidation of fatty acids (so is slimming), has synergistic properties with aspirin to reduce headaches and is a diuretic. It increases alertness and wakefulness. Negatives: can reduce bone density, increases blood pressure; not recommended for pregnant women. Is very toxic to dogs and horses.	Coffee, tea, yerba maté, cola, guarana, chocolate.

Theobromine

Similar to caffeine, though is much weaker. Acts as a stimulant and relaxes bronchi muscles in lungs: has been used for coughs. Is also a diuretic. Can increase heart beat, but also dilates blood vessels, which lowers blood pressure. Very toxic to many animals, e.g. dogs.	Cocoa beans, mate, tea, coffee.

Phyto-oestrogens

Isoflavones

Plant compounds that have mild oestrogenic and/or anti-oestrogenic activity. Soya beans (including textured vegetable protein, miso, tempeh) contain the greatest amounts and most occur as an isoflavone called genistein. Their activity within the plant is much less than that of mammalian oestrogen, so large amounts of food would need to be consumed to equal that found in humans. Regular, smaller intakes of isoflavone-rich compounds are recommended. The ability to digest of isoflavones varies from person to person, probably due to variations in the bacterial species present in the gut: Asian people seem to digest these compounds more effectively to produce more oestrogen-like compounds.

Isoflavones take the place of oestrogen when binding to oestrogen receptors on cells in tissues such as breast, prostate, uterus and ovary, and also within bone, liver, brain and heart. They either mimic the activity of oestrogen or are antagonistic. They can alter the biological activity of oestrogen and testosterone, and affect cell proliferation. These compounds can inhibit an enzyme that otherwise could increase breast-cancer cell proliferation. They also inhibit uncontrolled growth of cancer cells.

Phyto-oestrogens may reduce osteoporosis and are taken to relieve menopause symptoms (particularly hot flushes and night sweats). It is thought that phyto-oestrogens at pre-menopause block the action of mammalian oestrogens therefore inhibiting over-expression of this hormone. At post-menopause, phyto-oestrogens can top up other hormones and so may relieve some menopausal symptoms. There is some evidence that inclusion of phyto-oestrogens in the diet may prevent bone loss and increase bone density of post-menopausal women, though seems to affect spinal bones more than limb bones. There is evidence that regular consumption of phyto-oestrogens along with reduced consumption of meats and fats reduces the occurrence of prostate cancer. There is more evidence that they reduce the risk of breast cancer. An epidemiological study of women in Singapore found that pre-menopausal women consuming soya bean products had a lower risk of breast cancer. A long-term diet that included phyto-oestrogen rich foods, and also included high fibre, with low meat and fat consumption, further lowered the risk of breast cancer at both pre- and post-menopause. It is also thought that the earlier in life this diet is begun, the greater its efficacy. These compounds may also reduce the occurrence of colon cancer.

Phyto-oestrogens may reduce cardiovascular disease by decreasing cholesterol levels, i.e. lowering the ratio of LDLs to HDLs, and increasing elasticity of blood vessels, therefore reducing blood-clot formation. In China preparations rich in these compounds are used to treat alcohol addiction because they seem to remove the desire for another drink.

Negative effects of these compounds are that they can depress thyroid activity and may lower male fertility.

Sources: Soy, alfalfa sprouts, red clover, chickpeas, peanuts, other legumes.

Lignans

These are found abundantly just beneath the husk layer of cereals and seeds. Linseed (flax) contains more lignans than any other plant food. They have good bioavailability. When ingested, they are metabolised by gut bacteria to enterodiol and enterolactone (antibiotics can inhibit this process), which are thought to attach preferentially to oestrogen receptors and therefore block or suppress the effects of oestrogen in some tissues. They may reduce the development of hormonal cancers, i.e. breast, prostate, uterus, ovarian. Although research results are mixed on the efficacy of lignans to prevent hormone-related cancers, lignans, with other nutrients such as omega-3 oils, can reduce cancer development as well as cardiovascular and heart disease. Lignans may also help maintain bone density. The lignan sesamin (in sesame seed) is also believed to promote fat loss and is often included in diet foods; its benefits are enhanced when taken with vitamin E.

Sources: linseed (flax), sesame seeds, rye bran and meal, oat bran, poppy seeds, strawberries, blackcurrants, olives, brassicas, wheat bran, sunflower seeds, pumpkin, blueberries, cranberries, carrots.

Good sources of lignans

Linseed   oats   strawberries   pumpkin   blueberries

Coumestans

These compounds strongly interact with oestrogen receptors in the body, thus may have more activity than isoflavones at reducing hormone-related cancer risks.

A type of coumestan is glabridin, found in liquorice. This has strong oestrogen-like activity and can inhibit growth of human breast-cancer cells. It also has anti-inflammatory, antioxidant and antimicrobial properties. It inhibits melanogenesis and is used as a skin-whitening agent. It also has neuroprotective effects and may help improve cognitive function, including memory. Reduces weight gain by inhibiting abdominal fat storage. With vitamin D, it may help prevent bone loss in post-menopausal women.

Sources: red clover, liquorice, alfalfa sprouts, soya beans, peas, Brussels sprouts.

Isothiocyanates and allicin

These sulphur-rich compounds are only activated when a plant is injured. They rapidly release hot burning compounds via enzymatic systems as a defence mechanism to deter predators; consequently, much resides in the leaves and roots of these plants.

To humans, though, these compounds confer many health benefits. Humans, with their omnivorous diet, seem to have evolved to 'cope' with these molecules, and further, to derive benefits from them. They help reduce cancers, cardiovascular disease, diabetes and are antiviral. Also have antifungal, antibacterial and anti-allergic properties. Many of their activities work synergistically with other compounds, such as vitamins C and E and flavonoids.

These compounds are most effective when consumed fresh and uncooked. Heating for extended periods, freezing or microwaving reduces their activity by deactivating enzymes. Therefore, if possible, eat them fresh, or only cook them minimally, i.e. steam or quick stir-frying is best. Once prepared or cut, these compounds are only active for a short time, so cut and use within a few hours.

Allicins

Sulphide allicins are found in large quantities in garlic, but also in onions, chives, shallots and leeks. Allicins have proven antioxidant, antibacterial and antifungal properties. They are effective against many pathogenic bacteria, including *Staphylococcus* species and *Helicobacter pylori* (which cause stomach ulcers and cancer), and some pathogenic fungi that produce aflotoxins. They have antiviral activity (e.g. against human cytomegalo-virus, influenza B, herpes, human rhinovirus and, possibly, HIV).

Allicins reduce the formation of cancers: they seem to interrupt the development of cancer cells and can kill them. They act as anticarcinogens in the breast and prostate, but also liver, skin, stomach, colon and small intestine; reducing cancers of the digestive tract. Garlic has particularly potent anticarcinogenic properties. Studies show an inverse relationship between consumption of these foods and the incidence of some cancers. A meta study showed that garlic reduces development of stomach cancer by ~50% and colorectal cancer by 30%. If these plants are also grown in selenium-rich soil, these effects are increased.

Allicins also inhibit inflammatory processes and enhance the immune response. They help decrease blood pressure, reduce the formation of clots in vessels, lower serum LDLs, total cholesterol and triglyceride levels, and increase HDLs, thereby reducing development of cardiovascular diseases such as atherosclerosis. Research suggests that allicins are a safer way to reduce blood-clot formation than taking aspirin, with the latter linked to causing stomach ulcers.

Sulphides also reduce blood-glucose levels by either increasing the release of insulin or by increasing the removal of glucose from blood: thus, they may reduce development of type-2 diabetes.

Isothiocyanates

These are mainly found within the brassicas (cress, mustard, cabbage, etc.) and are only activated when the plant is cut or injured to form pungent, hot isothiocyanates (e.g. in wasabi and mustard). Their activity is greatest in young plants, particularly freshly sprouted seeds.

Much research confirms isothiocyanates are effective at reducing several types of cancer. They can kill cancer cells and may inhibit their multiplication. Like allicins, these compounds are most effective against cancers of the oesophagus, stomach, small intestine, colon, rectum, bladder and lung, but also breast. Sulphoraphane, found in abundance in broccoli, can reduce the development of breast tumours in lab animals by more than 40%, even in their later stages of growth. They seem to work by interfering with cell cycles that produce cancerous cells, but also indirectly alter oestrogen metabolism in a favourable direction. Reduced risk of colorectal cancers has been also observed in those who regularly consume brassicas.

Good sources of isothiocyanates

    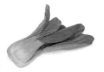

horseradish   mustard seeds   kale   broccoli   pak choi

Isothiocyanates also have antibacterial and antifungal activities, e.g. against *Staphylococcus aureas*, *Escherichia coli*, *Helicobacter pylori*. They also act as anti-asthmatics by inhibiting allergic-reaction compounds.

However, isothiocyanates can interfere with the thyroid gland's activity, though this can be usually reversed by supplementing the diet with extra iodine.

Sources: horseradish, mustard, wasabi, cabbage, kale, land cress, broccoli, Brussels sprouts, mustard greens, pak choi, radish, turnip.

Betaines, cholines and lecithin

Found in very high quantities within beets, but also in spinach and broccoli, betaine is produced commercially as a by-product of sugar beet processing. Closely linked to choline within the body, a deficiency can cause fatty liver and is linked to development of liver cancer. Several trials indicate that betaine protects against fat build up around the liver. It is also intimately linked with folate; newly pregnant women who had greater choline and betaine intake had children with a 72% lower risk of neural tube defects.

Choline is also an important precursor for a neurotransmitter involved in muscle control, memory and many cognitive functions. In the body, choline (and betaine) work with folate, B6 and B12 to increase elasticity of blood vessels and inhibit production of homocysteine (which causes vessel stiffening). Reduction in production of homocysteine reduces development of atherosclerosis.

Lecithin is found in seeds such as soy, sesame, sunflower, linseed, but also in eggs. It is intrinsic to every cell membrane in the body, it is particularly important within the brain. It keeps membranes supple and protects cells from oxidation, and is being trialled to treat patients with dementia and Alzheimer's. Plant-based lecithins can reduce serum-cholesterol and triglyceride levels.

Coenzyme Q$_{10}$

A fat-soluble compound produced by the body and found in all cell membranes. Vitamin B6 is needed for its biosynthesis within the body. It can also be obtained in the diet, commonly from meat and fish, but also from seeds and oils. It is essential for energy production and is an antioxidant. Because levels of internally produced coenzyme Q10 decline as we get older, extra added to the diet may provide anti-ageing properties. It may reduce the development of atherosclerosis, possibly coronary heart disease and relieve angina, reduce blood pressure, may improve elasticity of blood vessels, and is used to treat the early stages of Parkinson's disease. Needs selenium for its activity. Sources: beans, seeds, nuts.

Oxalic acid

A crystalline substance that can be irritating in larger amounts and prevent uptake of calcium, magnesium and iron from the gut and blood. It forms crystals with these, which can form kidney stones. Those with kidney disorders, gout and rheumatoid arthritis are advised to avoid foods high in oxalic acid, though in modest amounts it should not cause problems. Cooking removes little of this acid. Sources: amaranth, cassava, parsley, purslane, spinach, rhubarb, tea, sorrel, buckwheat, beet leaves.

Essential oils

These volatile, secondary plant products are powerful substances. They have wide-ranging medicinal activities, and are used in cosmetic and cleaning products, as aromatics and as food additives.

Many of the species described in this book can be distilled to extract their essential oils. They comprise only a small proportion of the plant, i.e. 0.5–1.5 %, and are usually very powerful, aromatic substances. However, a few species are so rich in essential oils that the plant material needs only to be crushed to remove its oil (e.g. citrus species). Because essential oils are so potent they should always be diluted before application to the skin using a carrier oil, such as almond, hazelnut or grapeseed, and diluting to ~5% essential oil to carrier. In addition, some oils, such as those derived from citrus and Apiaceae species can irritate the skin and cause dermatitis-like reactions, particularly if the skin is also exposed to direct sunlight. Ingestion of all essential oils should be undertaken with extreme caution.

Part Three:
A–Z of
Power Foods

Descriptions of nutrients within the following foods apply
to the fresh product unless stated otherwise, or unless the
food obviously needs to be cooked, e.g. dried beans. If you
want to find out more about a specific nutrient mentioned,
check the index for its location within Part Two.

RDA means recommended daily allowance.

Most of the raw nutrient data (though not secondary
plant compounds) were obtained from USDA Nutrient Data
Laboratory at http://www.nal.usda.gov/fnic/

Good levels of a nutrient within a plant are marked by the
following symbols:

F Fibre **M** Mineral **O** Oils **P** Protein
S Secondary plant compound **V** Vitamin

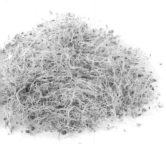

Alfalfa
(lucerne)

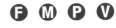

Alfalfa seeds are popular for sprouting and are delicious added to salads. Originally native to Iran, the Arabs gave it its common name, al-fac-facah, meaning 'father of all foods'. This plant has been long valued as a food for horses and was later grown by the Greeks for their horses. Although most alfalfa is still grown for this purpose, the increased interest in its nutritious seeds has meant that people too are eating this plant.

What it contains

The seeds are rich in **protein** (10–15%), **fibre** (10–20%) and contain good amounts of **minerals**. Are very rich in **vitamin K**, with only a little fat, and contain **carotenoids**. The seeds (and other plant parts) contain **L-canavanine** (an amino acid also found in other legumes). Also contain **phyto-oestrogenic isoflavones** and cholesterol-lowering **phytosterols**. Sprouted seeds are also nutrient rich.

What it does

The seeds promote pituitary gland function and have antifungal and anti-bacterial properties. There is ongoing research into L-canavanine's ability to treat certain neurological conditions, to lower cholesterol and to treat inflammation (see Warning). Its isoflavone properties have been used to relieve menopausal symptoms and to increase breast milk production and it is often mixed with other herbs.

Eating just 100 g of sprouted seeds a day has a clear protective effect against oxidative damage to DNA within human blood cells, therefore reducing the risk of cancers.

Warning: Research on mice shows that large doses of L-canavanine may possibly induce autoimmune disease. Also, those taking immunosuppressive drugs should perhaps avoid alfalfa seeds as they may reduce these drugs' efficacy.

How it is used

Sprouted seeds are great added to salads, sandwiches, dips, etc. Though, as with all sprouted seeds, ensure they are thoroughly washed to remove any harmful bacteria. They are also a tasty accompaniment to smoked fish, capers and mascarpone, and cold meats. The crisp sprouted seeds are great mixed with tomatoes, onion and cheese. Add to grated carrot, a little cilantro and oil, and then insert into a halved, just-ripe avocado to make a flavoursome, quick snack. The young leaves and shoots can also be added to salads.

> ✿ Sprout alfalfa and broccoli seeds together and enjoy their wondrous health benefits and flavours on a salad or just as a garnish. They can accompany sardines covered with a rich tomato and garlic sauce.

Almonds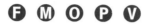

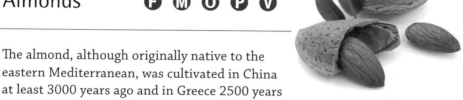

The almond, although originally native to the eastern Mediterranean, was cultivated in China at least 3000 years ago and in Greece 2500 years ago. In the Bible, almonds symbolised hope, and the Romans scattered them on newly married couples to represent happiness, good health and fortune, and future children. Almonds come in two main types: bitter and sweet. Bitter almonds were grown widely, but now, with selection, sweet almonds are preferred for their flavour but also, unlike bitter almonds, they contain very little cyanide-like compounds within their skins.

What they contain

Almonds are an excellent, healthy food. They contain ~50% **oil**, of which ~80% is **monounsaturated oleic acid** (15–20% is omega-6 linoleic acid, plus a little omega-3 oil). Almond oil has a similar composition to olive oil. Because of its oil, together with its good quantities of **dietary fibre** (~12%), almonds are digested slowly and so sustain and normalise blood-sugar levels.

Almonds are very rich in cholesterol-lowering **phytosterols**, and are wonderfully rich in **minerals**, particularly **calcium** and **magnesium**, but also **manganese, phosphates, potassium, copper, iron, boron, zinc**. Almonds are rich in **protein** (~20%) and this contains **all the essential amino acids**, though not large quantities of methionine. They are hugely rich in **vitamin E** (**tocopherol**), conferring powerful antioxidant and cardiovascular-protective properties. The nuts are a good source of **B vitamins**, particularly **biotin**, and **folate, niacin** and **riboflavin**.

Almonds in the diet have been shown to protect against damage to DNA, thus reducing development of cancers, even in those who smoke.

What they do

It is rare to get such a good protein and vitamin E source within one food. Almond's exceptionally rich vitamin E content helps decrease the risk of cardiovascular diseases and certain cancers. Studies have shown that almonds help prevent heart disease by lowering serum LDL levels. This vitamin is intrinsic in maintaining the integrity of cell membranes, is involved in the formation of DNA and RNA, is needed to form red blood cells and promotes wound healing. It may also help reduce development of some neurodegenerative diseases by helping stabilise and balance cell membranes. It helps reduce the incidence of eye cataracts and damage done to skin by UV light.

Vitamin E benefits the liver by neutralising certain toxins and enhances the immune system and inflammatory reactions. It may help protect against arthritis, diabetes, and bowel and renal disease. Regular intake of vitamin E may benefit those with type-1 or type-2 diabetes.

Almond oil is used to treat inflammatory problems, and aches and pains. It is also used in sedative medicines and health preparations. Its high calcium levels are beneficial to children and post-menopausal women: regular consumption has been shown to reduce development of osteoporosis. Finely crushed almonds make an excellent face scrub and emollient, and its oil works wonderfully in a range of skin creams to soften and moisturise.

Warning: As with all nuts, some people may be allergic to almonds. In addition, bitter almond skins contain cyanide-based compounds. If eaten in large quantities, bitter almonds can cause convulsions and death. However, these poisons are broken down at high temperatures, so cooked dishes containing bitter almonds are not dangerous. Sweet almonds have very low levels of these compounds and are not toxic.

How they are used

Sweet almonds can be dry-roasted at ~150° C for ~10 min or until they begin to change colour. Sprinkle with a little salt, tamari or sweeten with a little honey. Do not over-roast. Almonds are a popular snack and are added to desserts, cakes, confectionery, breakfast cereals, vegetable and fish dishes, and to stir-fries. They mix well with spices such as cinnamon. In Indian cooking, they are fried together with spices and then mixed with yoghurt to make a flavoursome sauce, and may be added to curries. They are also the main ingredient within marzipan, which is made by kneading ground almonds, sugar and essences. Almond oil is used as a flavouring in cakes and cosmetics.

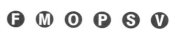 Mix chopped almonds and dried fruits into melted 70% cocoa chocolate. Allow to cool and become firm. Serve with fresh kiwifruit slices and a drizzle of fresh yoghurt.

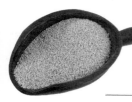

Amaranth   F M O P S V

Many think of amaranth as a decorative annual; however, its seeds and leaves are edible and nutritious. Of the amaranth species, *Amaranth caudatus* is probably the most popular. Native to Central and South America, amaranth has been utilised by indigenous populations for 6000 years as a staple, nutrient-rich crop. The seeds are a rich source of protein and contain several amino acids not commonly found in plant foods.

What it contains

The seeds are very rich in **protein** (15–18%), more so than most grains. This contains a balanced range of **essential amino acids**, in particular **lysine**, which is lacking in most cereals, and **methionine**, lacking in legumes. Its protein quality is as good as that from cow's milk or soy beans. The leaves are also one of the richest 'green' sources of protein. The seeds lack gluten and, therefore, although not good for bread-making, are an excellent substitute grain for those with gluten allergies. It is also easy to digest.

The seeds contain 5–15% **oil** content, of which ~35% is **omega-6 linoleic acid** (with some monounsaturated oleic and palmitic acids). The seeds contain good amounts of **vitamin E** (much as **tocotrienols**), which helps reduce serum-cholesterol and LDL levels, and are very rich in **squalene** and cholesterol-lowering **phytosterols**.

The seeds and leaves contain good amounts of **calcium, potassium, phosphates, iron, sodium**. The leaves are very rich in **vitamin A** and **vitamin C**, and **folate**. They are hugely rich in **vitamin K**, and are very rich in **antioxidants**. The leaves and seeds have good **fibre** content. The plant also contains **betalains**, which give it much of its red colouring.

What it does

Amaranth provides gastro protection and, in rats, helps the healing of mucosal injuries of the gut, thus could be a good food for those with digestive diseases. Amaranth also contains squalene, a powerful antioxidant that has been used to boost the immune system, to treat hypertension, skin problems and metabolic disorders, and is used in the cosmetics industry as a skin softener. It, along with tocotrienols (vitamin E), can significantly decrease blood-cholesterol levels, improve and stabilise cell membranes, resulting in reduced blood pressure and cardiovascular disease. Its betalains have powerful antioxidant and anti-cancer properties.

The seeds have been used to regulate and reduce menstruation, to treat diarrhoea and for gastrointestinal disturbances. The seed oil is used in skin-softening and moisturising products.

Warning: Leaves contain quite high amounts of oxalic acid, so should be avoided by those with arthritis, gout or kidney stones. Oxalic acid also reduces calcium and iron absorption.

How it is used

The lightly steamed stalks are asparagus-like in flavour. Young leaves are tasty either lightly steamed or stir-fried, and have a mild, spinach-like flavour. To avoid losing flavour and nutritive content do not overcook. The leaves are added to curries and blend well in cheese and egg dishes. Can be blended with garlic, basil, onions and tomato sauce, mascarpone, and then served with pasta. The grain, when prepared, has a nutty, sweet taste. It can be toasted or popped (like sweet corn), to give it more flavour, and then used in confectionery, bread, pancake mixes. It can be made into a porridge to which fruits such as raspberries, strawberries and banana are added. Sprouted seeds mix well in salads and are very nutritious. They can also be ground to a flour and added to bread and cakes, used as a thickener and made into a beverage. The seeds take <20 minutes to cook and rapidly become mushy if overcooked.

🍃 Undervalued, the seeds are very rich in protein. Toast a few sesame and mustard seeds, then add amaranth seeds and a little oil and stock, and then simmer until just cooked. Add chopped parsley and pinenuts and serve with a rocket, watercress, tangerine and kiwifruit salad, sprinkled with a tahini dressing.

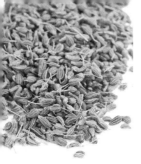

Anise

(aniseed, sweet cumin)

Anise, related to carrot and fennel, has seeds and leaves that are used to flavour pastries, cakes and beverages. Its distinctive aroma is popular in many parts of the world. Thought to originate from Mediterranean regions, it is now grown in Europe, India, China and Mexico. Anise has been used medicinally in China and in Indian Ayurvedic medicine for thousands of years. Its essential oil has virtually identical properties to that of star anise, though the latter is a completely unrelated species.

What it contains

The seeds, **protein** and **fibre** rich, are also very rich in **iron**, **calcium**, **manganese**, **zinc**, **magnesium**, **potassium** and **phosphorus**. Seed extracts have **powerful antioxidant properties**, more so than vitamin E, and they contain various **flavonoids** (e.g. **rutin**, **quercetin** and **luteolin**) and **coumarin**-like compounds (e.g. **anethole, estragole**).

What it does

Historically, the seeds and leaves were used as an antidepressant, a sedative, to reduce muscle spasms, for heart problems and as a diuretic. Its muscle-spasm-reducing properties help reduce indigestion, flatulence, belching and nausea. Anise has traditionally been given to young children to relieve colic. It has also been taken to reduce menstruation cramps, to treat coughs,

> Mixing a little anise into a fruity sauce to accompany some lightly cooked white fish can help ease painful menstruation and aids digestion.

bronchitis, etc. Recent research has proven this plant's ability to relax smooth muscle, and verified its usage to relieve as an anti-spasmodic.

Its essential oil, very rich in anethole, has proven antifungal properties, including action against the yeast *Candida* spp. It has antibacterial properties, including against waxy-coated, difficult-to-penetrate bacteria, and potent insecticidal properties (it is effective against the larvae of several mosquito species). Historically, it was used to treat lice and scabies. Anethole also has mild phyto-oestrogenic properties, which are being researched as possible replacements for synthetic oestrogens. Consequently, these compounds may help alleviate menopausal symptoms

Anise mixes well with nuts such as almonds, pecans, walnuts and pinenuts. It also blends well with tangy citrus flavours, and a little adds interest to roasted carrots. However, it does have a strong liquorice-like flavour, so should be used with care as its flavour can dominate.

and prevent osteoporosis. The seeds were historically consumed to increase breast milk production.

Warning: As with all essential oils, it should be used internally and externally with care. It contains coumarins, which if applied to skin and then exposed to sunlight, can cause skin to blister. Anise, consumed in fairly large quantities, has anticoagulant properties; therefore, those taking blood-thinning medications should avoid excessive consumption.

How it is used

The seeds are a popular flavouring in many sweet cakes, pastries and beverages. A little can be added to meats such as pork and beef. The flavoursome, fresh young leaves are added to salads and used as a garnish. They have a sweetish flavour.

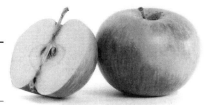

Apples

Apples have been appreciated since at least Neolithic times, and a myriad of cultivars have been selected since. Ranging in colour from green, yellow, orange to red, apples also range in size from more than 0.5 kg cooking apples to mid-sized red, sweet eating apples, to small fiercely sour crab apples, an ancestor of many modern types. Today, many are concerned that old orchards are disappearing; consequently, heirloom varieties are being saved and rediscovered. Although some old varieties may not keep as well, they are often more flavoursome and are richer in nutrients.

What they contain

There is strong evidence that regular consumption of apples reduces the incidence of cardiovascular disease.

Does an apple a day keep the doctor away? Most of the apple's nutrients are just under the skin, so don't peel them. They are a good source of **potassium**, have some **vitamin C**, and are rich in soluble **pectin fibre**. Apples are also rich in sugars (~10%), with more than half of this being **fructose**.

Apples also contain polyphenols (**anthocyanins**, and also **quercetin**), with most found in the skin of red apples. Cloudy apple juice contains up to four times more antioxidants than clear juice; it also contains lots of pectin fibre.

What they do

Pectin slows the release of sugars into blood, reduces blood-cholesterol levels and improves digestive health. They help prevent diarrhoea and constipation, act as a mucilage and encourage the growth of beneficial gut bacteria. In addition, apples are rich in organic acids (malic and tartaric acids), which may also aid digestion.

> 🐾 In one study pregnant women who ate a diet that included apple and fish produced children who developed less asthma and fewer allergies.

Green apples are said to act as a liver and gall-bladder cleanser: they may soften gallstones. Apples are a traditional remedy for joint pain and stiffness caused by rheumatism. Topical application of (acetic-acid rich) cider vinegar is an effective treatment for eczema. Eating fresh apples gives gums a healthy massage and cleans the teeth.

Warning: All members of this family contain cyanide-like compounds within their seeds. It is okay to eat a few, but note that a man who ate a cupful of apple seeds died! Also, due to the high fructose levels within apples, removal of fibre to make clear apple juice can cause diarrhoea in infants and young children: it is better to give the whole fruit or cloudy apple juice (which contains fibre).

How they are used

A fresh, crisp sweet apple takes some beating. Apples are eaten fresh and also widely used in pies, desserts, jams, sauces, apple butter, etc. They can be baked and stuffed with dried fruits. Apple juice is very pleasant and makes a good base for other juices. Apples also make a reasonable-quality wine. They are often mixed with dates, grapes, blackberries and bananas in desserts. They make a tasty compote and are great in oatmeal biscuits.

Cooked apple mixes well with warm spices such as cinnamon, cloves and nutmeg. Apple sauce can be served with pork and goes well with other meats. Fresh apple also livens up a pumpkin soup, and its crisp and tangy yet sweet flavour complements savoury dishes such as stir-fries, curries, pilafs and stews. Finely cut apple is wonderful with fresh salad greens and celery. Sour apples are used to make cider and for cooking and they make cider vinegar. The fruits can be dried or frozen for later use.

Apricots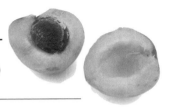

These oval, yellow, fuzzy fruits are popular, often in their dried form, for their dense flavour and wondrous health benefits. Apricots were native to north-eastern China, where their cultivation dates back 4000 years. Today, most are grown in Turkey and Iran. Within the rich, juicy flesh is a single hard stone, which, like other members of this family (e.g. almond, cherry), should be discarded due to the cyanide-like compounds it contains.

What they contain

The fruit is very rich in **carotenoids** (70–85% as β-**carotene**). They are virtually the richest source of this vitamin in everyday foods. Levels of carotenoids increase as the fruits ripen (canned apricots contain only about half of these levels). They are also rich in **flavonoids** (e.g. **quercetin**) and coumarin-like compounds (e.g. **chlorogenic acid**). Contain some **vitamin C** (12 mg/100 g) and have good levels of **soluble fibre**. Fruits are also high in **potassium**. The seed's oil contains both **monounsaturated** and **polyunsaturated fats**, and good levels of **vitamin E**. They contain a small amount of **lignans** (phyto-oestrogens).

What they do

The high levels of antioxidant carotenoids present in apricots have strong cancer-fighting properties. They help prevent skin, breast, lung and prostate cancers. These are involved in cell division and cell differentiation and are important for the proper formation of bones and teeth. Fat-soluble carotenoids (and vitamin A) help maintain the health of all cell membranes, and so help prevent infection and aid the immune system.

🍃 Apricots have been proven to enhance vision and seeing in the dark. The carotenoids are directly involved in the formation of rhodopsin, a compound needed by the light-sensitive rods in the eye that enable us to see in the dark.

The drug laetrile is derived from the seeds and is used as a controversial therapy for cancer; there are reports of tumour regression and pain reduction, and it is still used as a therapy in some alternative clinics. The cyanide-like compounds it contains are thought to specifically react with tumour cells. They have been used to treat tumours for ~2000 years. Warning:

Do not eat the seeds. The cyanide-like compounds can kill very quickly.

How they are used

Ripe apricots can be eaten fresh, though they are usually cooked and added to desserts, jams, chutney, ice cream and yoghurt. They go well in oatcakes and muffins. The fruits are puréed and given to young children, or added to biscotti, cakes and pies. Apricot strudel, with a little cinnamon and other dried fruits, topped with live yoghurt, is not too sweet but has an intense fruity flavour. Its beneficial carotenoid content is not damaged by heat. Puréed, it makes a tasty sauce to accompany meats such as pork and chicken. It can even be added to soups and vinaigrettes and makes a good juice or smoothie. The fruit dries well and is popular in breakfast cereals, trail mixes, etc. Drying concentrates the nutrient value of apricots several-fold. Apricot oil has the cyanide-like compounds removed and makes a fine-quality oil for salads, dips, etc.

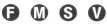

Asparagus

Who can resist fresh asparagus with a drizzle of fresh yoghurt or sour cream? Or perhaps accompanying salmon or pasta. The Greeks appreciated the shoots of this plant and named it 'asparagos', meaning swollen shoot. It was also valued and cultivated by the Romans. High in nutrients and vitamins, this popular vegetable features on many fine menus. It is versatile and is quick and easy to prepare.

What it contains

The fresh shoots contain excellent levels of the **B vitamin, folate**, one of the best of any fruit or vegetable, plus **carotenoids** (as β-**carotene**, **lutein** and **zeaxanthin**). Also contains some **vitamin C** and is very rich in bone-enhancing **vitamin K**. Is rich in **antioxidants**, particularly **rutin**, with **quercetin** and **kaempferol**. It has a greater antioxidant activity than broccoli, with green asparagus containing more than white asparagus. Are very rich in **fluoride**, and have good amounts of **potassium** and **iron**. Asparagus contains reasonable quantities of **fibre**, with much as **soluble inulin,** which benefits the digestive system and may explain why it has long been valued as a laxative. Are **very low in calories**. Asparagus is

> ❧ Rutin-rich asparagus has wondrous antioxidant and anti-inflammatory properties. It significantly improves elasticity and health of blood vessels, helping to strengthen capillary walls. It works most efficaciously when combined with hesperidin, so eat asparagus with a little grated citrus peel to get its full benefits.

particularly rich in the amino acids **glutamic** and **aspartic acid** (**asparagine**), with the latter named after this vegetable. Contains some **steroidal saponins**.

What it does

Folate, as well as being invaluable in preventing some neural-tube-related birth defects, also helps reduce heart disease by maintaining the transformation of homocysteine into cysteine. Levels of homocysteine rise if someone is deficient in folate (and deficiencies are very common in the general population). This can lead to a significant increased risk of heart disease by promoting atherosclerosis. Folate also seems to reduce the risk or effects of diseases such as Alzheimer's.

Glutamic acid is an important antioxidant that seems to protect against cancer, acts as an antiviral, enhances the immune system and partially regulates vitamins A and E. Its steroidal saponins are thought to be useful in treating nervous and rheumatic problems. These compounds also have anti-tumour activity, in particular in preventing colon cancers.

Warning: Hardly a warning, but those who eat asparagus will note that their urine develops a strange, not altogether pleasant smell which is caused by the breakdown of sulphur compounds, though these are harmless. Apparently, not everyone (genetically) can detect this smell. More seriously, a few people are allergic to asparagus: treat with caution at your first taste.

How it is used

The plump shoots are lightly cooked: they only need ~5 minutes of light steaming. Specialist tall, narrow pans have been designed so that the base of the stems stand in water while the tips are just steamed. They are delicious when young and tender. Asparagus spears can be served either on their own, or with a dip such as mascarpone, a vinaigrette dressing or garlic butter. They can be added to a multitude of dishes, such as quiches or pastas, they can accompany fish and meat dishes, or can be added to antipasto, risotto, frittatas and soups. They go well with egg and cheese (especially goat's cheese), and in menus that include mushrooms, smoked salmon or ham. They are great added to salads with garlic aioli, or can be served with a creamy mustard sauce.

Avocado Ⓕ Ⓞ Ⓢ Ⓥ

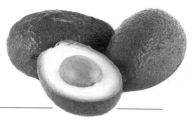

This delicious pear-shaped fruit has luscious, creamy flesh. Avocado trees were being cultivated in South America long before the arrival of the Europeans. Once 'discovered' this strange fruit was carried to many warmer regions of the world. Its thick, oily flesh is now hugely popular and is appreciated by people worldwide. Avocados also have excellent nutritional benefits, which have only recently become recognised.

There are three main types of avocados: Mexican, Guatemalan and West Indian. Mexican fruits are smaller and have thin skins that turn glossy green-black when ripe; Guatemalan fruits are oval or pear-shaped, with fairly thick, pebbled, dark-green skin (often the most popular and commonly seen); and West Indian fruits, which have a lower oil content, are the largest fruits, almost round, with thick, shiny, green skin.

What it contains

Have a **high oil** content, 10–35% (depending on cultivar), which is largely composed of **monounsaturated oleic acid**. Virtually the only other fruit with more oleic acid is the olive. The oil has excellent keeping quality if kept in a dark bottle. The fruits are rich in **vitamin E**, and in cholesterol-lowering **phytosterols**. Avocados are rich in **carotenoids** (much as **lutein** and **zeaxanthin**), and good amounts of the **B vitamins**, including **folate** (half a fruit ~25–50% RDA). They contain good levels of **vitamin C**, and much of the greenish colour of the flesh is from **chlorophyll**. They are high in dietary **fibre**, most of which is soluble, and are rich in antioxidant **flavonoids** (e.g. **catechins**).

What it does

A highly digestible food, recommended as a baby food and as a good, long-lasting energy source. Full of beneficial compounds. Avocado has significant anti-inflammatory properties. A mix of avocado and soya bean oil (known as piascledine) has been developed as a drug for osteoarthritis. It enhances synthesis of beneficial connective fibre, and inhibits the release and activity of compounds that are involved in development of

> Recent clinical studies report that avocado oil can reduce serum-cholesterol and triglycerides, while not increasing body weight, and retains beneficial HDLs, working better than a low-fat diet.

osteoarthritis. This drug results in decreased pain and reduces the need for analgesic drugs.

Phytochemicals within avocados inhibit the growth and selectively kill several pre-cancerous and cancer cell lines, particularly oral cancers: Hass avocados were the particular type tested.

The fruits also contain an unusual sugar (mannoheptulose), which may actually depress insulin production, thus levelling out the peaks and troughs of blood-glucose levels: thus are beneficial to those at risk for (or have) type-2 diabetes.

The seed, fruit skin and roots contain an antibiotic that prevents bacterial spoilage of food. A piece of the seed or leaf placed over an aching tooth may help relieve pain. The oil is included in hair-dressing products, facial creams, hand lotions and fine soaps. It may help filter out harmful UV, is non-allergenic and is similar to lanolin in penetrating and softening skin.

How it is used

A food for all ages – even children love its creamy flavour. The halved fruit is popular filled with a cornucopia of ingredients, though a favourite is mayonnaise and seafood: it is wonderful with smoked salmon or crab meat. Avocado is included in sandwiches and all types of salads. If blended with cream cheese and pineapple juice, it makes a creamy dressing for fruit salads.

Mexican guacamole – blended avocado and lemon or lime juice with finely cut onion, garlic, plus chilli or Tabasco sauce – is a delicious dip. Diced avocado can be added to hot foods, such as soup, stew, chilli, risotto or omelettes, but because the flesh becomes bitter if cooked, add just before serving. It goes beautifully with fruits and vegetables, such as papaya, courgette, cape gooseberry, pineapple, tamarillo and asparagus. Its mellowness complements tangy flavours. Avocado in freshly cooked Turkish bread, with sweet cherry tomatoes, a scattering of broccoli sprouts, a sprinkle of olive oil and black pepper, topped with crumbly feta or mozzarella cheese is delicious.

In Brazil, avocado is used more as a fruit and is mashed and added to sherbet, ice cream or milk shakes. In Hawaii, avocado is sweetened with sugar and combined with fruits such as pineapple, orange, grapefruit, dates or bananas. In Java, avocado flesh is thoroughly mixed

🌿 A New Zealand recipe for avocado ice cream blends avocado, lemon juice, orange juice, grated orange rind, milk, cream, sugar and salt. This is frozen, beaten until creamy, and frozen again.

with strong black coffee, sweetened and eaten as a dessert. Avocados are eaten with soy sauce or grated horseradish in Japan. Warning: Unripe avocados may be toxic, though they are hardly edible then anyway.

Bananas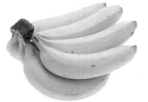

Bananas and banana plants have been valued by humans since before recorded history for a wide range of uses, including as a valuable food source, as a building material, medicinally and for clothing. The earliest mention of the domestication of the banana dates back almost 7000 years. Today, they are grown around the world in almost every tropical and subtropical area, and are the fourth-largest fruit crop worldwide, after grapes, citrus fruit and apples. Modern varieties have creamy-white, yellowy flesh, which becomes sweeter and softer as it ripens, though some species, such as the plantains, do not.

What they contain

Fruits contain about 23% **carbohydrate**, 1% **protein** and 0.5% **fat**, with virtually no cholesterol. They contain sugars, as balanced amounts of **glucose and fructose**, with some **sucrose**. They contain **soluble fibre**, which aids digestion and acts as mucilage. They are a good source of **B6**, contain some **vitamin C**, and are a good source of **potassium**.

What they do

Potassium helps normalise heartbeat and regulates the body's water balance. The fibre aids digestion, relieves constipation, reduces diarrhoea and can help soothe and heal intestinal ulcers and heartburn, as well as reducing morning sickness. They act as a natural anti-acid, and are a useful food for those in convalescence.

Eating bananas can improve mental activity as well as reducing high blood pressure: the US Food and Drug Administration has recently permitted the banana industry to make official claims for the fruit's ability to reduce the risk of high blood pressure and stroke. Research reports that eating bananas as part of a regular diet can cut the risk of strokes by as much as 40%. A drink made from banana, honey and milk is a good hangover cure: the banana calms the stomach and builds up depleted blood-sugar levels. Its B vitamins improve health and this fruit may have a calming effect, improve mood and give a sense of well-being.

How they are used

Bananas have a wide variety of uses and are an important food source to many around the world. They may be enjoyed fresh, make an excellent baby food, are added to cakes and used in many desserts. They are also good added to curries and are delicious lightly fried and served with white fish. They can be dried and flour is made from both bananas and plantains. If overripe or frost damaged, they are tasty if lightly fried with a knob of butter, a sprinkle of cinnamon and a dash of brandy. Or they can be dipped into a rich batter, deep-fried and then sprinkled with sugar and lemon. Mashed or whole bananas (in their skins) can be frozen for later use in desserts. Liquidise frozen peeled banana with cream or thick yoghurt and mix in a little tangy fruit such as passion or kiwifruit to make a quick, delicious ice cream-like dessert. Grate a little 70% chocolate on top.

In the Philippines, a spicy banana ketchup is popular. In India, they are made into a cool refreshing drink with yoghurt called lassi, and a sweet yoghurt cheese is made with banana, pistachios and almonds, which is spiced with cardamom. Also, there is the banana split: a banana cut lengthways and served with ice cream, chocolate and strawberry sauce. The Brazilians mash bananas with brown sugar, grated ginger and cinnamon or cloves and cook the mixture slowly until it thickens. When cool, it is moulded into a roll, sliced, and served cold. Plantains can be fried and eaten like French fries. Ripe bananas ferment easily and make a good, sweet white wine.

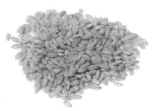

Barley

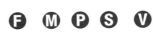

The fourth most commonly grown cereal, after wheat, rice and maize, barley is a staple food for many. Probably the first cereal to be harvested from the wild; it may have been gathered and eaten by pre-Neolithic man ~10,000 years ago: it was then one of the first to be cultivated. The Egyptians used barley extensively in breads and to make beer. Barley is particularly valued for its tolerance to cold, as well as its ability to grow in poor-quality soils, and is now widely cultivated in Russia, Canada, the Ukraine and other northern countries. Although much is now fed to livestock, its other main use is to make malt for beer.

What it contains

Barley grains are very high in **enzymes**, more so than most cereals, making it excellent for malting. Has a good **protein** content, though is short of lysine. Has excellent levels of **fibre**, much of it as β-**glucans**, of which it contains more than any other cereal. Has good levels of **B vitamins**, particularly **thiamine, niacin** and **B6**. Is rich in **manganese** (in particular), and in **selenium** (a powerful antioxidant), plus **iron**, **magnesium**, **phosphates** and **copper**. The latter may help relieve rheumatoid arthritis. As a whole grain, it is rich in **antioxidant** compounds, as yet largely unexplored, but which have many health benefits. Barley is rich in **phyto-oestrogenic lignans**. Pearled barley contains less of the above as it has had its outer layers removed. Malt contains ~75% sugars, mostly as **maltose**, and has a very high GI, but is rich in minerals, **calcium**, with good amounts of **folate**.

What it does

Barley's high fibre content is excellent for digestion, helps maintain healthy blood-glucose levels, reduces the risk of colon cancer (as well as haemorrhoids), lowers serum-cholesterol (reducing heart disease) and helps prevent (or manage) type-2 diabetes. Barley

> Barley has been recommended by the US Food and Drug Administration to help reduce coronary heart disease.

is more efficacious at this than most other cereals. It encourages beneficial gut bacteria (it works as a prebiotic); a by-product the bacteria produce, butyric acid, maintains healthy cells within the gut and lowers cholesterol. In addition, its lignans may protect against hormone-related cancers, such as breast cancer. Barley may also reduce the risk of gallstones.

The partially germinated seeds are highly nutritious and barley malt makes the best malt (compared to other cereals) due to its high enzyme content. Interestingly, barley contains an alkaloid (gramine) that can be converted to isogramine, which, in the 1930s, was discovered to have significant local anaesthetic properties. It was used to make lignocaine (xylocaine), a safe compound that has been widely used in dentistry ever since.

Warning: Barley contains glutens, which some people are allergic to, though the amount and reactivity are not as great as those within wheat.

How it is used

The grain is extensively used to make malt for beer and whiskey, malt vinegar and for sweet malt, with the latter used by bakers. To malt barley, the whole grain is soaked at ~16°C for <8 hours. They are then left in warmth, humidity and darkness for 2–5 days, until they sprout. The sprouted seeds are then roasted at 40–50°C for ~24 hours. This halts germination and 'captures' nutrients at a stage when they are partly activated by enzymes. Variations in roasting method affect the malt's characteristics and the consequent brew. The malted barley should have a crunchy, sweetish taste. This germinated grain can be crushed and processed to obtain a thick dark malt. Apart from beer, it is used to sweeten cereals, confectionery and to make malted-milk beverages. Whole barley grains can be cooked, though this does take about an hour. Pearled barley is quicker to cook, though has had most of its fibre-rich bran layer removed.

Barley can also be purchased as pot/scotch barley, which has been less processed. The cooked grains can be added, with other vegetables or meat, to soups and stews. They can be made into a pilaf or added to salads, and can replace the rice in risotto, or in stuffed peppers and marrow. The grains have a pleasant, sweetish, nutty flavour. If roasted and ground, barley can be mixed with lemon, honey and water, then chilled to make a refreshing summer drink.

Barley flour is added to cookies, breads, pancakes, waffles and scones. Barley is also sold as barley flakes, which are used in muesli, or the grains can be toasted and cracked to make barley grits, which are similar to bulgar, and are used in a similar way (see wheat). The sprouted seeds, if allowed to grow into 'grass', can then be used like wheat grass and added to juice. Or the sprouted seeds can be simply enjoyed in salads.

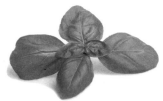

Basil

There are many species of basil, though *Origanum basilicum* is the best known and most widely cultivated. Historically, basil has, independently, become associated by many nationalities, such as the Egyptians, Indians and Europeans, to represent a gateway or passageway to God and heaven after a person has died. It is also revered by the Greek Orthodox Church, who add it to holy water. Known to cooks around the world, this wonderfully aromatic herb is highly-valued, particularly in Italian dishes, though is also used in Asian and Chinese cuisine, where it flavours soups. Basil also has many medicinal properties, including being a powerful antimicrobial, antifungal and insecticide.

What it contains

The plant contains an essential oil. The fresh leaves are hugely rich in **vitamins A** (**β-carotene, lutein** and **zeaxanthin**) and **K**, with good amounts of **vitamin C**. Has good amounts of **iron, manganese** and **calcium** (for a leaf). Basil is very rich in **antioxidants**; varieties with deep red/purple-coloured leaves are particularly rich in **anthocyanins**. It also contains **apigenin** and **rosmarinic acid**, many **terpenes** (e.g. **linalool, pinene, limonene**) and **coumarin**-like compounds (e.g. **eugenol**).

What it does

Compounds within basil leaves and seeds possess remarkable anti-inflammatory and antioxidant properties. Basil can inhibit and relieve pain, and has powerful wound-healing properties. Apigenin can repair disrupted cell-cycle checkpoints, thus acting as an anti-carcinogen for breast cancer. Research shows that other compounds (e.g. linalool) also have probable anticarcinogenic potential. A diet that included nutritious foods, such as basil, has been shown to benefit patients with advanced breast cancer. Its anti-cancer properties are being extensively investigated.

Basil leaves and seeds have wide-ranging antibacterial, antifungal, insecticidal and antiviral properties. For example, they are effective against certain strains of gonorrhoea that are becoming drug resistant, plus have some effect against bacteria such as *Staphylococcus aureus*. Eugenol has powerful anaesthetic and antiseptic properties, and is commonly used to ease toothache. Basil is effective at repelling flies, and shows great promise in repelling disease-carrying biting black flies. Uses for basil in internal and external medications, as well as to protect foods and incorporation in insect repellents, are being investigated.

> The awesome anti-microbial properties of basil are synergistically increased by as much as 20-fold when combined with eucalyptus oil. Apply a little of this mix (diluted with almond oil) on difficult-to-clear skin infections.

🌿 Mixed with balsamic vinegar and a little olive oil, basil makes a great dip for freshly cooked bread.

Historically, basil was used in Morocco to treat atherosclerosis. Recent research confirms that basil can reduce plasma cholesterol and reduce the risk for this disease in rats. The essential oil is used medicinally, and for perfumes and flavourings.

Warning: One of its compounds (estragole) has shown adverse health effects in rats and mice and may cause skin irritation in some. Its essential oil should be used carefully.

How it is used

The leaves are popular in Italian cuisine and go wonderfully with tomatoes, garlic, black pepper and olive oil. With pinenuts makes delicious, traditional pesto sauce and this has long been a way of storing basil, though it does oxidise and turn brown with time. Fresh basil makes a great garnish for pasta, pizza or lasagne dishes, and is mixed into quiches and tarts. A few leaves are used to flavour oily fish dishes, and can be added to green salads. The leaves have a strong but variable flavour, which depends on variety, but also on soil and climate, with plants grown in hotter climates often being stronger in flavour.

Asian varieties have a clove-like flavour whereas lemon basil (*O. americanum*) has a pronounced citrus taste. Basil is best eaten fresh; it should only be cooked briefly to retain its flavour. The leaves are even deep-fried. A few leaves can be mixed with dark, red berries in desserts to add an interesting flavour dimension. In Asia, basil is used to flavour soups, and soaked seeds are used to make a drink known as falooda.

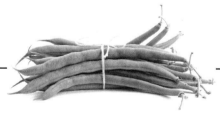

Beans   **F** **P**

Phaseolus spp., e.g. tepary, runner, lima, butter, black, brown, dwarf/French, flageolet, kidney, navy (Boston); *Vicia faba*, e.g. broad, fava, field; *Vigna* spp., e.g. azuki, urd (dahl), mung, pigeon peas, cowpea (blackeye, crowder, southern)

A very popular group of vegetables for their taste, nutrition and long-term storage benefits. Classed as legumes, they are within the same family as lentils and peas. The beans and pods of some *Phaseolus* species are eaten when still young, such as the runner bean. More usually, the beans are picked when mature, and are then dried for later use. *Vicia* bean species, native to North Africa and Southwest Asia, have been utilised for ~6000 years. One of the most popular is the broad bean, popular as an early-spring vegetable, but if left to mature further, is then known as the fava bean. Many *Vigna* beans are popular both in India and East Asia, as well as in the USA. Although some of these species are eaten when still young, they are more usually picked when mature and then dried for later use.

What they contain

Fresh beans are **vitamin** and **mineral** rich; unfortunately, levels of these are greatly reduced once cooked. Cooked beans are **protein** rich: 7–14%, having good quantities of most amino acids, though less methionine. Have good amounts of fibre (6–10%), much of it **soluble fibre**, contain virtually no fat, and have a low GI. Contain some of the **B vitamins**, with *Vigna* beans being rich in **folate**. Beans also contain **cholesterol-lowering phytosterols**. Contain some minerals, particularly **iron**. However, also contain **phytates**, which can reduce the uptake of some minerals. Many (e.g. red kidney, lima, navy) are rich in **saponins** and **lectins**. *Vicia* species also contain **vicine**.

What they do

Recent studies show that after 30 days of including *Phaseolus* beans in a carbohydrate-rich diet, human subjects had significantly reduced body weights, as measured by BMI, fat mass, adipose-tissue thickness and waist/hip/thigh circumferences, compared to subjects receiving a placebo. This loss was attributed to the slowness of digesting these complex carbohydrates. The beans' fibre, which is used by gut bacteria, may have enhanced these benefits. This result is reflected in beans' fairly low GI value, with wholegrain dishes having a lower GI than beans made into soups.

> Broad and fava beans have recently been found to be rich in levodopa, which can replace dopamine and is, therefore, of huge benefit to those with Parkinson's disease. This compound was first extracted from this species.

Warning: Water left after soaking and cooking dried beans should be discarded before beans are added to other ingredients (e.g. stew), as they (particularly red kidney) can contain high levels of lectins that affect absorption of nutrients and can cause red blood cells to stick together. Raw beans contain the most, though much is lost during cooking. However, cooking temperatures must exceed 80°C or toxicity can be worse; therefore, be wary of using 'slow cookers' for beans. Initially boiling the beans for 10 minutes at high temperatures, and then discarding the water should remove most toxins. Toxic levels of these compounds can cause intestinal discomfort or pain, and in some cases sickness and diarrhoea. *Vigna* beans (e.g. azuki and mung) do not cause abdominal gas or bloating like other beans can, and may therefore be fed to babies and those convalescing. They contain little to no lectins, though it may be prudent to discard water they are soaked or cooked in before adding other ingredients. Soaking these beans for a few hours before cooking makes them even more digestible.

A few people are genetically susceptible to vicine within *Vicia* species. It can cause severe haemolytic anaemia (known as 'favism'). Therefore, if trying these for the first time, treat with initial caution. In addition, *Vicia* beans contain tyramine, a compound that in some can increase blood pressure by causing vasoconstriction, which leads to increased heart rate. It may also be associated with migraines.

How they are used

Fresh, young beans, lightly cooked, are delicious – a popular vegetable to accompany traditional dishes. Try young runner beans, simply served with a dribble of yoghurt, a little grated parmigiano-reggiano and black pepper, served with fresh cherry tomatoes and minted new potatoes. Broad beans, apart from being steamed, are tasty lightly sautéed in garlic, or can be roasted and enjoyed as a snack.

Most dried beans need soaking for >6 hours before cooking, and then may need cooking for an hour or two, though use of a pressure cooker speeds this up. However, most *Vigna* beans, because they are smaller, take less time to cook: mung beans take only ~30 minutes. Cooked, dried beans can be used in many ways: stews, pies, soups, curries, ratatouille and salads. They mix well with tomatoes, sweet peppers, chilli, courgette, broccoli, cauliflower, kale, eggplant, pumpkin, potato, rice, herbs (e.g. parsley and thyme), lemon zest, garlic, onions, sausages and pepperoni, bacon, celeriac and olive oil. They can be added cooked, cold and spiced to salad ingredients, and can be 'refried' with spices to make a delicious filling for enchiladas. Beans, such as azuki, mung and urd, are great in soups, curries and stews; they make delicious dahl, and the flour is used in poppadoms, cakes and breads. Fava beans when cooked and mixed with olive oil, garlic, salt and lemon juice, make a delicious Mediterranean/ Middle Eastern dish. Add a pinch of epazote or asafoetida to reduce flatulence. Some add beans to lamb or seafood recipes. Navy beans,

🐾 Azuki, mung and urd type beans are popular in Ayurvedic cooking and are often mixed with rice to achieve a balanced protein food (called 'khichari'). They are combined with spices, such as turmeric, cumin, ginger and coriander. This tasty, nutritious dish is believed to restore balance to the body, mind, spirit, senses and emotions.

sometimes called Boston beans, are most commonly known as 'baked beans', which, when mixed with tomato sauce, provides a food that even the fussiest children seem to enjoy. Beans such as mung can be sprouted, and then mixed into salads and stir-fries. Germinating the smaller bean seeds changes the composition of their starches, etc., and makes them digestible uncooked. As with all sprouted seeds, particularly purchased sprouted seeds, wash thoroughly before use.

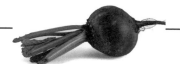

Beetroot

Root beets are generally divided into beetroot, mangels and sugar beet: these are also closely related to chard (see p. 136). Beetroot is probably the most interesting to eat, and was popular with the Romans, though was probably not as red then. The fully red beetroot may not have been selected until ~15th century. It seems people either love or hate beetroot, though this may be because many have only experienced it sitting in vinegar accompanying a salad. They can, however, be prepared in many other ways. Also, despite being a root crop, they are full of nutrients.

What it contains

Beetroots contain **soluble** and **insoluble fibre**, which are beneficial to the digestive system. Contain virtually no calories, and have good **folate** levels. Red beetroots are rich in powerful antioxidant **betalains** and **betaines**. These compounds are only found within a few plants, and red beetroot is the main edible source of betalains. Beets also contain cholesterol-lowering **phytosterols**. Beets, but particularly sugar beets, are very rich in sucrose, with a little fructose and glucose.

What it does

Research shows that beetroot juice reduces the risk of cardiovascular

🐾 Although completely harmless, it can be alarming if you are not aware that about one in ten people cannot break down the red compounds within beetroot: these are passed out with the urine, which takes on a blood-red colour.

disease. It is proposed that bacteria on the back of the human tongue interact with saliva and convert inert nitrate from beetroot into bioactive nitrite, which reduces blood pressure, blood-clot formation and reduces damage/injury to cells lining blood vessels. These processes probably work in parallel with other benefits obtained from antioxidants within beets to reduce cardiovascular disease. The beneficial activity of nitrites elsewhere in the body (particularly the digestive system) is also being researched: this evidence contrasts with what was previously known about nitrite and nitrates within the diet.

Betalains give beetroots much of their red colouring and are powerful antioxidants which have anti-cancer properties. Beets are also rich in betaine compounds, found at very high levels within beetroot. Betaines can reduce the multiplication of cancer cells. They may also help the body's hormonal system deal with depression; in fact, it has been claimed to work better for autistic children than pharmaceutical drugs. It stimulates the body to produce a compound needed to produce the neurotransmitters serotonin and dopamine, both natural mood enhancers. This compound also, indirectly, helps improve liver health; thus, recovering alcoholics are encouraged to take extra betaine. Levels of betaine naturally decline with age, so increasing betaine in the diet when ageing is likely to be of benefit.

How it is used

Sugar beet is an important source of sugar in colder, temperate climates. As well as refined sugar, it is also important commercially to make distilled alcohol. However, it can also be eaten as a vegetable, with roasting being recommended as a good cooking method.

Beetroots vary in sweetness, and are best eaten while still young; older beets become woody and less sweet. A little fresh beetroot is wonderful in salads – the outer skin is usually removed, and the flesh simply grated. Mixes well with grated carrot, though does colour the foods it is mixed with. Beetroots can be sliced and pickled in spiced vinegar, or can be roasted whole. Pickled beetroots retain their colour; roasting within their skins also keeps them red. Beetroots mix well with a range of foods, such as apple, onion, celery, orange, horseradish, potato, salmon, pears, celeriac, watercress, sweet potato. The very young leaves of beetroot can be used in salads and a few older leaves can be lightly steamed or stir-fried. They taste like mild spinach.

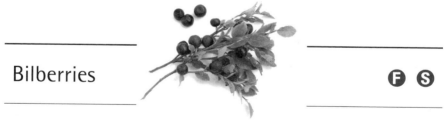

Bilberries

F **S**

Bilberries are picked from small, hardy bushes that grow in the cold mountainous districts of North America, the United Kingdom, northern Europe and Greenland. In some areas they are the dominant vegetation. The dried fruits have long been valued as a winter food source. In addition, their wide-ranging medicinal benefits have been recognised since at least the Middle Ages. They have been used to treat liver disorders, coughs and lung ailments. Many of these uses have now been validated – the nutritional benefits of these fruits are impressive.

What they contain

Although low in vitamin C, they are bursting with **antioxidants**, mostly as **anthocyanins** (25–36%), of which they contain more than most other foods. They also contain good amounts of **soluble fibre**.

What they do

Bilberry antioxidants reduce blood clotting; induce relaxation and improve elasticity of blood vessels and smooth muscles; and strengthen capillaries and connective tissues, thus significantly reducing the development of cardiovascular disease. Weak capillaries, common in ageing, are associated with poor blood circulation to connective tissues and are related to inflammatory conditions, such as arthritis, and to diseases related to fragile capillaries, such as arteriosclerosis, hypertension, varicose veins, liver disorders, peptic ulcers – bilberries have been shown to improve many of these problems. In Europe, preparations are used to treat micro-circulation, including eye conditions such as night blindness and diabetic retinopathy. Compounds within bilberries increase the regeneration rate of rhodopsin, the purple pigment intrinsic to rods in the eye and enable light and dark adaptation, thus improving night vision. Trials in Italy showed that 76% of patients with myopia (short- or near-sightedness) had marked improvement in retinal sensibility after eating bilberries and taking vitamin A daily for 15 days. The fruits have anti-inflammatory properties and can reduce development of chronic inflammatory diseases such as atherosclerosis, pulmonary emphysema and rheumatoid arthritis. Its anthocyanins also slow the growth of human colon cancer cells, *in vitro*.

> 🐾 Because the abundant flavonoids within bilberries work so well with vitamins C and A, consider mixing these fruits with strawberries, kiwifruit and apricots, and add some fibre-rich banana with a sprinkle of chopped walnuts for a truly healthy dish.

How they are used

The fruits can be stewed with a little sugar and lemon peel, and included within pies or tarts. The fruits have a rich, sub-acid taste and are juicy. They make an excellent preserve or jelly, or are added to fresh or cooked desserts, as well added to sauces, ice cream and yoghurt. They go well with stewed apples, a little cinnamon and some creamy yoghurt. Great within muffins and cakes. Or, simply scatter them on your breakfast cereal along with yoghurt and a little honey. Bilberry jelly can accompany meat and poultry dishes. In France, tcha-tcha is made from fresh bilberries, crushed with sugar, and then spread on buttered bread. They are delicious on pancakes. In the US they are added to chicken salads, with pears, and can be added to a dressing made with yoghurt, black pepper, a little honey or oil, and balsamic vinegar. The fruits make a rich, fruity wine.

Blackberries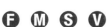

Blackberries are well known and appreciated by many in northern Europe. Often gathered from the wild, these tasty fruits are wonderful fresh, but also make excellent preserves, jam and wine. Cloudberries are closely related to the common blackberry, and are found growing wild in many colder regions of the northern hemisphere.

What they contain

Blackberries contain good amounts of **vitamin C** (30 mg/100 g of fresh fruit), though cloudberries contain even more (60–150 mg/100 g), and retain this if frozen immediately after picking. Have good levels of **folate**, plus good amounts of **vitamin K**. They are very rich in antioxidant flavonoids (e.g. **ellagic acid, catechins, anthocyanins, salicylic acid, quercetin**). The fruits are also rich in **soluble pectin fibre** (conferring many benefits to the digestive system) and **phyto-oestrogens**. They contain good amounts of **potassium, iron, copper, manganese**.

What they do

Blackberries reduce serum LDLs, contributors to heart disease, stroke and atherosclerosis. Ellagic acid is an antioxidant and flavour enhancer, and is found at 5–6 times greater levels in blackberries and raspberries than other fruits. In the human body, ellagic acid appears to impede cancer by blocking various hormone reactions and metabolic pathways.

Their high anthocyanin content, giving them their deep purple colour, is linked to improving vision, improving circulation, preventing cancer, controlling diabetes and even retarding ageing by preserving memory and motor skills. Quercetin and catechins are both antioxidants and anti-carcinogens. In addition, quercetin helps reduce allergy symptoms, possibly by reducing the release of histamines.

How they are used

Blackberries are delicious fresh and are often mixed with other fruits (e.g. blueberries, cherries, blackcurrants). They are added to many desserts to give a rich, distinctive flavour. They go well with apples in pies, and a blackberry and apple crumble with custard is a wonderful comfort food. They also mix well with strawberries, papaya, kiwifruit, pears, melon, other berries, and nuts such as almonds and hazelnuts. Serve fresh blackberries on top of an oat, dark chocolate and almond slice. The fruits make excellent jams, jellies and fruit sauces; their pectin gives them good thickening properties. They make a wonderful sauce to go with meats such as chicken. They freeze well for later use and can be added to ice cream and yoghurt. Cloudberries have a sweet/musky flavour that some say tastes like apple. They can be used in similar ways to blackberries and make a fine liqueur and wine. They have a wonderful colour when added to other fruits.

> Salicylic acid, found within blackberries, has the same protective value against heart disease and strokes as aspirin, without causing stomach acidity.

Blackcurrants   See 'Currants'

Blueberries

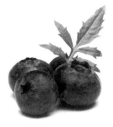

Closely related to cranberries, huckleberries, lingonberries and bilberries, blueberries are possibly the most popular of this group, though all have similar nutritional benefits. A North American plant, the fruits have been collected by indigenous peoples for thousands of years, and later by European settlers. The berries were eaten fresh, or were dried for use during the long winters. These delicious, tremendously health-giving fruits are now, deservedly, becoming increasingly popular. The rounded berries turn a dusky blue colour when fully ripe.

What they contain

The fruits have some **vitamin C** and **vitamin A**, plus good amounts of **vitamin K**. They contain **soluble fibre** and equal amounts of **glucose** and **fructose**. They are hugely rich in **antioxidants**, and are ranked first of all common fruits and vegetables for this – in particular they contain abundant **flavonoids**, particularly **anthocyanins**, but also **ellagic acid**, **quercetin** and **proanthocyanins**. Also contain **terpenoids** and **coumarin-like** compounds.

What they do

Blueberries' anthocyanins have impressive anti-inflammatory and anti-oxidant properties, with these progressively developing in riper fruits. The berries can potentially limit development and the severity of several types of cancer and vascular disease, including atherosclerosis and ischaemic stroke, but also age-related neurodegenerative diseases. The berries are very effective at lowering and reducing serum LDLs, which contribute to heart disease, stroke and atherosclerosis.

Blueberries also promote urinary tract health and reduce its infection. They appear to prevent bacteria from adhering to cells that line the walls of the urinary tract. In addition, in Sweden, blueberries have been used to treat childhood diarrhoea.

How they are used

The fruits can be eaten fresh – they are tart but tasty – and often mixed with other fruits to make flavoursome fruit salads. Can be added to a range of desserts and are used within muffins, breads, cakes, ice cream, sauce, yoghurt, preserves, chutneys. Blueberry pie or crumble, with ice cream, is delicious. Perhaps pancakes, made with rye flour, toasted wheat germ and coarse cornmeal, filled with a poached blueberry and strawberry sauce, topped with fresh yoghurt. They mix well with other berries, but also apricots, peaches, bananas and nuts such as pecans, hazels and walnuts. Blueberries can also go with savoury foods, perhaps as a sauce with chicken or lamb, or as a barbecue sauce with onions, a little chilli, mustard, wine vinegar, olive oil and a little sugar. They can also be added to rice and/or seafood dishes, to add a tangy component. Blueberries make a good-quality juice and wine.

> 🐾 Blueberries have been shown to improve and to actually reverse some of the effects of ageing, particularly loss of balance and co-ordination. A cup of blueberries a day enabled elderly people to develop 5–6% better motor skills than a control group and the women also reported improved mood feelings.

Bok choi   See 'Chinese greens'

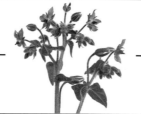

Borage

Borage, probably native to the Middle East, was widely used by the Celts, Greeks and Romans, and was believed to reduce melancholy and increase happiness. Nowadays, borage seeds are being appreciated for their high content of gamma-linolenic acid, which is greater in borage than in virtually all other plant species. Commercially it can be called starflower oil and has many health properties.

What it contains

When fresh, the leaves are very rich in **vitamin A**, with good amounts of **vitamin C** (~35 mg/100 g). They contain good amounts of **calcium** and **iron**. The leaves are also rich in other **antioxidants**, particularly **rosmarinic acid**. Borage seeds contain abundant (20–25%) **omega-6 gamma-linolenic acid** (GLA). Although the body can convert omega-6 linoleic acid to GLA, excessive linoleic acid consumption in Western diets reduces production of GLA. Thus, the ratio between these two fatty acids becomes unbalanced and, consequently, it is important to include extra GLA in the diet.

What it does

GLA has been shown, experimentally, to reduce rheumatoid arthritis and to reduce blood pressure (by widening blood vessels), inhibit cholesterol production and strengthen the immune system. In humans, it can decrease plasma triglyceride levels by 48% and increase HDL-cholesterol concentration by 22%. It also decreases platelet clot formation by 45% (see Warning). Borage oil has been used to treat various autoimmune diseases, such as multiple sclerosis, psoriasis and lupus. GLA is also converted to a precursor of an anti-inflammatory compound, which has been found to relieve premenstrual pain. The oil is used to reduce the effects of dermatitis and eczema, though its efficacy for this has been questioned. The oil, with antioxidants and fish oil, has significantly improved outcomes and reduced mortality rates in patients with severe sepsis and septic shock – the mix modulates the inflammatory response and reduces the risk of organ failure.

> Borage seed is super-rich in gamma-linolenic acid, which has many health benefits, including reducing weight re-gain in humans following major weight loss. It could therefore be important in the diets of those who are prone to obesity.

In addition, trials show that GLA suppresses a gene that causes over-production of a compound that otherwise increases the growth of cancer cells, particularly within the breast. GLA seems to target cancer cells without affecting healthy cells. In addition, when added to the drug Herceptin, it made breast cancer cells 30–40 times more sensitive to Herceptin. However, these are early results only performed on cells outside the body. Borage oil can also reduce the growth of some types of liver cancer. Note, though, that cooking and heating can reduce the effectiveness of this oil. Leaf extracts and the oil are added to skin creams – they are an effective moisturiser, help keep the skin elastic and are sometimes used as a skin rejuvenator.

Warning: GLA can increase bleeding time; therefore, those taking anticoagulant drugs (e.g. warfarin) should possibly not consume too many seeds.

How it is used

The flowers are candied and used in confectionery. The younger leaves have a mild, cooling, cucumber flavour. A few can be mixed with salad greens and the edible flowers make a good garnish. The leaves go wonderfully with lemon zest, cucumber and yoghurt. Can remove any outer roughness on the leaves before usage. Note that older leaves become tough and develop prickly, unpalatable hairs. The leaves can be lightly steamed and eaten as a vegetable, and can be combined with spinach or other greens, or be added to soups towards the end of cooking.

> 🌺 As a more unusual idea, the flowers and leaves are battered in an egg and flour mix and then deep-fried, before sprinkling with sugar and cinnamon.

Briefly scald chopped borage and nettle leaves, add roast garlic, olive oil, marjoram and a little nutmeg. Heat for a couple of minutes before adding ricotta and Parmesan. This mix is then used to fill ravioli.

Borage's bright blue, eye-catching flowers also make a great garnish. A few young leaves may be added to cold summer drinks, such as fruit juices, but also alcoholic drinks such as Pimm's, to add a refreshing, cooling note. The light oil can be used as a dressing or dribbled on toast instead of margarine.

Brazil nuts 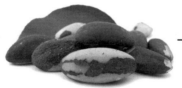 Ⓜ Ⓞ Ⓟ Ⓢ Ⓥ

These strangely formed nuts are delicious and healthy. The nuts grow on large, long-lived trees, naturally found in the rainforests of Brazil and neighbouring countries. About 20 hard seeds are produced within large, oval woody fruits. Within the hard outer seed covering is the white tasty kernel, or Brazil nut, as it is commonly known. As they grow poorly in plantations, and because of the many years it takes for trees to mature and the extensive deforestation that has occurred, the cost of these nuts is high. However, there are now some efforts being made to protect the forests they are found in.

What they contain

The nuts are very **protein** rich (~15%), containing **all the essential amino acids**. They contain ~70% **fat**, of which ~25% is saturated palmitic, ~40% is **monounsaturated** and 35% is **polyunsaturated** (much as **omega-6 linoleic acid**). They also contain good amounts of cholesterol-lowering **phytosterols**, and are rich in **squalene** and in **tocopherols** (**vitamin E**).

Selenium-rich Brazil nuts may be of benefit to those with conception and pregnancy problems.
Selenium is needed for human sperm maturation, sperm motility and may reduce the risk of miscarriage.

Brazil nuts are very rich in many minerals, including **copper**, **phosphates**, **iron**, **zinc**, **manganese** and **magnesium**. Their stand-out feature is that they have, by far, a greater amount of the **antioxidant selenium** than any other food (though levels do vary with where they are grown). They also contain good amounts of the B vitamin **thiamine**.

What they do

Selenium is a vital part of several enzymes involved with protecting cell membranes and producing lipids; it also works synergistically with vitamin E. There is evidence that selenium, with vitamin E, reduces the risk of prostate cancer.

Selenium is also a catalyst for the production of thyroid hormone; therefore, deficiencies result in a reduced capacity to fend off diseases, both bacterial and viral. It is also said to counteract the effects of heavy-metal ingestion – some practitioners recommend those with many amalgam fillings to regularly eat a few Brazils to ameliorate any adverse effects from mercury. Selenium is also vital for the activity of several antioxidant enzymes. It 'works' better when ingested in an organic form than taken as a supplement.

Squalene is a powerful antioxidant that has been used to boost the immune system and to treat hypertension, skin problems and metabolic disorders, and is used within cosmetics as a skin softener. Squalene, with tocotrienols (vitamin E), can significantly decrease serum-cholesterol levels – it improves and stabilises membrane fluidity, and so can reduce blood pressure. Thus, these nuts are a good food for those with cardiovascular disease.

The oil is used in skin and hair preparations.

Warning: As with all nuts, some people may be allergic to Brazil nuts.

Mix Brazil nuts with chopped hazelnuts and walnuts and sprinkle on a kiwifruit dessert – this contains good amounts of omega-3 oils due to the hazel and walnuts.

How they are used

These must be one of the finest-tasting nuts, with a rich, sweet nutty flavour. Their flavour is not unlike that of macadamias. They are often just eaten whole, or can be mixed with other nuts and dried fruits to make a highly nutritious snack – try them with dried apricots and prunes. Chopped, they are added to cakes, tarts, pies and breakfast cereals.

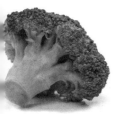

Broccoli

Broccoli has become one of the most popular vegetables in Western diets. It is valued for its taste, which most find agreeable, but also for its many health benefits. As a brassica, it is related to cabbage, cress and mustard. In has not been found for long in its present form and probably originates from vegetables such as purple sprouting and kale.

What it contains

Is wonderfully rich in **carotenoids** (**vitamin A**), much as **lutein** and **zeaxanthin**, which can slow the progression of age-related macular degeneration and cataracts, and help prevent cardiovascular disease. Also contains excellent amounts of **vitamin C** (~80 mg/100 g), though this is reduced by cooking. Is one of the best sources of **vitamin K**. It can contain good amounts of **selenium**.

Broccoli also contains **choline**, which is intimately associated with neurotransmitters and a lack of which can cause neural-tube defects and neurodegenerative disease. Also contains good amounts of **coenzyme Q10**, vital for energy production and a powerful antioxidant. Broccoli is very rich in sulphur-rich **isothiocyanates**, which have numerous health benefits. Also contains good quantities of the powerful flavonoid **quercetin**, and some **lignans** (**phyto-oestrogens**).

What it does

Many papers have reported the beneficial effects of the brassica vegetables and, particularly, on the isothiocyanates they contain. The ingestion of these compounds is inversely correlated with the incidence of cancer. They seem proven to reduce the risk of the development and spread of several types of cancer, including skin, lung, bladder, colon and prostate. They induce enzymes that repair damaged DNA. If broccoli is rich in isothiocyanates, then amazingly, fresh, 3-day-old sprouted broccoli seeds have 10–100 times more of these compounds than mature plants. It has been proven that eating just 100 g of sprouted seeds a day has a clear protective effect against oxidative damage to DNA, thus significantly reducing the risk of cancer.

Unfortunately, cooking broccoli 'destroys' most isothiocyanates, so just lightly steam or stir-fry, or even eat it fresh, finely chopped, in salads.

In addition, just-cooked broccoli tastes far better. Add a little broccoli to a turmeric-rich curry to reduce the development of and even help reverse prostate cancer – their combination is synergistic.

Broccoli can contain good amounts of the powerful antioxidant selenium, which reduces the incidence of colon cancer. When broccoli is digested, selenium forms a compound that is converted to a proven anti-cancer agent. Hybrids have been developed (known as 'super broccoli') that are a genetic mix between broccoli and a wild Sicilian relative; these have up to a hundred times more isothiocyanates than ordinary broccoli. Isothiocyanates also reduce serum-cholesterol, thus reducing the development of cardiovascular disease.

Broccoli sprouts significantly reduce populations of *Helicobacter pylori,* the bacteria that can cause gastric ulcers and stomach cancer. Broccoli is also unusual in being rich in lipoyllysine (a compound consisting of the amino acid lysine and α-lipoic acid (LA)). LA promotes production of several vital enzymes connected with energy production, is a powerful antioxidant, stimulates activity of other antioxidants, is involved in cellular communication and seems to enhance the insulin response.

How it is used

Delicious lightly steamed, or cut into small sections and stir-fried. It blends deliciously with soy sauce and other vegetables. It is a very popular side vegetable to accompany all types of meats and fish. To cook, just bring the water to the boil and let the florets stand in the hot water for ~5 minutes, or they can be steamed. Overcooking greatly compromises the flavour. If adding to soups or stews, add towards the end of cooking.

Add toasted sunflower and pumpkin seeds, chopped dried apricots, diced spring onions (scallions) and some crumbled goat's cheese to raw, finely cut broccoli and dress with a garlic aioli dressing. The young leaves are also tasty lightly steamed, though older leaves are tough and somewhat bitter.

Consider sprouting the seeds (though make sure they haven't been treated with fungicides), and add these to salads, sandwiches, or use them as a garnish.

🌿 Broccoli mixes wonderfully with garlic, tomato, black pepper and white cheese, but also with onions, lemon, almonds, peppers and creamy cheese sauces.

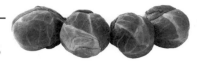

Brussels sprouts

A familiar vegetable in the United Kingdom, where it is typically served with the Sunday roast. The tightly folded, young leaf buds are widely enjoyed; however, they are often overcooked and so have developed a poor, undeserved reputation, which is a shame as they can be used in many ways. Brussels sprouts are also very nutrient rich.

What they contain

Being a shoot, Brussels sprouts are higher in nutrition than many leafy vegetables, and have good levels of **protein**. They are rich in both **soluble and insoluble fibre**, which benefit the digestive system, and contain very good levels of **carotenoids** (β-**carotene**, but particularly **lutein** and **zeaxanthin**), and excellent levels of **vitamins C** (~80 mg/100 g), and of **vitamin K** (a serving supply more than two times the RDA). Brussels sprouts are the most concentrated source of sulphur-rich **glucosinolates**: these, when cut or injured, are converted to **isothiocyanates**. Brussels sprouts are also very rich in cholesterol-lowering **phytosterols**.

What they do

Brussels sprouts are virtually proven to help prevent various cancers, including skin, lung, bladder, colon, prostate and breast. Research shows they can reduce DNA cell damage, in a short period, by as much as 28%. They induce enzymes that repair damaged DNA. Isothiocyanates inhibit cancer cell division and induce the death of some cancer cells. The ingestion of these compounds is inversely correlated with the incidence of cancer. The quantities of their beneficial compounds are much greater in fresh or only lightly cooked sprouts.

Warning: Compounds within brassicas can reduce thyroid activity in some susceptible people, though cooking is said to eliminate this effect. If you have thyroid problems, you may wish to eat less of these vegetables. Brussels sprouts can produce flatulence, though this is usually minor.

How they are used

Sprouts are usually prepared by removing the outer leaves, and some chefs cut a cross in the base of the stalk to speed up cooking time. They are delicious steamed (~5–7 minutes) and served with a traditional roast.

🐾 Take advantage of the synergistic benefits of Brussels and turmeric: add chopped Brussels sprouts (at the last moment) to a turmeric-rich curry to reduce the development of and even help reverse some cancers, particularly prostate cancer.

If overcooked, they become unpleasantly smelly and lose most of their flavour (and nutrients). They should be eaten while still green and a little crunchy. Sprouts can be finely chopped and added fresh to salads – they are very tasty fresh. Are delicious cut into quarters and stir-fried in a light oil, with sliced carrot, courgette, mushrooms, onions, a little bacon and soy sauce. Make great addition to bubble and squeak (fried-up leftovers of potatoes, veggies, etc.). Sprinkle with a little garlic and a tasty cheese, such as Parmesan, after steaming and then very lightly grill. They mix well with almonds, chestnuts, hazels, onions, artichokes, cauliflower, apples, pears, lemon zest, horseradish, mustard, rosemary, thyme and bacon.

Buckwheat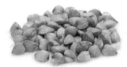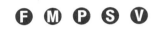

Though called buckwheat it is not related to wheat, but is instead more closely related to spinach. It originates from China and is likely to have been cultivated there for >6000 years. It is also grown in Korea and Japan. It is now popular in eastern and northern Europe, with 90% of cultivation in Russia, where it is a component of many traditional dishes. Buckwheat grains are very nutritious; its flour is valued in pancakes, noodles and many other foods. It is commonly sold as uncooked grain, though can sometimes be roasted, which enhances its nutty flavour.

What it contains

Very rich in **protein** – the whole grain contains ~12% (the inner seed has ~16%), which is more than most cereals. It also has a good balance of **all the essential amino acids** – it is particularly rich in **lysine**, which is often deficient in cereals.

Buckwheat is also **gluten free**. Contains good quantities of the **B vitamins**, particularly **thiamine** and **niacin**, and is rich in **soluble and insoluble fibre** (~10%), which significantly benefits the digestive system. Is rich in **copper, manganese, phosphates, iron, zinc** and **magnesium**. Has good amounts of **vitamin E**. It is **super-rich** in the **flavonoid rutin**

– some seeds contain up to 8%. Rutin improves membrane and capillary health. Also rich in other **flavonoids** (e.g. **quercetin**). The grain contains several **organic acids** and **choline**.

What it does

Fibre-rich buckwheat increases populations of 'good' gut bacteria, improves digestion, indirectly lowers serum-cholesterol, may reduce the incidence of gallstones and helps reduce the risk of colorectal cancers. Has a low GI and releases its food energy over a long period, meaning people feel fuller for longer. Consequently, it is also associated with reducing the risk of diabetes as it lowers blood-glucose levels. Also, as it is not a cereal, it makes an excellent substitute for those sensitive to glutens (e.g. coeliac disease).

The grain lowers LDLs while maintaining high levels of serum HDL, and reduces high blood pressure. These benefits have been partially linked with its high quantities of rutin. This compound works synergistically with vitamin C to reduce blood clotting. It also restores capillary health and elasticity – has been shown to reverse capillary damage in eyes. Damaged capillaries and their increased permeability are associated with many diseases, including cardiovascular disease, poor blood circulation to connective tissues, varicose veins, inflammatory conditions such as arthritis, diabetes and deteriorating vision. Abundant rutin may halt and even reverse some of these diseases.

Warning: Trypsin inhibitors in the seeds can cause indigestion; therefore, the seeds (or flour) should be thoroughly cooked before consumption.

> Sprouted buckwheat seeds are very nutrient rich. Trials show that at 8 days old they are at their richest in polyphenolics and quercetin. It is then that they then have their maximum antioxidant activity.

How it is used

The seeds develop a nuttier taste if roasted. They can be crushed or ground (in a blender) and added to cereals, soups, stews, etc. They are used instead of rice, or can be added to oats in porridge. Buckwheat whole grains cook quickly and just need simmering for ~15 minutes (groats only need ~7 minutes). Cook until they begin to soften then add salt, lemon zest, black pepper and perhaps a little grated Parmesan for flavour. More often, buckwheat is ground to flour for pancakes (blinis in Russia, galettes in France), muffins, bagels, tortillas. It may be added to wheat flour to make bread. It gives foods a light texture and an attractive brown colouring. Used to make Japanese soba noodles and can be added to pasta. The sprouted seeds are used in salads, sandwiches and stir-fries.

Capers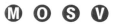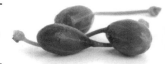

Capers are fairly closely related to brassicas, which explains why several of their compounds and flavours are similar. Capers are the immature flower buds, immature fruits or young shoots that are pickled in vinegar, oil or brine. They have long been used as a food and medicinally – remains of capers have recently been found in a Chinese tomb dated as 2800 years old. It is thought these plants were used for ritual as well as medicinal purposes. Capers are popular in a wide range of Italian dishes, as well as many fish dishes, with recent research verifying their significant medicinal properties.

What they contain

Capers contain many interesting compounds that can treat a wide range of medical conditions. They are rich in **vitamin K** and in **minerals**, particularly **calcium**, **potassium**, **phosphates** and **zinc**, though also sodium (particularly if they are in brine). Their seeds are rich in **oil** (~30%), most of which is **omega-6 linoleic acid**, and in **phytosterols**. The plant is rich in **antioxidants**, particularly **flavonoids** (e.g. **rutin**, **kaempferol**, **quercetin**). They are also rich in compounds that are converted to **isothiocyanates**; these give capers much of their flavour (similar to compounds found in brassicas).

What they do

Traditionally, capers have been used to treat rheumatoid arthritis. Caper extracts also have anti-allergenic and antihistamine properties in humans. It also interferes with the replication of the herpes simplex virus, so is a potential therapy for this condition.

> Capers have anti-inflammatory properties and can reduce inflammation around joints, even more so than indomethacin (an NSAID drug).

Traditionally, capers were used as a tonic for the liver and kidneys, to treat gout, as a diuretic and to reduce blood pressure. Capers are still used in herbal medicines to treat liver cirrhosis and other liver complaints and recent trials have shown capers to be liver-protective. They have potential as an anti-diabetic because they significantly reduce blood-sugar levels in diabetic rats, with this effect seeming to be independent of insulin secretion. In addition, the buds are rich in compounds that inhibit an enzyme that would otherwise increase the formation and progression of cataracts.

Warning: If applied to the skin, capers have been known to cause dermatitis.

How they are used

The young leaves, shoots and flowers can all be eaten fresh in salads. Occasionally, the younger leaves and flowers are cooked as a vegetable. However, fresh or cooked, they have a bland taste. Like olives they are usually cured and pickled in vinegar, oil or brine, though occasionally in crystal salt. Pickled capers are used as a flavouring in a range of dishes to give a sharp, tangy flavour. Younger, smaller capers are considered to have the best flavour. Usually, young flower buds are the most highly valued, though leaf shoots and almost-ripe berries can also be eaten. However, the flavour of capers is destroyed by too much cooking, so are best added just before serving.

🌺 Capers are popular in many Italian-style sauces and are great sprinkled on pizzas. They blend wonderfully with traditional Italian ingredients such as sun-dried tomatoes, artichokes, olives, garlic, basil and anchovies. They are also delicious with smoked fish, and are often included in tartare sauce.

Capsicums: sweet and chilli peppers

There are about 25 species of *Capsicum* and thousands of varieties. Their fruits come in a wonderful range of bright colours and range from large sweet peppers to the multitude of chilli peppers. Thousands of chilli varieties have been selected over many years and most are still valued and available today. The world's favourite spice, chilli is particularly popular in South and Central American, Asian, Indian, eastern European and Italian cuisines. Of the many sizes and shapes of chillies, those with the smaller fruits are often the hottest. Some varieties are more often used fresh, including jalapeño, pepperoncini, pimento, serrano, wax and New Mexican, and also tend to be milder (relatively!). Other varieties are more usually dried. It is said that people who eat a lot of chilli begin to want hotter and hotter varieties: some even claim to be addicted to chilli.

Numerous varieties of sweet peppers are found too. These colourful, less spicy veggies have increased in popularity hugely in a short time, with yellow, orange and even dark purple sweet peppers available for sale next to the older-style green fruits.

What they contain

Fresh (particularly red) chilli is tremendously rich in **vitamin C** – red chilli has ~180 mg/100 g and green chilli ~250 mg/100 g. They also have good levels of **carotenoids** (i.e. β-carotene, lutein and zeaxanthin). Dried chilli is phenomenally rich in carotenoids and is also very rich in **minerals** and **vitamin B**, **vitamin E** and **vitamin K**. Fresh and dried, they are also super-rich in other **antioxidants**. Chillies are virtually unique in the plant world in containing **capsaicinoid alkaloids**. Of these, **capsaicin** gives chillies most of their burning hotness: the smaller and redder the chilli, the more capsaicin it contains. Similar in composition to black pepper (though no relative), it can be detected by the tongue at 10 parts/million. It activates heat sensors, and has a relatively long-lasting effect. Chilli peppers are also rich in **oleoresin**, an ingredient in pepper sprays used by the military, police and for self-defence.

Sweet peppers, unlike chilli peppers, contain very little hot capsaicin. They are virtually fat free and contain some **soluble fibre**. Sweet peppers are tremendously rich in **carotenoids**, with red and yellow peppers having 125–190 mg/100 g of flesh (compared to ~50 mg/100 g in oranges), particularly β-**carotene**. Sweet peppers are rich in other **antioxidant** compounds too, with these being particularly abundant within red peppers. Because cooking reduces vitamin C and other antioxidants, if possible, eat them fresh, and go for red for the greatest benefits.

What they do

Capsaicin, not surprisingly, has some health benefits, but also attracts some health warnings. It stimulates flow of saliva and gastric juices. Historically, chillies were used to treat toothaches, coughs, sore throats and asthma – a few drops of hot pepper sauce in water is still considered by many to be an excellent treatment for sore throats, and chilli extracts are used commercially in warming lotions to soothe aching muscles, etc. Chillies seem to react with a neurotransmitter to reduce the feeling of pain and have been used topically to reduce pain from damaged nerve endings after limb surgery, for amputees, for shingles sufferers and to alleviate certain types of headaches. Capsaicin is sold as an over-the-counter drug to ease the pain of psoriasis, shingles, osteoarthritis and

Chillies seem to induce the release of endorphins in the brain, which act as pain killers and give a sense of well-being. Many claim that eating chillies has a calming, tranquillising effect.

rheumatoid arthritis. Its compounds seem to reduce the pain of arthritis by working as anti-inflammatories.

Red chillies can decrease appetite and subsequent protein and fat intake. They also stimulate carbohydrate use, at rest and during exercise, so are good for those on diets.

Capsiate esters found within sweet peppers (compared to capsaicins found in chillies) have inhibitory effects on cancers and are very effective at reducing inflammation.

Warning: Remember to wash hands after handling chillies, as the juice can burn sensitive skin. Prolonged contact may cause dermatitis and blisters. Excessive consumption can cause gastroenteritis, kidney damage, stomach ulcers and aggravate duodenal ulcers, though there are conflicting reports about this. In rats, it has been found that eating capsaicin reduces the efficacy of aspirin.

How they are used

Most chilli heat comes from glands situated close to the chilli seeds on the central core, so the removal of seeds and central core makes them less hot. If food is too hot, sugar can reduce the burning sensation and more so than drinking water. Fresh chillies are usually chopped finely and added to a multitude of cuisine styles, particularly in sauces, salsas and curries. They are the main ingredient in many fiery sauces, including Tabasco. A little adds depth and interest to a dish; a lot can smother all other flavours. Milder chillies are delicious stuffed with cream cheeses or feta and served as a starter. Their flavours are affected by cooking – raw chilli is the hottest. A beer is brewed from chillies.

🌿 Chilli varieties have different flavours, with many aficionados able to clearly distinguish the variety and quality, much in the same way as tasting wines or cheeses.

Sweet peppers, unlike their hot relatives, can be freely sliced and added to salads, stir-fries, quiches, roasts, bakes, etc. Perhaps scatter tamari-roasted chopped hazelnuts and pumpkin seeds on sliced sweet peppers placed on fresh watercress with a little avocado for a phenomenal starter? They are delicious stuffed with rice, other vegetables and cheese, and then roasted. They are popular on pizzas and in other Mediterranean dishes (e.g. ratatouille) as well as being an ingredient in many Central and South American dishes, such as salsa. Their crisp flesh is juicy and sweet. They can be stored by drying, and are often pickled. Paprika and pimento, derived from sweet peppers, are used as mild spices and colourings, and are added to many ketchups, meat products, snacks and sauces.

Cardamom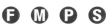

(cardamon)

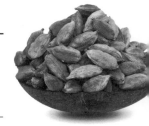

Cardamom is related to ginger and turmeric, with green (true) cardamom considered to have the finest flavour. In southern India, where most is still grown, it is known as the 'queen of spices'. It is popular in Indian, but also, oddly, in Scandinavian, cuisines. Cardamom is popular mixed with ground coffee to make an Arabian beverage. Because of its tricky cultivation it is the third most expensive spice in the world, after saffron and vanilla. However, because of its strong aroma and flavour, only a small amount is needed in a dish.

What it contains

The seeds contain very good amounts of **fibre** (~30%) and **protein** (~11%). They are very rich in **manganese**, **iron**, **zinc**, **potassium**, **magnesium** and **calcium**. They also contain **phytosterols** and are rich in **oleoresin** – a mix of oil and resin – which gives cardamom much of its aroma, flavour and medicinal properties. This compound is also used in pepper sprays. **Terpenes cineol** and **limonene** add to its aromatic properties.

What it does

Its essential oil has antibacterial properties and is used to preserve foods, particularly meats such as sausages, with only a small amount being needed to be effective. Historically, cardamom was used for digestive problems, including food poisoning. In China, cardamom is given to children suffering from coeliac disease (intolerance to gluten found in wheat, etc.) to help relieve symptoms.

Cardamom extracts have proven analgesic, anti-spasmodic and anti-inflammatory properties and help relieve gastrointestinal disorders, such as flatulence, indigestion and irritable-bowel syndrome. Cardamom can also lower blood pressure and help prevent formation of blood clots, so could reduce the risk of cardiovascular disease. Studies also show that cardamom has protective effects on experimentally induced colon carcinogenesis.

The seeds are chewed to cure bad breath and have been used to treat sore throats. The diluted essential oil is used to treat various skin conditions, and modern skin creams and soaps sometimes include it.

Warning: Its essential oil, like all others, should be diluted and used with care.

How it is used

The seeds are often removed from their pods before use and the pod, which some find too woody, is discarded. The seeds can be used whole or are ground to a powder, which is best done just before usage. Cardamom is richly, sweetly and deeply aromatic, and has a distinctive, warm flavour a little like ginger, nutmeg and cinnamon. This spice is used in both sweet and savoury dishes. It is combined with other spices in curry sauces, in pilau dishes and in dahl, as well as various vegetable, chicken and meat recipes. It is also added to betel pan. In India, it may be coated with sugar and used in confectionery. In Scandinavia, it is used as an ingredient in and on scones, cakes, waffles and other bakery products. Can be added to whipped cream and used as a dessert topping, added to rice puddings, and one recipe recommends mixing it with mango, yoghurt and ice to make a smoothie. The seeds, either whole or ground, are used to flavour tea, often with other spices. Its essential oil is used to flavour various foods and drinks, including liqueurs and mulled wine.

> ✿ Cardamom seeds have many diverse culinary uses – one of its main uses is mixed with ground coffee beans to make the very popular Arabian beverage 'gahwa'. Or how about a Swedish recipe for an alcoholic, spicy punch, called 'glögg', which includes brandy, wine, sugar, cinnamon, cardamom, orange peel, almonds and raisins.

Cardoon   See 'Globe artichoke and cardoon'

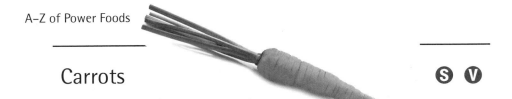

Carrots   Ⓢ Ⓥ

Older-style carrots, as eaten by the Egyptians, are likely to have been yellowish or white in colour, and they were almost certainly more woody. The sweeter, more succulent, bright orange carrot was not cultivated until the 1600s, probably first by the Dutch. Carrots, like cabbage, have sometimes received a poor reputation, mostly due to being overcooked, resulting in a bland, tasteless vegetable. But young, fresh carrots are quite a different thing.

What they contain

Carrots are loaded with α- and β-**carotenes**. They contain almost no calories and some **fibre**. They are rich in **polyacetylene** compounds. Heirloom-type purple carrots contain much more carotenoids and **anthocyanins**.

What they do

Carrots are well known for improving vision: their carotenoids are involved with the formation of rhodopsin, which is needed by the light-sensitive rods in the eye: so they really do help us see in the dark. Carotenes are also powerful antioxidants with strong cancer-fighting properties, and may help prevent skin, breast, lung, bladder and prostate cancers. Polyacetylenes are natural pesticides and have pronounced activity against certain types of cancer cells (e.g. leukaemia). Carrot extracts reduced the formation of cancers in rats by 33%. These compounds are also highly toxic to fungi and bacteria. In us, they act as anti-inflammatories and help prevent formation of blood clots. Purple carrots have been developed with higher levels of antioxidants and have even greater cancer-inhibiting activities. Carrot seeds may inhibit egg-implantation after sex, if taken at the correct dosage for several days. Carrot juice has been used to stop diarrhoea in young children.

How they are used

Young carrots are the sweetest, crispest and tastiest. Do not peel carrots unless you need to. Carrots are great juiced especially when mixed with apple and celery, and they are a main ingredient in vegetable stock (*mirepoix*). They make delicious, moist carrot cake and biscuits; are added

🐾 Carrots can be used in a multitude of ways in savoury or sweet dishes. They are delicious lightly sautéed with butter and honey; sliced and added with other vegetables to stir-fries; and freshly grated in salads, with beetroot, apple and parsley. They roast well in oil and a little soy sauce.

to soups with other vegetables or meat; and are included in sushi rolls. More unusually, they can be cooked and puréed and made into a mousse with cream, nutmeg and salt and pepper; or they can be pickled. They also make a sweetish, reasonable-tasting wine and, in Germany, have been added to beer. Carrots lose little of their nutrients during cooking.

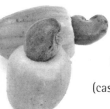

Cashews

(cashew apple)

The cashew is bizarre, consisting of a colourful two-piece fruit. The nut is kidney-shaped, thick-shelled and borne beneath a yellow/orange fleshy pseudo-fruit, known as a 'cashew apple'. Between the nut and fruit is a layer of thick, caustic, toxic oil that has to be removed using gloves before the nut can be accessed. The cashew apple, although forming a pear-sized fruit with very juicy, fibrous, tangy, refreshing yellow flesh, is seldom seen or used due to its short storage time.

What they contain

Of the 45% oil within the nut ~40% is **monounsaturated oleic acid**, with the rest being a mix of **omega-6** and **saturated oils**. The nuts also contain 14–20% good-quality **protein**. They are rich in **minerals**, particularly **phosphates, copper, iron, zinc, magnesium**. They are rich in **vitamins K** and **E**, and cholesterol-lowering **phytosterols**. The 'apple' fruit is very rich in **vitamin C**. One of this plant's most active compounds is **anacardic acid**, with greater quantities found in the nut shells.

What they do

Cashews make a good, sustaining energy food, releasing their energy slowly over time and therefore reducing peaks and troughs in blood-sugar levels. Their rich oleic acid content helps reduce serum LDLs, total cholesterol and raises HDLs, thus deterring development of cardiovascular disease. These oils, plus vitamin E, act as anti-inflammatories and assist wound healing. The nuts are also rich in several minerals and in protein.

Anacardic acid has proven antibiotic activity against many bacteria; a recent study showed it to be effective against 13 of the 15 micro-organisms tested. It can also control *Streptococcus mutans*, partially responsible for tooth decay – chewing cashew nuts may help control this bacteria and has even been reported to cure an abscessed tooth. It is a powerful antioxidant and may have anti-cancer properties.

Warning: A few people are allergic to cashews, and they may cross-react with pistachios

How they are used

🍂 Enjoy a snack of roasted cashews and dried fruits, such as apricots, prunes and raisins, to give you a quick burst of energy (from the fruits) but also sustained energy to last you through the day.

Cashews are one of the most delicious nuts, particularly when roasted. They are used in stuffing, confectionery and baking. Cashews are tasty mixed with other ingredients to enhance a mild, creamy korma curry, or added to a stir-fry. A few cashews complement a salad and, being less hard than many nuts, they blend in well. They go well with chicken, particularly in many Asian-style dishes, and are delicious with vegetables such as carrot, broccoli and asparagus. Cashews mix well with other diverse ingredients too, such as beans, citrus zest, cabbage, mushrooms, corn, tomatoes, ginger, pinenuts, berries, chocolate, tuna, prawns and other seafoods.

Celery, celeriac, lovage

It was not until the 17th century in Europe that tastier, less bitter celery varieties were selected and it then became popular as a vegetable. Celery is also popular in China where varieties with a stronger flavour are used. Now more popular, celeriac is grown for its swollen basal crown, rather than its stems. Very similar to celery, it has a pleasant but milder flavour. Lovage, similar to celery, is very popular in southern Europe – it has edible roots and its seeds are often used instead of celery seed as a flavouring.

What they contain

These vegetables have very few calories and are great for weight watchers. Indeed, they have so few calories that they are said to take more metabolic energy to chew and digest than the calories they contain. Contain some **fibre**, some **vitamin K** and are rich in the **flavonoid apigenin** and **coumarins**. The seeds are **protein-** (~18%) and **fibre-rich**, contain good amounts of most minerals, particularly **calcium**, **iron**, **magnesium** and **manganese**, and are rich in **phthalides** and **omega-6 linoleic acid**. They also contain **polyacetylenes**, which have anti-cancer properties. Lovage is also tremendously rich in the **flavonoid quercetin**.

What they do

Polyacetylenes within celery can be highly toxic to fungi and bacteria and in humans display anti-inflammatory effects and help prevent blood-clot formation, though are also responsible for adverse skin reactions. They are being researched for their ability to reduce tumour formation. Celery's flavonoids and coumarins have anticarcinogenic properties. Apigenin helps repair disrupted cellular reactions, thus halting further damage that could lead to more serious conditions. Apigenins also possess remarkable anti-inflammatory and antioxidant properties. The seeds reduce the formation of liver cancer in rats.

> Interestingly, celery juice seems to be good at repelling mosquitoes (though see Warning), being particularly efficacious when mixed with vanilla, and gives greater protection than many commercial repellents.

Phthalides within celery and celeriac allow vessels to relax and dilate, therefore decreasing blood pressure. This makes these vegetables excellent foods for people with high blood pressure. The effects are compounded by their ability to increase bile acid secretion, which results in decreased serum-cholesterol. Phthalides are also effective at relieving gout symptoms, may help those with arthritis and may act as a mild tranquilliser.

Warning: Some people develop adverse skin reactions when handling these plants, particularly if the skin is subsequently exposed to sunlight. The consumption of seeds is not recommended during pregnancy, as they may induce uterine contractions.

How are they used

The outer stalks and leaves of celery are usually discarded and the tender inner stalks preferred. A popular ingredient in stocks, with carrot and onion, it often makes the base for stews and soups. Popular also with apple in soups (hot and cold) and salads. Celery stalks are great for dips. It goes well with roast parsnips and potatoes, and also with spicy brassica ingredients such as horseradish, mustard, watercress, radish, cilantro and fennel. The seeds can be used as a spice, or crushed and mixed with salt to make celery salt.

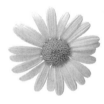 ✿ Fresh, crisp, young celery stalks are wonderful in salads or eaten just on their own with cheese, particularly tasty blue-veined cheeses such as Stilton. The celery heart is the best, being particularly tender and delicious.

The outer tough, knobbly skin of celeriac is usually removed, while the inner white tissue has a crunchy texture that is excellent finely sliced in salads, particularly with apples, watercress and walnuts. Rinsing in a little lemon juice prevents discolouration. It is also added to soups, stews and stir-fries; can be roasted with other vegetables or can be baked in its skin, with the skin later removed when cooked. It mixes well with potatoes, cheese, fish, seafood and mushrooms.

Chamomile

(English, Roman and German)

These herbs are familiar to all, usually for the soothing tea that is made from the dried flowers. English chamomile is often considered to be the most popular and fragrant species. This is commonly grouped with German (or Hungarian) chamomile, though the latter is from a different genus and is a larger, erect, coarser plant which is used in many of the same ways.

What it contains

English and German chamomiles have similar properties. The flowers contain some **vitamin A**, plus **manganese** and **copper** in particular. They contain good amounts of **flavonoids** (e.g. **apigenin, luteolin, quercetin**). German chamomile may contain more of these compounds, particularly apigenin and luteolin. Are also rich in **terpenes**.

What it does

Apigenin acts as an anticarcinogen, including against breast cancer. Compounds within these plants have anti-spasmodic and anti-allergenic properties and have been used to treat Parkinson's disease, hay fever and asthma. They also reduce nerve pain in neuralgia and are used to treat shingles. The terpenes reduce spasms of smooth muscle, so help with flatulence, non-ulcerative digestive ailments, including colic, stomach cramps and irritable-bowel syndrome. Extracts can also lower blood-glucose levels in rats, without affecting insulin output, and so may have potential in treating diabetes.

> Chamomile possesses remarkable anti-inflammatory and antioxidant properties. These plants can also reduce the growth and kill a range of human cancer cells.

Chamomile is widely used in skin-care products to reduce skin inflammation and dermatological diseases. Its antiviral properties are reported to effectively treat genital herpes infections, including herpes strains that don't respond to the antiviral drug acyclovir. Their essential oils can control the yeast infection *Candida albicans*. The liquid from soaked flowers makes a good wash for skin infections, sores, wounds, sunburn, burns, ulcers and insect bites, and is an insect repellent. The oil from German chamomile is used to relieve mouth ulcers (and in other mucous tissues) – extracts are given to teething babies. The liquid or oil can be used on swellings and painful joints as an analgesic. The apple-scented flowers are popular in pot-pourri, and are used as a hair rinse, particularly for blonde hair.

Warning: Skin allergies to chamomile have been reported, and a minority show allergic symptoms after ingestion.

How it is used

The flowers are popular infused in hot water to make a soothing, fragrant tea. The younger leaves can also be used. The flowers and leaves can be dried for later use. A few sprigs can be added to sauces as a seasoning, and go well with poultry and shellfish, though the sprigs should be removed before the food is served. However, the flowers do not taste as they smell – they have a bitter flavour. The whole plant is used to make herb beer. Its essential oil is used to flavour some liqueurs. The fresh flowers also make a pretty garnish.

> 🐾 In aromatherapy, the light-blue essential oil from chamomile is used to relieve stress and insomnia and to induce relaxation. A tea made from the flowers is used for similar purposes. A few flowers can also be added to bath water.

Chard, beet leaves

(Swiss chard, silver beet, spinach beet, perpetual spinach)

Chard (also known as silver beet in New Zealand) is closely related to the beets and spinach. Its taste is milder and its oxalic acid content is lower than that of spinach. Easy to grow, it is a popular garden vegetable.

What they contain

Beet and chard leaves are very rich in **carotenoids** as β-**carotene**, **lutein** and **zeaxanthin**. They contain virtually no fat or calories but abundant **vitamin C** (~30 mg/ 100 g) and are hugely rich in **vitamin K**, with one serving providing 12 times the RDA. They are also rich in **betalains** (as in beetroot), showing as ornamental deep yellow or red stalks.

What they do

Its powerful antioxidant carotenoids are excellent for improving eye problems and can reduce serum-cholesterol levels, which lowers the risk of cardiovascular disease and reduces the risk of developing several types of cancer. Betalains reduce multiplication of cancer cells and is indicated to help the body's hormonal system deal with depression and may help reduce cardiovascular disease.

Chard has been traditionally used by diabetics in Turkey; recent studies found that the leaves, in a rat model, protected the liver and kidneys from damage caused by diabetes mellitus.

Warning: The leaves contain some oxalic acid, so should be eaten in moderation, particularly by those at risk of arthritis, kidney stones and gout. Its super amounts of vitamin K may antagonise anticoagulant medications.

How they are used

The very young leaves are great in salads. Older leaves

Chards' rich vitamin K content helps maintain normal bone growth and development: in trials, elderly people who regularly ate more green leafy veggies suffered from significantly fewer bone fractures. It is also likely to help combat osteoporosis.

🌿 Try lightly steamed chard mixed with mascarpone, garlic, black pepper and cooked wholemeal penne with a little Parmesan grated on top. A very simple, quick, yet tasty nutritious meal.

can be lightly steamed or stir-fried. Some cooks serve the green leaves and diced stems separately. The stems are crisp and juicy, with a celery-like texture and a mild flavour. The leaves taste a little like spinach, but are not as acidic. When cooked, they do not reduce in volume as much. It can be added to soup and goes well with white fish and cheese and egg dishes.

Cherries: sweet and sour

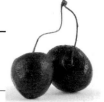

Modern cherries originate from two wild forms, the sweet and the sour cherries (e.g. morellos). Both species probably originate from Asia, though are now found growing wild in many countries. Sweet cherries, as their name suggests, are delicious fresh; whereas sour cherries are more often added to cooked desserts. As well as being tasty, they are very nutritious. The fruits are usually shiny, rounded and red, though there are varieties with yellow fruits. Their flesh is juicy, rich and succulent, surrounding a central hard stone, which should be discarded.

What they contain

Fresh sweet and sour cherries contain some **vitamin C**, and are very rich in **antioxidants** – they contain large amounts of **anthocyanins** and **proanthocyanins**, which are most abundant within dark red sour cherries. Sour cherries are also rich in the **flavonoids epicatechins** and **quercetin, chlorogenic acid** and **phyto-oestrogen isoflavones**. They are also very rich in **vitamin A**, particularly β-**carotene**. Cherries contain **perillyl alcohol**.

Warning: Like all members of this family, the seeds contain cyanide-like compounds that are toxic if eaten in quantity, though one is unlikely to eat too many cherry stones by mistake!

> Tart cherries have huge and dose-increasing antioxidant capacity and strong antineuro-degenerative activity.

What they do

Their anthocyanins protect arterial walls from plaque build-up and heart disease. Cherries are very effective at reducing build-up of LDLs, a contributor to heart disease, stroke and arteriosclerosis. A survey showed that cherry growers have a lower incidence of cancer and heart conditions than the general public, with growers eating, on average, ~3 kg of sour cherries per year. Cherries' neuroprotective activities may help improve memory. However, anthocyanin levels deteriorate during processing and freezing, so fruits are best eaten fresh.

Perillyl alcohol can switch tumour cells to less-malignant forms – clinical studies indicate that it can shrink pancreatic tumours, as well as help prevent tumours of the breast, lung, liver and skin.

The new nutrient-packed Bing cherry variety, developed in North America, is claimed to be particularly beneficial in relieving arthritis and gout, and to lessen the severity of other inflammatory conditions, such as cardiovascular disease and cancer.

Tart cherries significantly lower insulin and fasting glucose levels, so if included regularly in the diet they are likely to reduce development of type-2 diabetes. Cherries can speed healing: cherry juice given to athletes significantly reduced the time it took muscle to heal compared with those just taking a placebo.

🌿 Cherries go gorgeously with dark chocolate: for an easy treat, pit fresh cherries and roll in melted chocolate, then allow to set and cool in a fridge (guard against all potential pilferers until ready to enjoy).

How they are used

Sweet cherries are delicious just on their own. They can be added fresh to desserts, ice cream and make a good garnish. Sour cherries are more usually stewed and added to various pies, conserves and sauces, though to avoid reducing their health benefits it is best not to cook them for too long. Both sweet and sour cherries complement many savoury dishes, such as duck, fish or meat: a few dark, lightly cooked cherries go wonderfully with lamb. Cherries can be made into delicious rich liqueurs, and make a fruity, rich wine or juice.

Chicory, endives, Jerusalem artichokes 🕒 🅥

(witloof, radicchio, Belgium endive)

These are members of the sunflower family and have long been popular in Europe, particularly in France and Italy. Chicory has long taproots that are used as a flavouring and as a coffee substitute, and several varieties are cultivated for their salad leaves. The leaves are often blanched, with the white leafy shoots known as witloof or chichons. Radicchio is another type of chicory, very popular in Italy, and comes in several shades of red.

Endive is a less well-known salad ingredient, usually with very curly leaves that have more taste than lettuce, but are also more bitter (though are less so if blanched). Jerusalem artichokes are grown for their odd knobbly tubers, which are surprisingly tasty. Its flowers are like small sunflowers. These little-utilised vegetables deserve to be more widely appreciated due to their highly nutritious properties, and are often found at farmers' markets, or grow your own.

What they contain

The roots of chicory and Jerusalems are wonderfully rich in **inulin** and **oligofructose** – very important sources of soluble fibre – with oligofructose being more soluble and sweeter. Chicory is widely used in the production of many processed foods. Their roots also contain iron and potassium, plus the B vitamins.

Chicory and endive leaves are nutrient rich – they have very good levels of antioxidant **carotenoids**, much as β-**carotene, lutein and zeaxanthin**, and also **vitamin K** (100 g gives 3–4 times the RDA), **vitamin C** (10–24 mg/100 g) and good amounts of **folate**. Green leaves are the most nutrient rich, but are also more bitter.

What they do

Chicory and Jerusalem artichokes are particularly important sources of inulin. This increases populations of 'good' gut bacteria and increases absorption of calcium. Eating this prebiotic fibre after a course of antibiotics is particularly beneficial as it encourages the replenishment of 'good' bacteria – when eaten with probiotic live yoghurt these benefits are further enhanced. Inulin prevents constipation and, consequently, may reduce the incidence of bowel cancer. It also binds with compounds that are involved with the production of cholesterol, so indirectly helps lower cholesterol levels. However, because inulin is not digested, but is instead fermented by bacteria, it can have the side effect of causing flatulence. However, not harvesting the tubers until after a frost (or placing them in a fridge) or leaving them in the sun for a few days, initiates the conversion of inulin into sweeter oligofructose, which decreases flatulence. Because inulin is not absorbed by the body, it is often added to diet foods. It is excellent for diabetics and those worried about weight gain – it gives a feeling of fullness without absorption of any carbohydrates. Chicory roots also contain anti-malarial compounds.

Compounds formed when artichokes are wounded have a significant ability to kill tumour cells while not affecting normal cells in plants, humans and animals, including human breast tumour cells.

In India, chicory is a traditional treatment for diabetes – a recent study has shown that chicory reduces glucose production within the liver in a non-insulin-dependent way, therefore confirming its possible usage for diabetes.

The rich carotenoid content of unblanched endive and chicory leaves slows progression of age-related eye conditions, acts as a cancer inhibitor and is protective against heart disease. Chicory also has antibacterial and antifungal properties, and its seeds have marked liver-healing properties.

Warning: A few people are allergic to inulin. A minority also suffer an adverse skin reaction when handling these plants. Jerusalem artichokes can cause severe flatulence, although this seems to vary from plant to plant, and with sweetness. The addition of asafoetida or cardamom may counteract this.

How they are used

Endive leaves are popular within Mediterranean salads, to which they add flavour and ornamental value. Fresh blanched leaves are also popular in salads, or served with carrot or tomato, with a little olive oil. Older leaves can be lightly cooked as a vegetable.

The roots of chicory can be dried, ground and added to coffee to make it go further, but also to add an interesting flavour. Some find that adding chicory to coffee neutralises its acidity and stomach-irritating properties. Its roots are also used as a flavouring in soups and stews, or can be roasted. Its young leaves and flower heads are used in salads, as can the forced winter leaves. Older leaves and stems can be steamed or stir-fried as a vegetable. Witloof chichons can be eaten fresh in salads, or braised. Chichons go well with creamy cheese.

🌺 Endive and chicory leaves are very nutritious, particularly if not blanched. Radicchio, red-leaved chicory, is very popular in salads, particularly in Italy, and its ornamental leaves are also added to pasta and risotto, though cooking reduces their colour.

Although fiddly to clean due to their knobbly shape, Jerusalem artichokes have a delightful, sweetish, nutty taste and many uses. They can be boiled, sliced and fried, cut finely and eaten raw in salads, or can be roasted and are delicious served with a sprinkling of Parmesan and a squeeze or two of lemon or lime juice. They are used in salads and added to roasts, curries, Mediterranean dishes, sometimes instead of potato. Only cook until just soft – any longer and they turn to mush, though can be added to soups. Make a delicious soup with cream, veggies, mashed potatoes and herbs. Their nutty but neutral flavour complements many foods. The tubers can be fermented to make a good-quality liquor, and have been used in wine and beer.

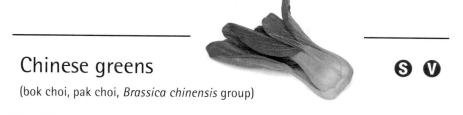

Chinese greens

(bok choi, pak choi, *Brassica chinensis* group)

S **V**

As brassicas, their nutritional properties are highly valued, with claims that the greater longevity and reduced development of many diseases (including many types of cancer) in Asians compared to those in the West, is largely due to consumption of these vegetables.

What they contain
They are rich in **vitamin C** (45 mg/100 g), **folate**, **vitamin K**, and varieties with dark green leaves are wonderfully rich in β-**carotene**. They are also very rich in **isothiocyanates**.

What they do
Isothiocyanates have been shown to reduce the risk of a range of cancers as well as reducing blood cholesterol. They also reduce skin cancers and the spread of lung and stomach cancers. They seem to beneficially affect oestrogen–metabolite balance, so thus may reduce some hormone-related cancers (e.g. breast, uterus, prostate). In China, research shows that isothiocyanate-rich greens reduce the risk of breast cancer by 45%. They may also relieve symptoms associated with premenstrual syndrome and menopause. Studies into their ability to reduce uterine fibroids and prostate hypertrophy are under way. Their compounds may also help relieve irritable-bowel syndrome and long-term muscle pain and fatigue.

Warning: Brassicas contain thyroid inhibitors, so those with thyroid problems may wish to moderate consumption of these veggies, though cooking should largely nullify this effect.

How they are used
The dark green leaves and wide white leaf stalks of pak choi types are

♨ Remember not to cook Chinese greens for too long to avoid destroying their nutrients and flavours: are best lightly steamed or stir-fried, or better still, eaten fresh, finely chopped, in a salad.

delicious lightly stir-fried or added to soups. They can be lightly steamed as a vegetable, or young leaves can be shredded and eaten raw. They can be braised with oil, soy sauce and oyster sauce and are delicious with sesame oil, ginger and garlic. A popular dish is kimchi, in which the leaves are fermented with carrot, spring onions, daikon, soy sauce, vinegar, honey, ginger, garlic and peppers. The stalks and leaves of Chinese greens vary in texture and flavour and may be served separately to add different components to a dish. They have a fairly mild flavour, and mix well with other Asian vegetables.

Chives   See 'Garlic'

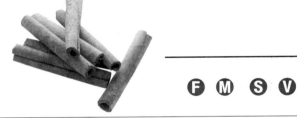

Cinnamon   Ⓕ Ⓜ Ⓢ Ⓥ

From China, there are two main varieties of this warming aromatic spice, which is obtained from the inner bark of Ceylon cinnamon and cassia. Of the two, Ceylon cinnamon is lighter in colour and has a sweeter, delicate flavour; however, cassia is the more commonly available. Ceylon cinnamon forms fine, pale-coloured rolls ('quills') with a more delicate, sweet flavour; whereas cassia is coarser and darker in colour and its flavour is somewhat bitter.

What it contains

Cinnamon is very rich in **fibre** (~50%), **calcium**, **manganese** and **iron** and **vitamin E** and **K**. It is very rich in secondary plant compounds, particularly **coumarins**, gum, tannin and **mannitol**. Its essential oil contains **eugenol** and **pinene** – the leaves yield 70–95% eugenol, which is used as a clove substitute.

What it does

Cinnamon has been used to ease all types of digestive problems. Research has now confirmed that it can reduce smooth-muscle spasms of the gut, and so reduces indigestion, irritable-bowel syndrome and flatulence.

Cinnamon oil has antifungal and antibacterial properties, and is added to foods such as meat to act as a preservative. It is also effective at killing the bacteria that cause tooth decay and gum disease, so can be added to toothpaste. It can help clear up urinary tract infections caused by *Escherichia coli* bacteria and *Candida albicans* yeast infections. It may help prevent stomach ulcers, possibly by controlling the bacteria *Helicobacter pylori*.

Recent studies show that cinnamon has anti-diabetic properties, could improve sugar metabolism in type-2 diabetes and regulate blood pressure. Rather than decreasing blood-glucose levels it seems to lower circulating insulin concentrations – it may reduce the amount of insulin necessary for glucose metabolism (although this research is still not conclusive). Its coumarins have blood-thinning properties, increase blood flow in veins and decrease capillary permeability, thus are likely to be of benefit in relieving some effects of diabetes, as well as reducing cardiovascular disease. However, it should probably be avoided by those taking anticoagulants.

Warning: A minority are allergic to cinnamon. Cinnamon oil applied to skin can cause redness and burning. Taken internally, the oil can cause nausea and vomiting; there are even reports of it causing kidney damage. Coumarin, in its pure form, should only be ingested in small quantities as it is moderately toxic. However, it is much more toxic to rodents and is often included within rat and mouse eradication preparations (e.g. as warfarin and brodifacoum).

How it is used

Cinnamon has a fragrant aroma and a spicy yet sweet flavour. It is used in a diverse range of foods, such as cakes and other baked goods, milk and rice puddings, chocolate dishes and fruit desserts – particularly with apples and pears – and in French toast, eggnog, pickles and steamed puddings. It is popular within many Middle Eastern and North

> If you have persistent problems with cystitis or similar problems, perhaps a dessert of lightly stewed blueberries and cranberries, sweetened with honey, sprinkled with cinnamon and served with coconut cream might do the trick.

🌿 In India, cinnamon quills are used whole – they are fried in hot oil until they unroll (which releases the fragrance). The temperature is then reduced and other ingredients such as tomatoes, onions and yoghurt are added. The cinnamon chunks are usually removed before serving.

African dishes to flavour lamb stews or in stuffed aubergines. It is added to curries and rice pilau dishes and in garam masala spice mix. Cinnamon is used to spice mulled wines, creams and syrups. In Mexico it is drunk with coffee and chocolate and brewed as a tea.

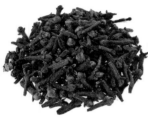

Cloves

Cloves are the unopened flower buds from a small tree that originates from Indonesia. They have long been used for their aromatic and medicinal properties, and many are familiar with their usage to reduce the pain of toothache.

What they contain

Cloves have good amounts of **fibre**, are hugely rich in **vitamins C, K and E**, and also in the minerals **magnesium**, **manganese**, **iron** and **calcium**. They are rich in **essential oil**, ~15%, which is greater than in most plants. This contains mostly **eugenol** (~80%), but also **caryophyllene** and **vanillin**, plus **oleoresin** (a mix of oil and resin, which is used in pepper sprays).

What they do

The oil has one of the highest synergistic rates when given with antimicrobial drugs to treat *Staphylococcus aureus*. Its oil is one of the strongest inhibitors against a wide range of pathogenic bacteria, yeasts and moulds, including *Enterococcus faecalis*, *Listeria monocytogenes*, *Escherichia coli*, *Salmonella choleraesuis* and *Candida albicans*. It also reduces the growth and activity of herpes virus and may have some activity against hepatitis C virus. It also has proven 100% repellent action, for 2–4 hours, against the three mosquito species it was tested with – more so than the other 37 plant oils tested.

The oil has antioxidant and anticarcinogenic properties – it contains compounds that dramatically reduce the mutagenic potential of several carcinogens. However, another trial found that eugenol is also a weak tumour promoter, so the oil needs to be used with caution.

Cloves have been researched for their ability to treat

> Cloves are particularly used as an analgesic and anaesthetic for toothache and other oral problems, and are still recommended by professionals as an effective short-term remedy.

(and reduce) the occurrence of type-2 diabetes. In India, cloves have long been a traditional medicine for this disease and a recent study suggests that cloves do act as an anti-diabetic and also that their antioxidant properties help ameliorate damage caused by free radicals formed in diabetes. Clove oil has also been used as an aphrodisiac, with recent experiments showing that it does lead to a significant and sustained increase in the sexual activity of normal male rats, without any adverse effects. The buds are used in perfumery and have long been used inserted into oranges to make a fragrant pomander, and are used in incense. In Indonesia, they are popular in a type of cigarette known as 'kretek' and are sometimes mixed with marijuana.

Warning: Clove oil should be treated with caution because in large amounts its actions are unpredictable. In particular, eugenol, in large quantities, has serious and damaging effects on health.

How they are used

Cloves have a strong, warm to hot taste, with a distinctive flavour. Only a small amount is needed to flavour foods. Cloves are either used whole or are ground and used as a powder, with the latter meaning they do not need to be removed after cooking. Cloves are commonly added to fruit pies, particularly with apple, and are cooked with the fruit to impart their warm, spicy flavour. They are also added to cakes and desserts, and are a main ingredient in many pickling spices. Cloves are popular in Indian cuisine, and are added to a range of curries – in southern India they are added to biryani. They also complement pumpkin and squash dishes.

🐾 A wonderful recipe mixes a little powdered clove with 70% dark chocolate and double cream; the set chunks are then served with fresh figs, candied orange peel and vanilla poached pears.

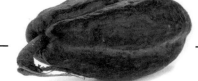

Cocoa beans

(chocolate, cacao)

Ⓜ Ⓟ Ⓢ Ⓥ

Traditionally, cocoa beans were used as a spice. Native to tropical South America, the beans were used to make a bitter drink by both the Maya and Aztecs, though the latter did sweeten it. The beans were also used for medicinal purposes, and were valued as an offering in spiritual ceremonies, with its botanical name, *Theobroma*, being Greek for 'food of the Gods'. In the mid 1500s, the beans were taken to Europe where they were soon considered a delicacy, along with the similarly introduced coffee bean. Chocolate houses became popular in Europe during the 17th century. In the early 1800s, Dutchman Conrad J. van Houten discovered and patented a new method for pressing the fat from the roasted cocoa beans. This was mixed with salts, water and sugar to produce rich, dark, gorgeous eating chocolate.

What they contain

Cocoa is very rich in **fibre** (~33%) and **protein** (~20%), and is rich in **all the amino acids** (though somewhat less in tryptophan and methionine). The cocoa bean is very rich in **minerals**, particularly **iron**, **copper**, **magnesium** and **manganese**, but also **zinc**, **phosphates** and **potassium**. Cocoa butter contains some **vitamin E** and is rich in **vitamin K**. The centre of the bean, also known as the 'nib', contains ~54% cocoa butter, of which two-thirds is **saturated palmitic** and **stearic acids**, with one-third unsaturated, which is mostly **monounsaturated oleic acid**. Chocolate beans are rich in the alkaloid **theobromine**, which is a similar compound to caffeine, plus **phenethylamine**, and some **caffeine**. The beans are incredibly rich in **antioxidants** particularly **phenolic gallic acid** and the **flavonoid epicatechin**, of which they contain more than any other fruit, vegetable or nut. The beans are also rich in cholesterol-lowering **phytosterols**.

Theobromine has a soothing effect on coughs – greater than that of codeine. A beverage made from cocoa, a little chilli and manuka honey could relieve chest infections and irritating coughs.

What they do

Research has confirmed the benefits of eating chocolate. Theobromine and phenethylamine affect the pleasure centres of the brain, increasing serotonin levels, which results in people feeling happier and seems to increase verbal and visual memory. They also act as a mild stimulant. Its powerful antioxidants can reduce the incidence of several debilitating illnesses, such as heart disease and cancer. Dark chocolate contains more antioxidants than virtually all other common foods, including all berries, red wine and green tea. Dark chocolate also exerts a protective effect on the cardiovascular system and reduces blood pressure by relaxing the smooth muscle of the arteries and veins. It reduces inflammation, blood clotting, helps blood flow, increases HDL and decreases LDLs. Daily consumption of chocolate has been recommended for lowering cholesterol and improving blood pressure.

Its flavonoids can ameliorate insulin sensitivity, so may help prevent type-2 diabetes (though note that chocolate also contains large quantities of sugar!). In addition, a trial showed that eating chocolate decreased the risk for pre-eclampsia during pregnancy. It has even been claimed to increase life span, though as with most of these claims, there are two sides to the story, with moderation being the best policy.

On the negative side, chocolate has gained a bad reputation for weight gain and tooth decay, and some consider it to be addictive, though this is largely unproven. Cocoa butter is rich in saturated fats (~65%) and is very high in calories (~98%). Cocoa powder contains less fat and fewer calories. However, cocoa itself is not sweet, so sugar must be added. Chocolate has also long been associated with triggering migraine headaches; however, a recent study on humans showed that chocolate did not play a significant role in triggering headaches in most typical sufferers and was no more likely to provoke headaches than carob.

Cocoa butter is used in cosmetics and as a lubricant for chapped lips, skin, etc., and in suppositories and pessaries.

Warning: Has been linked with increased acid reflux. A recent trial showed that older women who consumed chocolate daily had lower bone density and strength. Theobromine can be very toxic and causes death to dogs, cats, horses, parrots and other animals who have difficulty metabolising this alkaloid (symptoms are also delayed).

How they are used

Traditionally, cocoa was used in beverages, often mixed with hot or warming spices such as chilli, to make mole, or with vanilla, cinnamon, allspice and mace, sometimes with a sweetener such as honey. Citrus and jasmine could also be added; later, milk was included, and the start of modern chocolate drinks and confectionery began. Today, cocoa-rich products are increasingly popular, with the richness and bitterness of cocoa being appreciated at contents of 65–75%. Chocolate is indispensable in a vast number of wonderful desserts, soufflés, ice cream, tarts, puddings, accompanying fresh fruits and sauces, as well as being used in a huge number of confectionery products, often

If you've got that chocolate craving but are worried about the fat content have a cocoa drink. It contains all the active agents but is not high-calorie like the cocoa butter in chocolate.

along with ingredients such as nuts, lemon, raisins, peppermint, and many exotic chocolate fillings. It can be added to stronger-tasting foods and drinks such as beer, some savoury fish and seafood dishes, chicken dishes and pasta.

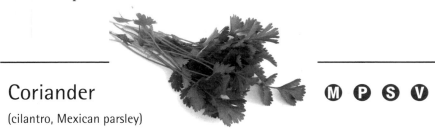

Coriander
(cilantro, Mexican parsley)

Ⓜ Ⓟ Ⓢ Ⓥ

Related to parsley, dill and fennel, the distinctive aroma and flavour of coriander's leaves and seeds have been valued for thousands of years. A Mediterranean plant, it is believed to be one of the oldest known herbs. The leaves have a distinctive pungent taste that many love and include in a wide range of dishes, though some find its aroma too strong and unpleasant. It is often called or compared to parsley, though its flavour is quite different. The name 'coriander' may be given specifically to the seed, whereas the fresh leaves are commonly known as cilantro.

What it contains

The leaves are hugely rich in **carotenoids** (particularly β-**carotene**) and **vitamin K**, and contain lots of **vitamin C**. They are also rich in other **antioxidants** and in **phytosterols**. Dried, the leaves are very rich in **protein** (~20%), **calcium**, **manganese**, **copper**, **potassium** and **iron**. They contain huge amounts of **vitamin C** (~560 mg/100 g), the **B vitamins** and **carotenoids**, and mega amounts of **vitamin K**. The seeds are rich in **protein** (~12%), **fibre** (~40%), **calcium**, **iron**, **selenium**, **zinc** and **magnesium**. Its essential oil is very **terpene** rich and is composed mostly of **linalool**, **pinene**, **geraniol**, **myrcene** and **limonene**. It also contains **coumarins**. The seed oil (20%) is mostly **monounsaturated petroselinic acid**.

What it does

The leaves have anti-mutagenic and antibacterial properties – they are particularly effective against *Listeria* species. Cilantro is also a natural chelator, and may help bind and remove heavy metals, such as lead, mercury and aluminium, from the body. The leaves are also eaten to reduce halitosis.

The seeds can significantly decrease the triglycerides, total cholesterol and LDL levels of rats, while increasing the HDLs. In addition, the activity of antioxidant enzymes is increased. Thus, may inhibit development of cardiovascular disease.

Warning: Its essential oil should, like all essential oils, be used with care. Its coumarins can cause adverse skin reactions in some.

In India, coriander is a traditional treatment for diabetes: recent research confirms that coriander has blood-sugar lowering and insulin-like activities.

How it is used

The leaves are best used fresh and are popular in salads and as a flavoursome garnish. They have a strong distinctive flavour that, in Asian cuisine, is often mixed with galangal, garlic, chilli and lemongrass. Its flavour also complements fish and eggs and it is added to bean dishes. Coriander leaves are an ingredient in various chicken and lamb recipes. It is popular in Indian, Asian and Chinese cuisine, and in Mexican dishes such as salsa. The seeds are a main ingredient in Indian garam masala. They are also used commercially to flavour tobacco products, liqueurs and beverages, and their flavour is used to disguise the taste of bitter medicines.

Coriander seeds have a sweetish, nutty, orange-like flavour and are used in both sweet and savoury foods. Roasting increases their flavour and are included in cakes, candies, rye breads, soups, stews, curries, pickles and chutneys.

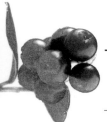

Cranberries

Cranberries are native to the United States and southern Canada. The acid bogs where they grow have long been harvested for these tasty fruits, which are a valuable source of vitamin C and were used as a diuretic. Today, their popularity has hugely increased, as demand for their rich flavours and nutritional benefits has expanded.

What they contain

Is fairly rich in **soluble fibre** (~7%). Has good levels of **vitamin C** (~20 mg/100 g of flesh) and also good amounts of **manganese**. Are very rich in **anthocyanins**. The fruits also contain **benzoic acid**, **flavonoids**, **cinnamic acids**, **stilbenes** and **terpenoids**.

What they do

Cranberries have numerous health benefits. Containing abundant anthocyanins, they are particularly effective at strengthening capillaries.

Synergistically, with vitamin C, cranberries help prevent age-related progressive loss of sight. They also help the absorption and use of vitamin C and assist in maintaining intercellular collagen, which forms connective tissue throughout the body. Cranberry extracts reduce the incidence of many cancer-associated processes related to epithelial origins (e.g. in breast, colon, prostate, oesophagus). Cranberries can also lower LDLs and exert potentially beneficial effects on the heart which help prevent cardiovascular disease. The juice also seems to lower blood-glucose levels, so could be beneficial to those susceptible to diabetes.

They also have powerful antioxidant properties and are well known for their ability to prevent and relieve urinary problems, such as cystitis. This effect may partly be due to the high levels of benzoic acid present, which seems to acidify the urine and thus reduce infection. In addition, the anthocyanins are thought to prevent *Escherichia coli* bacteria from adhering to cells on the urinary tract wall, which is a critical step in the development of infection – the bacteria are simply flushed out with urine. These antibacterial properties also seem to work against *Helicobacter pylori*, which can cause stomach ulcers and cancer. Historically, cranberries were used as a poultice on wounds and infections.

Warning: Cranberries can reduce the efficacy of anticoagulant drugs such as warfarin.

How they are used

The berries are fairly sour and are usually added to pies and other desserts, stewed and made into preserves or a popular sauce to accompany turkey.

🐾 Cranberries reduce bacterial populations found in the mouth that are a leading cause of tooth decay, so eating a few cranberries after a meal could reduce dental caries.

They are also tasty with chicken and meat recipes. A delicious vinaigrette for salads or chicken can be made by mixing puréed cranberries with wine, a little sugar, mustard, garlic, black pepper and oil. Their rich fruity flavour goes well in muffins, cakes, tarts and bakes. They can be added to ice cream or to smoothies. Because cooking largely destroys their vitamin C content, they could be added to other sweeter fruits and eaten fresh in this way. They can be dried easily, and become sweeter with an intense juicy flavour. Dried cranberries are great added to cereals, trail mixes, muffins and cakes.

Cress   See 'Garden Cress'

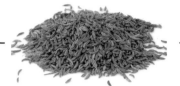

Cumin

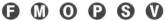

Cumin, related to fennel, parsley and dill, is popular in India, where its seeds are used to flavour many curry dishes. It is also popular in Middle Eastern cuisine, parts of Europe, North Africa, China and Mexico. It has long been a valued spice and has many medicinal properties.

What it contains

The seeds are rich in **fibre** (~10%), **protein** (~18%) and **fats** (~23%), mostly as **monounsaturated oleic acids**. Contain good amounts of **vitamins C and E**, and are rich in the **B vitamins, thiamine, riboflavin, niacin** and **B6**. They are very rich in **iron** and also **calcium, magnesium, manganese, zinc** and **potassium**. The seeds produce a good-quality **essential oil** (~2.5%) which has the main aromatic compound **cuminaldehyde** and also several **terpenes**.

What it does

This plant has similar properties to coriander. The seeds also reduce liver complaints – they decrease lipid levels caused by alcohol intake, and thus reduce damage to the liver. They also have significant antioxidant properties.

> Cumin seeds are widely used to treat digestive problems – they contain compounds that relax spasms within smooth muscle of the gut, so relieve intestinal problems and flatulence.

The seeds can reduce blood-glucose levels and may aid in the treatment of diabetes mellitus. Its terpenes, in particular, have strong potential to reduce the formation of carcinogens (e.g. colon, pancreas). Cumin extracts are particularly effective at controlling *Helicobacter pylori* bacteria, which can cause stomach ulcers and cancer. Cumin does this without risking antibiotic resistance, as can occur with conventional treatments. The seeds are also effective against other bacteria (e.g. *Staphylococcus aureus*). Extracts, if chewed, can relieve the pain of toothache.

Warning: Its terpene compounds can cause allergic-type reactions. The essential oil should be treated with caution.

How it is used

Pleasantly aromatic cumin seeds are used to flavour many recipes. They have a fairly hot, rich, slightly bitter flavour, which, when added to dishes, tends to draw out the flavours and sweetness of foods. They may be roasted or fried beforehand to release their full flavour. They are very popular in Indian cuisine, added to curry sauces, dahl, poppadoms and chapatis, as well as to cooling yoghurt.

The seeds are also popular in Middle Eastern cuisine to flavour dips, breads and meat dishes. They are used in Europe to flavour sausages and cheeses, to which they add a distinctive flavour. Their flavour mixes well with vegetables such as potato, cauliflower and carrot, and they are a popular ingredient within many dried bean and chickpea dishes and as a flavouring for chicken. They are sometimes used in cakes and sweet foods.

> 🐾 Grind cumin, coriander and pumpkin seeds together with pinenuts, and a little black pepper, to make delicious dukkah, which is gorgeous served with virgin olive oil and fresh, warm bread.

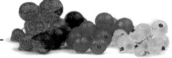

Currants: blackcurrants, redcurrants 🄵 🄾 🅂 🅅

These small, tasty fruits are full of nutrients and are now becoming increasingly re-popularised. They come in colours of black, red, pink and white, though blackcurrants are the most commonly encountered, as well as the most nutrient rich. Note that dried currants are not actually black-currants, but are the dried fruit of the Zante grape.

What they contain

Blackcurrants have close to the highest **vitamin C** content of all temperate fruits (~180 mg/100 g), with redcurrants having about half this quantity. They are also very rich in **flavonoids**, both **anthocyanins** and **proanthocyanins**, and also **quercetin** – all are linked to inhibiting many cardiovascular diseases and cancers. The oil from blackcurrant seeds is rich in **unsaturated oils**, particularly **omega-6 linoleic acids**. They also contain good amounts of **pectin fibre**.

What they do

Its rich antioxidant vitamin C content helps reduce the development of cancer and eradicates free radicals that could cause cell damage. Vitamin C also protects against heart disease and stress, is involved with energy production in cells, helps boost the immune system, binds with certain poisons to render them harmless, works with antibodies, helps to increase the absorption of nutrients (e.g. iron) in the gut, thins the blood and is essential for sperm production. It is needed for the production of collagen, which is widely needed for cartilage, joints, skin, and blood vessel formation and maintenance. Its flavonoids also have powerful antioxidant properties, synergistically adding to the benefits of vitamin C.

Blackcurrants have powerful antibacterial and antiviral properties, including proven anti-influenza virus effects, so eat some fruits if flu is in the 'air'. Currants reduce the incidence of *Helicobacter pylori*, which can lead to stomach ulcers and cancer. Compounds within the seeds block the adhesion of these bacteria to the gastric membranes. They also significantly inhibit the growth of the herpes simplex virus. The oil is often used to reduce the effects of dermatitis and eczema, though some question its efficacy for skin ailments.

Although currants are rich in omega-6 linoleic acid, they also contain some gamma-linolenic acid (GLA), which does have anti-inflammatory properties and seems to help treat autoimmune diseases such as rheumatoid arthritis.

How they are used

Currants are tart, but sweeten when fully ripe and are then very juicy and flavoursome. They can be eaten fresh, but are added to various desserts, often with other fruits, where they contribute flavour and rich colour. Blackcurrants are delicious sprinkled on breakfast cereals and then topped with live yoghurt. Currants also make good jellies and jams, as they are rich in pectin, and are good in pies, sauces and cheesecakes. They can also be added to savoury dishes, such as curries. However, heat destroys much of the vitamin C and damages the flavonoids. Black- and redcurrants are also used to make wine, which has been compared to Graves or Rhine wines. Blackcurrants are a traditional source of juice, and of the French liqueur Cassis, as well as the brandy Noir de Bourgogne.

To balance the omega-6s in these excellent fruits enjoy currants with sliced kiwifruits and chopped nuts.

Dandelion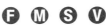

(pissabed)

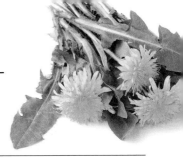

Although many consider it a weed, dandelions are a species that have long been eaten in Europe and Asia and used for their medicinal properties. Its bright yellow flowers are also gorgeous en masse. Dandelion's other name, 'pissabed', is derived from its diuretic properties. This plant is found growing wild in many parts of the world, but because of its many useful compounds, dandelions are now being grown commercially in Europe, the United Kingdom and the United States, with ongoing research into its many uses being undertaken.

What it contains

The leaves are extremely nutritious. They are very rich in **carotenoids**, as β-**carotene**, and also **lutein** and **zeaxanthin**, which help slow the progression of age-related macular degeneration and cataracts. They have good **vitamin C** (~35 mg/100 g) and **vitamin E** contents, and are very rich in **vitamin K** (a serving can provide 10 times the RDA). Dandelions are also rich in **iron** (contain more than spinach), **calcium** and **potassium**. The leaves and flower heads are rich in **flavonoids** and **coumaric acid**. Being a member of the sunflower family, its root contains mostly **soluble inulin** and the amounts of this are greater in autumn, with much being converted to sweeter oligosaccharide compounds in spring and summer. Roots also contain the bitter compounds taraxacin and taraxacerin.

What it does

A proven diuretic, dandelion has the advantage that its high potassium levels replace that lost with urine. It seems to improve disorders of the urinary tract and gall bladder, helps reduce liver damage (is used to treat cirrhosis), reduce high blood pressure and relieve painful joints. Dandelion extracts also have potential anti-cancer properties (breast and prostate). Other trials have shown it to have anti-inflammatory and pain-relieving activities. All parts of the plant can be used.

Inulin, within the root, acts as a prebiotic, therefore encouraging populations of 'good' gut bacteria. It has many beneficial effects on the digestive system, including reducing the risk of developing colorectal cancers. Because it is not digested, but is fermented by bacteria, it can cause flatulence, though roots richer in oligosaccharides cause fewer problems – harvest the roots in spring. Also, because inulin is not absorbed by the body, it is good for those on diets.

Dandelions have antifungal and antibacterial properties, so inhibit the growth of several bacteria (e.g. *Staphylococcus aureus* and *Candida* infections).

The white latex within all parts of the plant can be rubbed on warts and verrucae. It has been used in skin preparations and is said to moisturise and soften the skin, particularly dry skin. Test for allergies before usage because some find it a skin irritant (as with other members of this family).

Dandelions are very rich in lecithin, which is needed by every cell in the body for cell membrane flexibility and structure. It also prevents oxidation and is incredibly important for the brain. Lecithin speeds up the metabolism of fats and reduces serum-cholesterol and triglycerides, so may help with weight loss and reduce cardiovascular disease. Although it can be produced by the liver, additional dietary lecithin should be eaten.

Warning: A few people are allergic to inulin, so eat the roots with caution. Due to their very high vitamin K levels, those on anticoagulant drugs (e.g. warfarin) should be wary of eating too many leaves.

How it is used

The young leaves are used in salads, though some find them a little bitter. The plants can be blanched to reduce bitterness; however, much of their nutrients are then reduced. Older leaves can be lightly steamed, added to soups, stews, etc., and used with or like spinach. Nettles also go well with poached eggs and in cheese dishes. They can be added to stir-fries. Historically, the roots were dried, ground and roasted to make a reasonable-tasting coffee substitute. Summer- and spring-harvested roots can be roasted and eaten as a vegetable, though they may be a little bitter. The sweet-smelling flowers make a light, delicate wine, with a little orange or other citrus added. The roots and leaves are added to beer and also make the famous dandelion and burdock drink. Young, unopened flower buds can be pickled.

🍃 For soup, lightly cook young nettle leaves in a stock to which is added oats and butter. After a short time of further cooking, add chervil, chives and black pepper to flavour and serve with halved hard-boiled, free-range eggs.

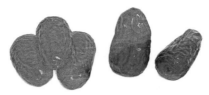

Dates

The date palm originates from the Persian Gulf and in ancient times was especially abundant between the Nile and Euphrates Rivers. There is archaeological evidence of its cultivation in eastern Arabia 6000 years ago. It was highly revered and regarded as a symbol of fertility, and was depicted in relief carvings and on coins. Much literature is devoted to its history and romance. It has also long been grown ornamentally along the coastlines of the southern Mediterranean. Iraq has always led the world in date production. Presently, there are 22 million date palms in Iraq producing nearly 600,000 tons of dates annually.

What they contain

Dates are very rich in **potassium** (as high as 0.9% of the flesh). Also have some **boron, calcium, cobalt, copper, iron, magnesium, manganese, phosphates, selenium, zinc**, some **sodium** and good quantities of **fibre** (6–12%), much of it as **soluble pectin**. Contain virtually no fat, and are low in calories, but **high in energy**, being rich in sugars (40–90% of balanced amounts of **fructose** and **glucose**). Contain some of the B vitamins, particularly **pantothenic acid**. The fruits are rich in **flavonoids**, particularly **luteolin, quercetin** and **apigenin**. Fresh dates also contain **anthocyanins** and **carotenoids**, and some **tannins**. The seeds are rich in **monounsaturated fatty acids**.

What they do

Potassium-rich dates maintain nerve and muscle activity and can reduce hypertension. They help normalise heartbeat, send oxygen to the brain (which improves neurone activity) and regulate the body's water balance. Consequently, eating potassium-rich foods improves mental activity and reduces high blood pressure. Because potassium is not stored within the body, eating a few dates a day can supply this need.

Dates' rich antioxidant flavonoids reduce cardiovascular disease and the development of some cancers. The fruit's tannins are used as an astringent for intestinal ailments and it was traditionally used to relieve gastric ulcers. Historically, it was given to treat sore throats, colds, bronchial catarrh and fevers, but also for cystitis, gonorrhoea, oedema and liver troubles. It is said to counteract the effects of alcohol intoxication.

How they are used

Dry or soft dates are eaten out-of-hand, may be seeded and stuffed, or chopped and used in a wide variety of ways on cereals, in puddings, breads, cakes, cookies, muffins and in ice cream. Date and walnut cake is a favourite – the two flavours complement each other. They also mix well with the sharpness of oranges and tangerines.

Dates are popular in Christmas cakes and puddings and within snack bars. They are blended with bananas to make a rich yet healthy dessert. A few chopped dates can be added to a stuffing and are popular in chutney. Surplus dates are made into cubes, paste, spread, powder (date sugar), jam, jelly, juice, syrup or vinegar. Dates can make a sweet juice or syrup, or are fermented to make an alcoholic drink.

In India, date seeds may be roasted, ground, and used to adulterate coffee. In Ghana and the Ivory Coast, date palms are tapped for their sweet sap, which is converted to palm sugar, molasses or alcoholic drinks.

> 🌿 One of the sweetest fruits, they make a good alternative to produced confectionery for those craving sugar. They are also nutritious and their fibre helps balance out peaks and troughs in blood-sugar levels.

Dill

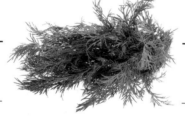

Dill, closely related to fennel, coriander and carrot, is native to western Asia, though is now found growing wild in many other regions. Traditionally, it was widely used in colder European countries to flavour winter-stored foods, when little else was available. The whole plant is aromatic and the leaves and seeds are used in many dishes, but are also well known for their medicinal purposes, most effectively for eliminating flatulence and easing digestion – its name may originate from 'dylle' meaning to calm or lull.

What it contains

The fresh leaves are rich in **vitamins A** and **C**. Both leaves and seeds are rich in minerals, particularly **iron, calcium, manganese** and **potassium**. Its essential oil is rich in **terpenes**, containing mostly **carvone** (~50%) and **limonene** (~40%).

What it does

Dill's ability to effectively relieve wind is particularly useful for lulling young children to sleep and it is still used for this purpose. Its anti-spasmodic action is used to ease digestive ailments and to reduce menstrual cramps. It has been used by nursing mothers to increase milk supply. Recent research has shown that it affects regulation of hormones and the menstrual cycle of rodents.

Its terpenes initiate production of an enzyme that has powerful anti-cancer properties. Dill also reduces serum lipid levels, so could be useful in reducing cardiac disease. The crushed leaves have been used as a poultice to reduce swelling and pain, and its essential oil is used in the perfumery industry.

Warning: Some people have adverse skin reactions after handling this species, particularly if the skin is then exposed to sunlight.

> Dill has significant antimicrobial properties: in one trial, it was tested against eight pathogenic bacteria that cause human disease. Dill oil was effective against all the bacteria tested, including difficult-to-kill waxy-coated bacteria, and was equally or more effective than standard antibiotics, even at very low concentrations.

How it is used

The young leaves and ripe fruits are used to flavour a range of dishes. They have a sweetish anise-like flavour, and are added to potatoes, bean dishes, soups, stews, sauces, chicken and dips. They are used as a flavouring in breads and mix well with vegetables such as asparagus, artichokes, beans, citrus, mustard, carrot and parsley. The seeds have a stronger flavour and are used in moderation in the same types of dishes. The leaves and fruits can be steeped in vinegar, which is then used to flavour pickles, particularly gherkins, to which they add a depth of flavour. The spicy vinegar in Europe, particularly France, is used to flavour cakes and pastries. The seeds can be sprouted and used in salads. Its essential oil is used as a flavouring – the variety 'Dukat' is particularly rich in this oil and is grown commercially for this product.

> 🐾 Dill butter is made from the young leaves and is popularly served with meats, fish or chicken. Dill is particularly good on smoked salmon – it makes the famous gravlax sauce – and is also popular with seafood.

Elderberries

(common or European)

F S V

European elderberries are popular, often picked from the wild, for making juice, preserves and wines, and the flowers too are sought after to make delicious cordial or bubbly white wine. They also have medicinal properties. There is an old saying: 'He who cultivates elderberry will die in his own bed.'

What they contain

They have very high antioxidant scores, more so than most fruits and vegetables – more than even cranberries or blackcurrants. Have good levels of **carotenoids**, **vitamin C** (~35 mg/100 mg of flesh), and are a good source of **dietary fibre**, much of it as **pectin**. The fruits are super-rich in many **flavonoids**, including **quercetin** and **rutin**.

What they do

The berries and flowers have long been known to cure colds, fevers and flu. Recently, the fruits were shown to inhibit the replication of several human influenza viruses. A trial in Israel showed that >90% of people who ate elderberries and who had contracted flu found relief from fever and other flu symptoms several days sooner than people who just took a placebo. Elderberries successfully treated influenza A and B, which no other standard medication was able to do. Elderberry fruits can also significantly inhibit enzymes that could otherwise initiate and promote the development of cancers.

Warning: Although the fruits and flowers of black varieties are perfectly safe, if gathering from the wild, particularly in North America, check the species. Red-fruited types, or unripe fruits, may be dangerously purgative and should not be eaten. The leaves are toxic, containing cyanide-like compounds.

> The flowers have anti-inflammatory properties: they reduced the inflammatory activities of all peridontal microbes tested, so would make a tremendous mouthwash. The fruits may help with weight loss and are added to slimming products.

How they are used

The berries and flowers of black elderberries are used in cordials, and elderberry wine is an old favourite and is easy to make. The flowers make a splendid, light, refreshing, fizzy cordial for hot summer days and are also used to make a popular bubbly white wine. The fruit can be used in pies, sauces and jelly – their abundant pectin gives them excellent setting properties. They are added to desserts, such as apple and blackberry crumble. They also mix well with rhubarb and are used in muffins, cakes and make a sauce to accompany meat or chicken. A vinegar is made from them. The flowers have a mild floral aroma and flavour, and are used in pancakes or are dipped in batter and fried. Try adding them to cooked gooseberries.

Endives   See 'Chicory'

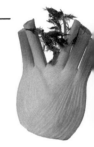

Fennel, Florence fennel, Sicilian fennel
(sweet fennel, finocchio)

The fennels originate from southern Europe and are related to celery, dill and parsnip. They were popular with the Greeks, who discovered their appetite-suppressant properties. In the Middle Ages fennel was a popular herb and was used to repel insects and to flavour food that was beginning to spoil. It is still popular in southern Europe, the Middle East and is used widely in India as a food and medicinally.

Although herb fennel is the most familiar, and is popular for its strongly aromatic feathery foliage and seeds, Florence fennel is becoming increasingly valued for its swollen, densely layered basal stem, or bulb. Sicilian fennel, most popular in southern Italy, is grown for its young celery-like stems.

What it contains

All parts of fennel have some **vitamin C** (~10 mg/100 g), and some **B vitamins**, particularly **folate**. The seeds are rich in **protein** and **fibre**, are very rich in **minerals** (**calcium, iron, magnesium, phosphates, potassium, copper** and **manganese**), some of the **B vitamins** and **monounsaturated oleic acid**. Fennel plants are rich in **antioxidant** compounds and many **coumarins**. Most of their characteristic anise-like flavour is derived from **anethole**, the same compound found in anise. This compound is much sweeter than sugar and is perceived as pleasant even at high concentrations. The seeds are rich in **monounsaturated petroselinic acid**, an unusual oil that is common in this family.

What it does

Fennel can also suppress appetite, so is excellent for those on diets. Other promising research shows that fennel indirectly increases levels of a neurotransmitter, which has promise in reducing the effects of mental retardation and it significantly aids the treatment of dementia and Alzheimer's in mice, and perhaps could be used to treat the autoimmune disease myastheria gravis.

Fennel has been used as an oestrogenic – recent research reports that topical application significantly reduced the growth of unwanted hair in women. It also significantly reduces symptoms of painful menstruation and is reported to be a safe and effective herbal drug for this condition. Historically, it was used to increase the milk supply of breast-feeding mothers. Fennel also has a potent effect on the regeneration and protection of the liver.

> Research confirms that fennel reduces intestinal discomfort and flatulence, and can significantly decrease the intensity of infant colic. This is a promising finding, as some pharmaceutical remedies have serious side effects, whereas fennel does not seem to. This efficacy is due to anethole.

It has very strong antibacterial properties against many food-borne pathogens, which explains its common usage as a food additive to meats and the like during the Middle Ages. It is also added to toothpaste and chewing the seeds is said to freshen the breath. Fennel has antifungal activity and can repel several insects, including mosquitoes. Compounds within fennel are precursors for the party drug ecstasy. Historically, many nationalities have used fennel as an eyewash and to improve eyesight, though see warning.

Warning: As with other members of this family, skin contact can cause adverse reactions, particularly with exposure to sunlight.

How it is used

Fennel leaves and seeds are used in Mediterranean cuisine to flavour stews, soups and fish recipes. Its distinctive aniseed/liquorice flavour can be quite powerful, so use in moderation because its flavour and aroma, although wonderful, can dominate a dish. The leaves are also used in many Indian and Asian recipes. Mixes well with potato, beets, pinenuts and orange. The finely cut leaves make an attractive garnish on fish dishes or in sauces. Any tough fibres are removed from Sicilian fennel and the stalks may be then soaked in vinegar and black pepper before serving as a salad. The seeds are added to both savoury and sweet dishes (such as pastries and candies), and are added to breads, though in moderation due to their strong flavour. They are an important ingredient in Chinese five-spice and in Indian spice mixes. Traditionally, fennel was included in the flavouring Absinthe. The pollen is also collected as a luxury-item food, with many food connoisseurs considering this to be the finest-flavoured part of the plant – it is sometimes called 'spice of the angels'. However, because pollen collection takes a long time it is very costly to buy.

> 🐾 Florence fennel bulbs are delicious, with a milder flavour than fennel leaves – they work well when finely chopped and added to salads, and mix wonderfully with goat's cheese or feta. Is also great added to soups and, in Italy, it is marinated and served as part of an antipasto. Can also be baked or steamed, then served with butter to accompany pasta. It is sometimes served with chicory and avocado.

Figs

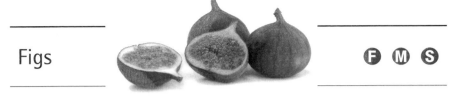

F **M** **S**

Figs have been valued for a long time – Classical, Eastern and Biblical mythology are full of references to figs. There are many varieties, but they are best fully ripened in the sun and are often eaten dried.

What they contain

Dried figs are rich in **fibre** (~10%), most as **soluble pectin fibre**, and are very rich in **glucose** and **fructose**. Dried figs are also quite rich in **minerals**, particularly **iron** and **potassium**. In addition, they contain abundant flavonoids (e.g. **anthocyanins**), **terpenes** (**lupeol**) and **coumarins**. These are found mostly in dark-skinned varieties, particularly near to the skin. But figs are low in vitamins. Their seeds contain 30% oil, which is rich in **omega-3 α-linolenic** and **omega-6 linoleic**. The oil is used for cooking.

What they do

Pectin-rich figs aid the removal of toxins from the gut, lower plasma LDLs, decrease blood-sugar levels and help stabilise insulin levels, thus reducing cardiovascular disease and improving the health of the digestive tract. They provide a very effective treatment for constipation. The fibre also helps balance the figs' high sugar levels, ameliorating potential rapid rises in blood-sugar level.

Their antioxidant polyphenols have been shown to reduce the development of cancer and cardiovascular disease – these compounds are still active in dried fruits.

Lupeol has significant antioxidant, anticarcinogenic, antidiabetic, anti-inflammatory, antiarthritic and antimalarial properties, and is being widely researched. Lupeol, in mice, combats testosterone-induced changes in the prostate, causes cell death of prostate cancer cells and helps restore damaged liver and skin cells (which could otherwise become cancerous). Its coumarins have also been used to treat prostate and skin cancers. In Latin America, the fruits are used as a poultice on tumours and abnormal growths.

The figs' latex is dried and used to coagulate milk to make cheese and junket. It also contains a protein-digesting enzyme (ficin), which is used to tenderise meat, to render fat and to clarify beverages.

Warning: The latex from unripe fruits, leaves and stems can severely irritate the skin – it may break down proteins within mucous membranes.

How they are used

Figs are wonderful ripe and fresh and are usually peeled. They are added to pies, crumbles, puddings, cakes, etc., as well as jellies and preserves. Whole fruits can be preserved in syrup and they can be made into jam, marmalade or chutney. Figs can be added to biscuits, puddings etc. They can be stewed with honey or stuffed with other fruits and make an excellent dried fruit, which increases many of the nutrients. Dried figs are used in trail mixes, but also in many dessert recipes. In Mediterranean countries, low-grade figs are converted into alcohol.

🌰 Figs aren't just for sweet recipes – they can be used in pastas, are stuffed with tasty creamy cheese and a dash of white wine, or are added to chicken recipes. Figs also mix excellently with Parma ham and a strong cheese such as Gorgonzola, and with chicory, radicchio and mozzarella.

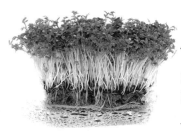

Garden cress
(pepper cress)

Garden cress, which is now naturalised in many parts of the world, has been gathered and appreciated for hundreds of years. Although related to watercress, garden cress can grow in ordinary soil. Today, in Europe and the United Kingdom, it is more usually consumed as the young sprouted seeds, harvested from small tubs, and is the 'cress' in 'mustard and cress'.

What it contains

Garden cress is extremely rich in **vitamins**. It has excellent levels of **carotenoids**, i.e. β-carotene, and even more **lutein** and **zeaxanthin**; is rich in **vitamin C** (~90 mg/100 g) and very rich in **vitamin K**. It is also very rich in **chlorophyll** (the photosynthetic molecule in plants), more so than most vegetables. This has anticarcinogenic and wound-healing properties. Similar to other brassicas, much of its distinctive flavour is derived from **isothiocyanates**. The oil in its seeds is one of the richest sources of **omega-3 fatty acids**, of which ~32% is α-**linolenic acid**.

> The isothio-cyanates within garden cress have a greater ability to prevent damage to DNA (and thus prevent formation of cancer) than most other brassicas.

What it does

Isothiocyanates have been shown to prevent cancers and cardiovascular disease. Compounds within cress can strongly inhibit the formation of liver, breast, lung and colon cancers. Isothiocyantes also significantly decrease blood-glucose levels in diabetic and non-diabetic rats, and this occurs without affecting basal plasma insulin concentrations: thus seems to have anti-diabetic benefits. The leaves also seem to reduce high blood pressure, plus act as a diuretic.

Its seeds are being investigated as an important source of omega-3 fatty acids. Their abundant α-linolenic acid significantly reduces serum LDLs, while HDL ('good' cholesterol) remains unchanged. The seed oil also lowers liver-produced cholesterol by ~12%, serum- triglycerides by ~40% and has several other significant benefits to the cardiovascular system. In Arab countries, consumption of these seeds is associated with bone healing: recent experiments have confirmed that bone heals significantly faster if seeds are included within the diet. Warning: Some report that eaten in quantity the seeds can induce abortion.

How it is used

The sprouted seedlings are popular in salads and as a garnish, often with egg or potatoes, and sometimes in sandwiches. They have a pleasant, mild, peppery flavour. Leaves from mature plants are mixed with cottage cheese and fruit to make a delightful, light salad, or can be added to soups, stews, etc. Note though that isothiocyanates are mostly nullified by extended cooking – add leaves to dishes just before serving, or only lightly steam them. Some eat the leaves with bread and butter, lemon and vinegar or sugar.

> 🍃 Create a base of garden cress leaves with slices of creamy avocado, a couple of slices of smoked salmon, and a few pumpkin seeds then dress with a drizzle of virgin olive oil.

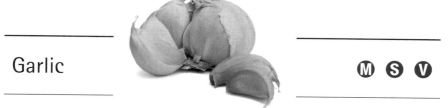

Garlic Ⓜ Ⓢ Ⓥ

Related to onion and leeks, garlic has been used by virtually every known civilisation, including ancient India, Egypt, Rome, China and Japan. Garlic has a wealth of varied medicinal benefits and has long been valued as a unique and delicious flavouring, added to a multitude of dishes.

What it contains

Garlic contains good quantities of **vitamin C** (~32 mg/100 g of bulb) and of **vitamin B6**. Also has good amounts of **manganese** and the **antioxidant selenium** and contains some **phyto-oestrogens**. Garlic is particularly rich in **sulphur-rich compounds** (e.g. **allicin, diallyl sulphide**).

What it does

More than 3000 scientific papers have confirmed the efficacy of garlic in preventing and treating many diseases and have acknowledged and validated its traditional uses. More than most foods, garlic's powerful antioxidant properties and ability to increase the activity of several antioxidant enzymes have been repeatedly shown to prevent and actually fight a wide range of cancers. The sulphur and high selenium content reduced the incidence of colon cancer by 50–70% in rodents. Daily consumption of garlic, particularly by the elderly, is recommended. Garlic exerts its anticarcinogenic effects through multiple mechanisms. For example, cooked meats release compounds that are suspected carcinogens (e.g. for breast cancer); however, diallyl sulphide (found within garlic) inhibits the effects of these compounds, thus inhibiting formation of some cancers.

In addition, garlic has also long been valued for its ability to fight off colds, coughs and other similar infections. It is valued for 'purifying' the blood.

Recent research reports that raw garlic reduces cholesterol and triglyceride levels and lowers blood sugar, therefore reduces development of heart disease. It also significantly reduces fluctuations in heart beat. Remarkably, garlic can reduce the symptoms of human fatigue, including physical fatigue. Eating raw garlic also reduces development of dementia. Garlic may even help relieve the symptoms of sickle cell anaemia and helps reduce damage caused by fungal aflatoxins.

Garlic has been used to expel intestinal worms, is used externally to treat various skin complaints (e.g. eczema) and is diluted with warm oil to treat earache.

Warning: Some people's skin is sensitive to garlic and large internal doses can cause intestinal discomfort. Garlic is also not good for dogs.

How it is used

Young garlic leaves can be eaten and have a mild flavour. The curled flower stalks can also be eaten. The tall green or white fresh stems of some garlic varieties are valued in Asian cuisine and have a fresh but fairly strong garlic flavour – they are excellent finely chopped and lightly fried, which sweetens their flavour. They make an attractive garnish on stir-fries and soups and go wonderfully with fried mushrooms, fresh lemon juice on fresh, warm bread. Garlic cloves are delicious in a wide range of foods, including many Italian, Asian, Chinese and Indian dishes. They are a common ingredient in curries, pastas, pizza, ratatouille, soups and dips. When roasted, garlic's flavour becomes sweeter and less intense. It can also be gently fried (too much heat destroys its flavour). It is added raw to dressings, such as wonderful garlic aioli for salads, and roasted garlic can be mixed with horseradish and creamy yoghurt and served with smoked fish or chicken – delicious and very quick to make. Garlic soup can be easily made: simmered roast

> ✿ Garlic is most efficacious when eaten fresh: even mincing garlic changes some of its compounds and roasting and drying changes them further. However, slicing and then leaving for ~10 minutes before cooking reduces this loss somewhat.

garlic in stock with a little olive oil and sliced spring onions and parsley sprinkled on top. Because much of its activity is destroyed by cooking or microwaving, reduce cooking time to a few minutes. Although garlic has a divine aroma when it's cooking, its effect on the breath is infamous. Parsley is meant to counteract this somewhat.

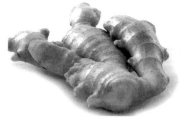

Ginger

Ginger is the root tuber of an attractive tropical plant that has been used for >4000 years for its medicinal properties and as a flavouring in many food and drink recipes. Today, it is cultivated in many tropical regions of the world and is particularly popular in many Asian-style recipes.

What it contains

Contains ~3% essential oil, which gives ginger its flavour and medicinal properties. The oil consists mainly of **terpenes** (spicy **zingerone** and aromatic **bisabolene)**, plus the alkaloid **farnesene**, which gives it much of its flavour. These three compounds are also the main compounds that ease nausea. It contains abundant **flavonoids**, adding to ginger's distinctive flavour and aroma, plus **oleoresin**, a mix of oil and resin, which is also used in pepper sprays.

What it does

Its flavonoids have anti-cancer activity – colorectal may help prevent and also possibly fight existing cancers. Ginger also has antibacterial and antifungal properties, which are being investigated as a safe and cheap treatment for bacterial-caused diarrhoea. Zingerone appears to block a toxin produced by *Escherichia coli* which causes diarrhoea. It also has antibacterial reactions against other bacteria (e.g. *Staphylococcus aureus*).

Ginger is a strong antioxidant and anti-inflammatory – it may reduce heart disease by preventing platelets clotting together and seems

Ginger has been used for thousands of years to ease digestive problems and feelings of nausea, either brought on by motion sickness or pregnancy. Recent trials confirm its usage for motion sickness and, so far, it has been shown safe to take for morning sickness. It can also be taken to reduce post-operative nausea and vomiting.

to reduce cholesterol levels. Ginger has relaxant and analgesic properties – it can soothe coughs and inflamed bronchial passages. Research suggests ginger may also have the ability to treat diverse complaints such as arthritis, diabetes, Crohn's disease, osteoporosis and Alzheimer's. It has been used externally to treat rheumatism, psoriasis, migraines and strains. Its wonderful warm aroma means it is used in cosmetic scents and fragrances.

Warning: Ginger can cause skin sensitivity in some.

How it is used

The fresh, young roots are juicy and have a mild flavour; older roots are drier and hotter. Grated or finely diced it is used in a multitude of Asian and Indian recipes, including curries, marinades, soups and stir-fries. It is usually not added until the meal is nearly cooked to prevent ginger losing its freshness and flavour. It is pickled in Asia and is used as a relish on many dishes, including tofu-based recipes. Ginger goes wonderfully with garlic and lime, and is great added to fish and chicken recipes. It mixes well with vegetables such as carrot, citrus and pumpkin and can be preserved in syrup or sugar to make a sweet candy – a traditional Christmas treat in the West. Some add ginger to drinking chocolate, coffee or tea. Candied ginger in dark chocolate is delicious, as are ginger cake, ginger snaps and gingerbread.

🦐 Cold, 'real' ginger beer is terrific. You will need to source a ginger beer plant – a yeasty culture that is fed with sugar and ginger, and then share it with friends.

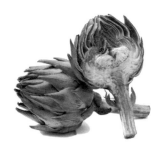

Globe artichokes, cardoons

The strange flowers of globe artichoke were eaten and enjoyed by the ancient Greeks and Romans, with the Greeks believing that artichokes had aphrodisiac properties and could encourage the formation of male rather than female children. It has long been popular in French and Italian cuisine. Although fiddly to eat, with much of the large immature flower head being discarded, the flesh at the base of the flower bract, particularly the succulent heart of the flower, is delicious. Very similar in appearance is its close relative the cardoon. Although it has small edible flowers, it is more valued for its leaves, which are usually blanched.

What they contain

Globe artichokes and cardoons are rich in **soluble** and **fermentable fibre**, with much of this being **inulin**. The flower heads also contain good amounts of **antioxidants**, particularly **cynarin**, and several **flavonoids** thought to be responsible for much of their liver-protective properties. Cardoons are similarly rich in **fibre**, **flavonoids** and **cynarin**, plus **chlorogenic acid**.

What they do

Globe artichoke is valued for its ability to reduce serum-cholesterol and to treat liver and gallbladder complaints. This plant was traditionally used to treat hepatitis and other liver complaints. Cynarin has long been believed to 'purify the blood', in particular it is thought to increase bile production in the liver, and bile flow within the gallbladder. Research has confirmed its liver-protecting properties, as well as it reducing many liver and digestive disorders, such as sensation of fullness, loss of appetite, nausea and abdominal pain. Eating globe artichokes can ameliorate the

> Globe artichokes improve blood-vessel health, which is particularly important for the elderly, reducing the risk of cardiovascular problems. In trials, when it was fed to older rats, it restored their vascular 'suppleness' to that of young rats.

symptoms of irritable- bowel syndrome, and improves health-related quality of life. Artichokes are also eaten to treat gout, stomach ulcers, diarrhoea and for high blood pressure.

Recent trials show that cynarin can lower serum-cholesterol by ~10–15%, particularly LDLs. Extracts also have antibacterial, anti-yeast, but particularly antifungal properties.

Inulin improves digestion and reduces the risk of colorectal cancers. Even better, eat your globe artichokes or cardoon leaves with some live yoghurt. The probiotic effects of yoghurt then combine with the prebiotic inulin to further enhance beneficial bacteria within the gut – these microbes are intrinsic to our health in many ways that are only just being realised. Inulin within cardoons may be as good as or better than that within Jerusalem artichokes. Additionally, because inulin is not digested, it has no calorific value, but gives the sensation of having just eaten, so is great for those concerned about weight gain. It can cause flatulence.

Warning: A minority are allergic to inulin, so treat with caution until this is ascertained.

🌸 To prepare globe artichokes, boil in a stainless steel pan (to avoid discolouration) for ~30 minutes, then remove and thoroughly drain. Just the base of the fleshy bracts are eaten, with the harder parts being discarded. However, the central 'heart' within the bracts is the most highly prized. This is found below the immature flower – the 'choke' – whose fine 'hairs' need to be thoroughly removed or they are very irritating (hence their name). Below the 'choke' is the delicious fleshy heart – wonderful dipped into creamy yoghurt, garlic butter, olive oil or balsamic vinegar, or even tomato-based dips.

How they are used

Globe artichoke is an unusual vegetable that many love, though some find it too fiddly to eat. Along with being braised, the flesh may be eaten raw and, in Italy, they deep-fry young globes. Cooked, they can be served on their own as a starter, are great in Mediterranean-style recipes (e.g. pastas, antipastos), and also in fish dishes. The hearts can be stored in olive oil with herbs and are delicious when roasted with a little garlic. They can also be smoked.

Although cardoon flower heads are edible, they are usually considered too small. However, young cardoon leaves can be eaten fresh in salads and treated in the same way as celery. They can also be lightly cooked. For blanched leaves, the older, outer leaves are removed to leave the younger leaves, the stems and the tender central crown. This is often sliced into sections horizontally and then simmered for a short time. They have juicy, tender midribs. They can be added to soups, ratatouille, pasta, etc., though are best when their pleasant flavour can be appreciated. Drizzle with garlic butter, or crumble white cheese over. They mix deliciously with Mediterranean ingredients such as olives, eggplant, courgettes, garlic and tomatoes. Their flavour is slightly reminiscent of celery.

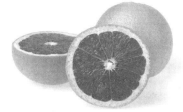

Grapefruit

There are a few types of grapefruit, though the common grapefruit (*Citrus* x *paradisi*) is the main species cultivated. It is a natural hybrid between pummelo and orange, hence its botanical name. It became known as a grapefruit when it reached Europe, which is strange because it does not look or taste like a grape. It is most traditionally known as a breakfast fruit, though it has many other food and medicinal uses.

What it contains

The pulp is a good source of **vitamin C** (~35 mg/100 g of pulp) and the fruit skin and pith, in particular,

have good levels of the **soluble fibre pectin**, which is beneficial to the digestive system. There is an oil in the outer layer which contains **nootkatone** (used as a flavour enhancer in fruit juices) and **terpenes**, particularly **limonene**, and **coumarins**. Pink and red grapefruits also contain abundant **flavonoids** (e.g. **hesperidin**, **apigenin**), and are rich in **carotenoids**, particularly **lycopene** – a very powerful antioxidant which can reduce the development of prostate, lung and mammary cancers, and β-**carotene**. The seeds are used medicinally and contain many **flavonoids**.

What it does

Its flavonoids may reduce development of cancerous tumours. These flavonoids also regulate and steady heart rhythm and help block the secretion of hepatitis C virus from infected cells, thus reducing its virulence and spread.

Grapefruit, but particularly its peel, has antibacterial, antidepressant, antiseptic, astringent, digestion-aiding, diuretic, mild-stimulant prop-erties and is valued as a general tonic. It seems to stimulate fat digestion and improve liver health. Many of grapefruit's benefits may be linked to limonene. This compound improves digestion by neutralising gastric acid secretions and helps regulate normal movement of the gut, which can relieve heartburn and gastro-oesophageal reflux. Limonene also has well-established activity against many types of cancer (e.g. breast and colorectal). The seeds are known for their antibacterial, antifungal, anti-protozoan and antiviral properties: they can kill many pathogenic species, and have been used as an antibiotic and antiseptic.

How it is used

Grapefruit has long been included on weight-reduction menus. It is

🐾 Grapefruit juice makes a terrific marinade/tenderiser for raw fish. Leave fish pieces, such as fresh salmon, in grapefruit juice for about 45 minutes. The juice imparts a delicious flavour and gives the flesh a soft texture. Add seasoning and simply serve with rocket or watercress, a few slices of kiwifruit and a baked sweet potato topped with a little coconut cream.

traditionally eaten for breakfast, cut in half and sprinkled with sugar, honey or cinnamon. The fruit sections are used in fruit salads and various desserts, often to balance the sweetness of other ingredients. It also mixes well with vegetables such as carrots, avocado, artichoke, and with fish and seafood. Grapefruit flesh can be added to various preserves, including marmalade, or can be made into jelly, or into a juice. They can be lightly grilled and served as a savoury with bacon, fish or vegetables. Grapefruit broiled with maple syrup and cinnamon is delicious. A good-quality vinegar or even a wine can be made from grapefruit and the peel may be candied. The oil from its skin is used commercially as a flavouring.

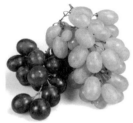

Grapes, muscadines

There are two main commercial subgenera of grape (*Vitis*): *Euvitis* and *Muscadinia*. *Euvitis* are the 'true grapes' (or 'bunch grapes'), where long clusters of fruits remain on their stalks at maturity. Within this group are two main types: the Old World or European grape and American bunch grapes. The European grape accounts for >90% of world production. The American bunch grape, because it is resistant to fungal disease, is mostly used as rootstocks for European grapes. It is also used to make grape juice, jam, preserves and some wine. *Muscadinia* includes the muscadine (scuppernong) grapes, which have smaller, sweeter fruits that readily detach when mature. They are native in the south-east of the United States, where they have been cultivated for more than 400 years.

What they contain

In red wine, non-flavonoid **caffeic acid** is found in the flesh and antioxidant **flavonoids** and lots of **anthocyanins** in the skin. White wine only contains non-flavonoid polyphenols (it has no contact with skins or seeds). Grapes contain the flavonoid **quercetin**, which protects against cancer and strengthens connective tissues, and are very rich in **resveratrol**. Resveratrol induces many actions which depend on cell type, cellular condition (normal, stressed, malignant) and concentration, and can have opposing activities. It affects whole pathways and sets of intracellular events rather than a single enzyme. Grapes also contain **ellagic**, **tannic** and **gallic acids**. Though relatively low in sugars, they contain balanced amounts of **glucose** and **fructose**. Muscadine fruits have similar health properties, but are richer in **vitamin C**. Raisins and sultanas (from white seedless grapes) are very nutrient rich, especially in **antioxidants**, and contain good quantities of **soluble fibre**, which is excellent for the digestive system. They are also very rich in **iron**, **boron** and **potassium**.

What they do

Red grapes are rich in the anticarcinogenic compound resveratrol only discovered in 1996, which can prevent DNA damage, slow/halt cancerous cell transformation and slow tumour growth. It also has anti-inflammatory properties and may help prevent colon and liver cancer. Resveratrol is being investigated as a potential anti-cancer drug. It seems to block several steps in the carcinogenesis process. In addition, resveratrol protects the cardiovascular system through many mechanisms, including defence, protection and maintenance of arterial membranes, promotes relaxation of vessels, has anti-atherosclerotic properties, inhibits production of LDLs and suppresses platelet aggregation – all which strongly support its role in preventing coronary disease.

The proven anti-blood clotting and antioxidant benefits to arterial health mean that daily intake of purple grape juice or moderate amounts of red wine can reduce the risk of developing cardiovascular disease. There are also data for the use of resveratrol for progressive neurodegenerative diseases such as Alzheimer's, Huntington's and Parkinson's.

The flavanols greatly enhance vitamin C activity within the body. Grapes also promote elasticity and flexibility of muscles, tendons and ligaments, help heal injuries, reduce swelling, bruising and oedema, improve peripheral circulation, strengthen weak blood vessels, protect against atherosclerosis and inhibit enzymes that lead to allergic reactions. Its compounds are rapidly absorbed and distributed throughout the body and have many anti-ageing benefits. Muscadines contain the same

🌿 A delicious fruit salad can be made with grapes, kiwifruit and strawberries, which boosts vitamin C and enhances arterial and body suppleness.

polyphenols as Old World grapes – both non-flavonoid and flavonoids – and good quantities of resveratrol.

How they are used

They are wonderful fresh just on their own or added to a fruit salad. They make a good garnish on sweet and savoury dishes, can be added to sauces, make a wonderful non-alcoholic juice and are delicious with cheese. Grappa, a powerful alcoholic drink (100% proof), is distilled in Italy from the fermented skins, seeds and stems, which are left over from pressing the juice. Vine leaves are tasty after blanching and can be stuffed with rice, vegetables, meat, etc. In the past, grape vines were tapped in spring, and the sap was drunk for its medicinal properties.

Wine-making is the crushing of grapes to produce the 'must' (juice, skins, seeds and stems for red; juice only for white); pH is assessed before sugar is added, if needed. The must is then either partially fermented with the skins to produce red wine, with lesser contact for a rosé, or with no skin contact for a white wine. Higher fermentation temperatures are used for red wine (24–28°C) compared to white (14–18°C). After a period of time, the wine is filtered and placed in oak barrels (or similar) in a cool environment. Red wine is usually aged for between 1–10 years, whereas white wine usually only needs ~1 year.

Muscadine grapes are very tasty eaten fresh, or added to jellies, jams, juice, sauces. They are added to various desserts and make an excellent dessert wine. The fruit has a distinctive fruity aroma. They are tasty eaten dried and can be used as other dried fruits.

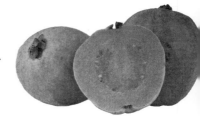

Guavas

(tropical and cattleya)

Tropical guava originates from Mexico and South America, and are now grown in many warmer areas of the world. Cattleya guava comes in two main colours – yellow and red. Those with yellow fruit have sweet, aromatic flesh, but are generally not very tangy, whereas red cattleyas have delicious, tangy flesh. Both guava types are filled with small, hard seeds. When ripe, the fruits have a delightful aroma.

What they contain

Vitamin C within tropical guavas is very high (200–300 mg/100 g of fresh fruit), being greatest in just-ripened fruits, and then declining with age. Most vitamin C is in the outer firm flesh. They also have good levels of **carotenoids**, particularly **lycopene**, a powerful anticarcinogen and pro-cardiovascular antioxidant. Tropical guava contain some **potassium**, the antioxidant **ellagic acid**, and good amounts of **soluble fibre**. The seeds contain ~14% of an aromatic oil. Cattleyas are not as nutrient rich, though they do have good levels of vitamin C (~35 mg/100 g).

What they do

The fruits have excellent antioxidant properties – ellagic acid can help prevent tumours and the fruits reduce serum-triglyceride levels (a risk indicator for heart disease), reduce hypertension, while increasing levels of HDLs. Quercetin has many activities including inhibiting spasmolytic activity of the gut, thus reducing diarrhoea and irritable-bowel syndrome. Lycopene is also an anti-cancer compound – it may prevent cancers of the prostate, pancreas, stomach, breast, cervix and lung. Consumption of lycopene is inversely associated with cancer of the digestive tract. It is also significantly associated with reduced prostate cancer, helps prevent cardiovascular disease and reduces the damage done to skin by UV light.

Guavas' wondrous antioxidant vitamin C content has many health benefits – it reduces development of cancer and protects against heart disease and stress. It is involved with energy production within cells, helps boost the immune system, binds with certain poisons to render them harmless, helps increase absorption of nutrients in the gut (enhances absorption of iron better than other fruits), and is involved in the production of collagen, needed for cartilage, joints, skin, and blood-vessel formation and maintenance. This vitamin is also needed for sperm production. The fresh fruits are an excellent remedy for coughs and colds.

How they are used

The best tropical guavas are delicious eaten fresh with firm, sweet/sub-acid outer flesh and juicy sweet inner pulp which has small, edible seeds. They are also used in desserts, puréed or are added to salads. The fruits are cooked to eliminate their strong odour, which some people do not enjoy, and they

> ✿ Try slices of guava in a green salad, perhaps with some sliced hazelnuts and almonds, served with fresh rye bread for a delicious lunch.

may be stewed, though this reduces their vitamin C. Guavas can be added to ice cream, sauces, jam, cakes, drinks, chutney and dressings. In South America, a thick guava paste and a guava cheese are made, as is guava jelly. The fruits go well with barbecued meats, including chicken. Some fruits have harder, larger seeds that are difficult to eat and may need to be removed. Cattleya fruits are usually eaten fresh and have a tangy yet sweetish flavour that some compare to strawberries. They do not have the musky flavour of tropical guavas.

Hazelnuts

(cobnut, filbert)

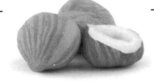

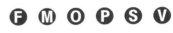

Hazelnuts have long been a popular food. The tree is associated with many mystical and occult rites, particularly from Celtic times, and is linked with ensuring fertility and happiness. Its branches were used for rituals, and dowsers still use them to find water underground. Most hazelnut cultivation now occurs in central and eastern Europe, with Turkey being a major exporter, but they are also cultivated in China, Oregon and New Zealand.

What they contain

Hazelnuts are a wonderful yet surprisingly undervalued food. They are rich in **protein** (~15%) and have excellent levels of **fibre** (~10%), most of it **soluble fibre**. They are very rich in powerful, heart-protecting **vitamin E**, and contain a rich and balanced range of healthy **oils** (~62%), of which ~55% is **monounsaturated oleic acid**, ~20% **omega-3 linoleic acid** and ~17% is **omega-6 linoleic acid**. Few foods are as rich in oleic acid with good amounts of omega-3s – hazelnuts have even more than olives. They are rich in **squalene** and related **phytosterols**, which have proven cardio-protective and anti-cancer benefits. Are also **mineral** rich, with more **calcium** than most other nuts, except almonds, and have large quantities of **copper**, **manganese**, **magnesium**, **potassium**, **phosphates**, **boron** and **iron**. They are very rich in **biotin**, with good amounts of the B **vitamins**, particularly **folate**. Hazelnuts are also rich in **coumarin-like** compounds (e.g. **ferulic** and **caffeic acids**), which have powerful antioxidant activities.

When 25 g of hazelnuts were eaten each day for 16 weeks by a group of people ranging in age from children to elderly, the nuts reduced serum-cholesterol by 2–10% and serum LDLs.

What they do

Hazelnuts are a wonderful source of minerals, vitamins, protein and fibre. They release their energy slowly, so are excellent for digestion, for those concerned about weight gain and for anyone at risk of developing type-2 diabetes. Their beneficial oils, vitamin E and phytosterols all work as anti-inflammatories, reducing the risk of many disorders, including age-related neurodegenerative and cardiovascular disease. Their oleic and omega-3 are crucial to cell membrane health.

Hazelnuts' abundant calcium and phosphates are excellent for bone health. Folate contributes to reducing the development of cancer, is good for the cardiovascular system and neuronal activity, and reduces the likelihood of birth defects. Warning: As with all nuts, hazelnuts can induce allergic reactions in some people.

How gorgeous are copped hazelnuts mixed with dark chocolate served with dark fruits such as raspberries and cherries and then topped with creamy yoghurt.

How they are used

Hazelnuts have lots of flavour and are included in many dessert and savoury recipes. They are eaten fresh as a snack, are roasted, and used in spreads (often with chocolate), muesli-type cereals, are added chopped to baked foods and can be mixed with toasted oats, honey and dried fruits to make a nutritious, tasty snack bar. They are delicious added to stuffing for chicken, aubergine, tomato and seafood dishes, etc. A few chopped nuts enliven a salad. Hazelnuts can be chopped and mixed with cumin and coriander seeds to make a tasty dukkah for dipping. They can be ground to a flour and then included in bread to add a nutty flavour. Chopped they can be added to cooked grains such as rice and quinoa.

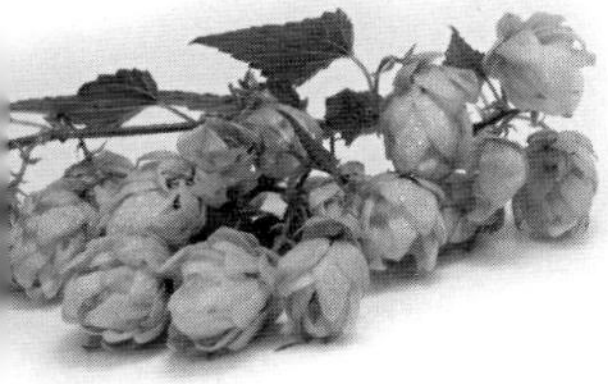

Hops

S V

(lupulin)

People have been using hops for at least 5000 years – possibly much longer. Ale has been drunk for many hundreds of years in England and throughout Europe and was, and still is, made using fermented malt. Today, beer is by far the greatest usage of this plant; however, the young stems and leaves are flavoursome, and the flowers have long been valued medicinally for their sedative and muscle-relaxing properties. The fruit (strobile) contains resinous and bitter compounds that give beer its characteristic flavour.

What they contain

Hops are rich in **vitamin C**. The flowers contain ~1% **essential oil** and 15–25% resinous bitter principles. They contain alpha acids (e.g. **humulone, valerianic acid**) and beta acids (e.g. **lupulone**). Together, the oil and bitter resins are known as **lupulin**. They also contain **tannins, flavonoids** (**rutin, quercetin** and the fairly unusual compound **astragalin**), **terpenes** and powerful **phyto-oestrogens**. The seeds are rich in **gamma-linolenic acid**.

Due to their phyto-oestrogens, hops have been also used to treat heavy or painful menstruation and to relieve some of the symptoms of menopause, with ongoing research into its modes of action.

What they do

Hops relax the central nervous system. They act as a sedative, a soporific, a hypnotic, an astringent and a diuretic; they reduce muscular contractions, dampen male desire (because of their phyto-oestrogens), and have been used to treat premature ejaculation. Hops can reduce smooth-muscle spasms which benefit nervous dyspepsia, irritable-bowel syndrome, diverticulitis, Crohn's disease, palpitations, nervous or irritable coughs and asthma.

Its flavonoids act as anticarcinogens by inhibiting an enzyme that can otherwise activate the cancer process. They have shown activity against prostate, breast and colon cancers. Its terpenes have anti-cancer activity against (e.g. colon and pancreas). Astragalin has antioxidant and anti-inflammatory properties and may reduce reactions to allergies and protect against liver damage.

Humulone and lupulone also have anti-inflammatory actions and are antibacterial, particularly against Gram-positive bacteria (e.g. *Staphylococcus aureus*). Hops are therefore used to treat infections of the upper digestive tract, ulcers, skin eruptions and wounds. Its antibacterial compounds also reduce *Porphyromonas gingivalis* (which causes gum disease and tooth decay), so perhaps hop extract could be included in toothpaste.

Beer, in moderation, has now been shown to reduce the risk of heart attacks. It is also good for dissolving kidney stones. Applied as a lotion, hops act locally as an antiseptic. Placed in pillows, the volatile oils and valerianic acid may help overcome insomnia. Warning: Hops can act as a mild depressive.

How they are used

The flower heads are used as a flavouring and preservative in beer and have a phenomenal aroma. The young leaves and shoots can be lightly cooked and taste like asparagus – they are definitely worth trying. Serve with a knob of butter, a little sautéed garlic, new potatoes and cherry tomatoes.

🐾 Hops are rich in oils and bitter resins. They have long been known to relieve nervous tension, anxiety and indigestion, and to increase appetite.

Horseradish

A member of the brassica family, this plant's deep taproots are enjoyed as a very hot relish, though they are also valued for their medicinal benefits. However, it has only become a popular flavouring, mostly within Europe, over the past few hundred years.

What it contains

Horseradish contains good amounts of **vitamin C** and some **folate**. Like other brassicas, horseradish is rich in glucosinolates, which are converted to strong-flavoured **isothiocyanates**. Horseradish also contains anti-oxidant **flavonoids**, particularly **kaempferol**.

What it does

Horseradish has powerful anti-mutagenic properties; it has been shown to reduce the prevalence of colon, lung and stomach cancer cells. It is similar in action and properties to wasabi. It has also long been used as a laxative, a diuretic and as a stimulant. Its hotness is good for clearing the nasal passages. Remedies include a mix of horseradish root with honey to clear passages of mucus. A mix of horseradish with nasturtium has been found effective and safe at treating people with chronic

The aroma from horseradish roots is so powerful that it can wake people who are in deep sleep – it is being researched as a spray to be emitted from activated fire alarms to alert deaf people.

recurrent urinary tract infections, acute sinusitis and acute bronchitis.

This plant combination is as effective as an antibiotic treatment, without the negatives associated with antibiotic therapy. The combination also results in a rapid reduction in cold symptoms and the authors of the trial concluded that the earlier this herbal remedy was started after initial cold symptoms were evident, the greater its benefits. Individually, but more so together, nasturtium and horseradish possess broad antibacterial activities against many Gram-positive and Gram-negative bacterial pathogens.

Horseradish has been used as a poultice for aches and sprains, bruises, etc, and applied locally to improve blood flow. The crushed root, in a cloth, laid on aching muscles or rheumatism, is said to be effective, with the poultice removed once heat is felt.

Warning: Take care that the juice in its pure form does not come into contact with eyes or other delicate tissues – it can irritate and burn. Eaten in large quantities (which is unlikely), horseradish can cause intestinal discomfort. As with other brassicas, it can reduce the efficiency of the thyroid gland in those who are vulnerable to this condition.

How it is used

Young spring leaves can be used in salads or lightly steamed as a vegetable. Blanching the leaves for 2–3 weeks, by covering with cloth, sweetens and tenderises their flavour. The fresh root is stunningly hot – much more so than any commercial horseradish sauces/relish. A small amount brings tears to the eyes. It is similar in taste and flavour to wasabi and is often used as a substitute. It is usually grated for this purpose.

🐾 Horseradish is great with sour cream or yoghurt and then used as a dip for corn chips, globe artichoke leaves or carrot sticks. Is also good with tomatoes, black pepper and a little olive oil to make a variation of salsa.

If not using straight away, store horseradish un-grated in a refrigerator to minimise loss of its active ingredients.

Mince the root with cream, a little vinegar, mustard and dill. It makes a terrific relish not only for roast beef, but also to accompany foods such as vegetable pie, mashed potatoes with cheese, roast vegetables, smoked fish (e.g. salmon, herring, trout), ham and lamb. A little can be added to soups just before serving. In Austria, horseradish is mixed with grated apple to make a relish.

Heating horseradish causes its active compounds to be largely nullified; therefore, it is best served with foods rather than cooked. A little is added to various cocktails to give them oomph.

Jerusalem artichokes   See 'Chicory'

Juniper berries
(common juniper)

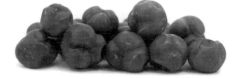

Ⓢ

Juniper is a member of the large cypress tree family, and is found growing in many parts of the northern hemisphere in a wider range of climates and over larger areas than almost any other plant species – from Iceland to Asia to New Mexico. The tree is known for its aromatic foliage and its berries, with the latter used to flavour many foods and drinks. These fruits are particularly popular in Hungary and southern Europe, especially Italy. They have a long history of usage as a flavouring and medicinally, and were used by the Greeks, Arabs and then the Romans. In the Renaissance, the fruits were used to treat plague and pestilence.

What they contain

The berries are rich in **terpenes** (e.g. **pinene** (~47%), **limonene**, **myrcene**), antioxidant **flavonoids**, tannins, and also the unusual **lignin podophyllotoxin**. Although a toxin in larger amounts, in smaller quantities podophyllotoxin is an ingredient in certain anti-cancer drugs and is used to treat warts. The berry oil is also rich in rare **eicosatrienoic acid**, a polyunsaturated fatty acid similar to that found in fish oil, but which is more stable. The fruits contain good amounts of **vitamin C**.

What they do

Most medicinal juniper remedies utilise the green berries, which are thought to be more potent. Historically, they were used to treat kidney and urinary tract infections and disorders, to promote healthy blood pressure and to treat gout. They have been used topically to treat warts. Today, the antiseptic properties of juniper are valued for treating urinary infections, such as cystitis, in the same way as cranberries, and also infections of the bladder, kidneys and prostate. In a trial, they were active against all 16

181

Juniper berries' podophyllotoxin has very important anti-cancer properties. This compound is used in many chemotherapy drugs (e.g. to treat lung cancer), and is used to treat genital warts. It has powerful properties to kill cancer cells and prevent DNA replication. The berries also reduce the growth and invasion of human breast cancer cells.

bacteria, 10 fungi/yeasts and four skin microbes tested. They were particularly effective against the yeast *Candida*.

The berries improve digestion by increasing the flow of digestive juices and help relieve stomach cramps and flatulence. They have also been used as a diuretic. Juniper has anti-inflammatory properties – it has been used to treat rheumatism and arthritis, and as a decongestant for chest infections. There is also evidence that it reduces blood-glucose levels, so it could play a part in the treatment of diabetes.

The berries are reported to have proven anti-egg-implantation effects, and have been suggested as a form of natural birth control. Its unusual fatty acids are beneficial to the liver and reduce oxidative stress.

Warning: Because it contains podophyllotoxin, pregnant and nursing women should avoid eating juniper berries. Use of the essential oil should be carried out with great care due to its strength and possible toxicities at higher doses.

How they are used

One of the best-known uses of these berries is to flavour gin. The berries are also added to strongly flavoured meats, to hung game and poultry dishes, where they counteract fattiness and strong flavours. They are often added to stuffing, where they blend well with other herbs such as rosemary, sage, bay leaves and thyme, and mix well with garlic, onions and shallots. They make a good addition to gravies and wine sauces and can be added to stews and casseroles. The berries are used with coriander in smoked meats and are added to pâtés, pickles and sauerkraut. They can be added, in moderation, to fruit desserts such as fruit salads, fruit pies and strudels. The fragrant foliage is used to smoke meat and cheeses.

🌾 Ripe juniper fruits have a sweetish but pine- or turpentine-like aroma and flavour. Their taste is strong and only a small quantity is needed. The soft flesh can be puréed or macerated, with all parts of the berry being edible, though they are usually cooked before usage. Added to foods, they freshen and improve overall flavour.

Kale and collards 🄵 🄼 🅂 🅅

(borecole) and (sprouts)

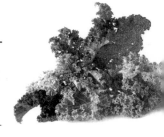

Both collards and kale are ancient brassica varieties and are probably ancestors of the modern brassicas, such as cabbage, kohlrabi, cauliflower and broccoli. These older-style brassicas are highly nutritious and have a delightful flavour if lightly sautéed, stir-fried or added to soups. Both deserve to be more widely appreciated. Several modern varieties have leaves that are sweeter and can be even incorporated in salads.

What they contain

They contain good levels of **fibre**, which promotes healthy digestion, reduces constipation and may prevent colon cancer. The leaves are very rich in **vitamin C** (~120 mg/100 g of leaf – much higher than most other leafy vegetables, oranges and limes). They are very rich in **vitamin K** (a serving providing ~700% of RDA), containing much more than any other common food. They are very rich in **carotenoids**, as β-**carotene**, **lutein** and **zeaxanthin**, which improve vision, slow progression of age-related eye problems, and are protective against heart disease. They contain more lutein than virtually any other food apart from spinach. Are rich in the minerals **manganese**, **potassium** and **iron**, and particularly **calcium**, containing more than most other vegetables.

Even when cooked, kale and collards retain much of these nutritional benefits. They are also rich in the powerful antioxidants **quercetin** and **kaempferol**. Also, like other brassicas, they are rich in **glucosinolates**, which are converted to **isothiocyanates** when the leaves are cut or chewed. Kale contains the **phyto-oestrogen lignan**.

What they do

The many vitamins, minerals and health-promoting secondary plant compounds in kale contribute to reducing the risk of many disorders, including cardiovascular disease and cancers. Their rich calcium content is beneficial for the bone growth of both young and old.

Consumption of their isothiocynates is inversely correlated with the incidence of cancer. Kale now seems proven to reduce the risk of a range of cancers (lung, breast, colon, stomach and bladder). They induce enzymes that are involved in the repair of DNA. The reduced risk of breast cancer may also be due to their lowering of oestrogen levels. In China, it is reported that isothiocyanates reduce breast cancer risk by 45%. These compounds also reduce development of skin cancers. Additionally, eating kale with turmeric (e.g. in curry) can reduce the occurrence of and even help reverse prostate cancers. Unfortunately, cooking at >50°C for more than ~5–8 minutes reduces the production of isothiocyanates, so leaves are best lightly steamed or briefly stir-fried.

Warning: Like other brassicas, kale and collards contain compounds that can interfere with thyroid function – those with thyroid problems may wish to consume these in moderation.

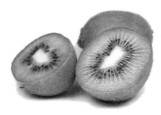

🌿 Old-style kale and collards are tremendously nutritious, being richer in many vitamins and minerals than most foods: they also taste delicious, if not overcooked.

How they are used

Their leaves can be shredded and are tasty stir-fried with other vegetables, though only cut/slice the leaves just before they are needed. Can be added to stews and are excellent in soups (e.g. minestrone) and vegetable pies. They work well in bean, lentil and chickpea recipes. The leaves are tasty stuffed with rice and other ingredients. They can be sautéed with a little butter, garlic, ginger and black pepper. Kale and collards mix well with apple, pumpkin, parsnips, mushrooms, bacon, potato, onion, tomatoes and ricotta cheese. They are delicious steamed, then sprinkled with soy sauce and a little sesame oil. When young, the leaves can be finely chopped and added to salads. Young leaves of both kale and collards can also be juiced, with other vegetables or fruits, to make a highly nutritious drink. The flavour of older varieties can be too strong to eat raw; however, most modern varieties have sweeter leaves. The flowers are edible and taste similar to purple sprouting.

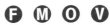

Kiwifruit

(Chinese gooseberry)

The Chinese collected these fruits from the wild for thousands of years, but did not domesticate the plant – it is New Zealand growers who have largely developed kiwifruit. There are many *Actinidia* species, which vary in shape and the colour of flowers and fruits. However, it is the fuzzy-skinned and green- and golden-fleshed kiwifruits that are most commonly available. These fruits store well, are delicious and are full of nutrition.

What it contains

Kiwifruit are wonderfully rich in vitamins and minerals. They are very rich in **antioxidants** and in **fermentable fibre** (~10%). The fruits are one of the best sources of **vitamin C** (75–100 mg/100 g), with the gold varieties containing even more (~120 mg/100 g). The fruits are also rich in **vitamin K**. They also contain a lot of **potassium, copper, manganese** and **folate** (rare for a fruit). They also contain good amounts of **chromium** (which is involved in controlling heartbeat and carbohydrate use). Kiwifruit also have very good levels of the **carotenoids lutein** and **zeaxanthin**, which improve eyesight and delay age-related vision problems, and contain high quantities of a proteolytic enzyme called **actinidin**, which is used to tenderise meat.

What it does

Its fibre is beneficial to the digestive system and also reduces serum LDLs and blood-sugar levels, as well as aiding insulin control. It has been used effectively in China to treat constipation. Actinidin aids digestion.

The powerful antioxidants in kiwifruit can reduce oxidative damage that occurs, ironically, after eating a meal; therefore, a few slices for dessert will have major health benefits. Another study shows that eating 2–3 kiwifruit per day for 28 days reduces blood-clot formation by 18% (compared to controls) and significantly lowers blood triglycerides levels, therefore conferring significant cardiovascular benefits. The fruits also have antibacterial and anti-cancer properties and were historically used to treat liver and oesophageal cancers.

Warning: A minority are allergic to the compound actinidin found within these fruits.

🐟 Unusually for a fleshy fruit, their many tiny seeds are rich in vitamin E, and are incredibly rich in omega-3 fatty acids, being the second-richest food source of this important essential fatty acid. Together, these are crucial to cell-membrane health throughout the body, reducing neurodegenerative and cardiovascular disease.

How it is used

The flesh is best eaten when still firm – it is tangy, sub-acid and zingy. When ripened further, the flesh softens and becomes sweeter. Kiwifruit are enjoyed simply on their own, added fresh to desserts, and can be used to garnish savoury foods. Kiwifruit make a great side dish to neutralise greasy foods: they lift the whole flavour of the dish. Can be added fresh to savoury ingredients such as ginger, garlic, onion, chilli, curry spices. Kiwifruit mixes well with avocado, salads, prawns and fish (e.g. trout, salmon), chicken and anywhere a tangy, but not sour, fruit is needed. They are very rarely cooked, but are made into juice, wine, jam and other products. They also go well with fruits such as bananas, lychees, strawberries papaya and mango. The peeled, whole fruits can be pickled with vinegar, brown sugar and spices. An enzyme in yoghurt conflicts with those in kiwifruit.

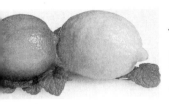

Lemons and limes

Lemons were appreciated during the time of the Roman Empire, and at the beginning of the 8th century the Arabs took them to northern Africa and Sicily (where many lemons are still produced). Columbus took them to the Americas, and it was during these long voyages that their curative properties were discovered to prevent the seafarer's disease, scurvy.

There are two main types of lime – the most popular and highly rated is the Mexican lime (West Indian or key lime). The other is the Tahitian or Persian lime, which is similar to Mexican lime, but is not as acidic. Lemons and limes are grown in many warm regions of the world and are highly valued for their juice and delicious peel, which are used in myriad sweet and savoury recipes, as well as medicinally and cosmetically. They are also added to numerous other diverse products.

What they contain

Lemon juice contains good amounts of **vitamin C** (55 mg/100 g of flesh) with limes having somewhat less. Both are rich in citric acid, though limes have more and a higher sugar content. Lemon and lime skins are wonderfully rich in **terpenes**, particularly **limonene**, and the skin and flesh contain the **flavonoids hesperidin**, **rutin**, **apigenin** and **quercetin**, all of which are powerful antioxidants, and protect cells from becoming cancerous as well as helping fight existing cancers. Lemon also contains **coumarins** and limes contain **citral**, **camphene** and **linalool**. Lemon oil, obtained from the outer peel, is pale yellow and has a wonderful aroma. The peel is hugely rich in **vitamin C** (~130 mg/100 g), and **flavonoids**. Their pith is edible and is rich in the **soluble fibre pectin** (~10%) and the **flavonoid limonin**.

What they do

Limonene has a beneficial action on digestion by neutralising gastric secretions and promoting healthy movement of the gut wall. It stimulates the digestive system and has been used to reduce heartburn and gastro-oesophageal reflux.

Limonene also reduces the risk of cancers, for example, stomach and breast cancers. In addition, a study reports that people who drank black tea with lemon peel were 70% less likely to develop skin cancer (drinking tea alone reduced the risk by 40%). Another study found a dose–response relationship between greater citrus peel in the diet and degree of lowered skin cancer risk. This has been found to be due to its limonene. Adding lemon juice to green tea increases the release of beneficial catechins from the tea.

Traditionally, lemon juice has been used as a diuretic, an astringent, a laxative and as a preventive for the common cold.

> Lemons and limes improve blood-vessel suppleness and health – they reduce high blood pressure, reduce varicose veins, reduce bleeding, and improve blood flow and capillary permeability. They reduce inflammation, are used to treat mouth infections and are highly recommended for acute rheumatism.

Apigenin has antidepressant activity and hesperidin may help prevent bone loss. Together, hesperidin, rutin and vitamin C have a synergistic effect – their efficacy is greatly increased to enhance the health of connective tissue, help wound healing and enhance the immune system.

The pectin from the pith, which has a mild flavour, aids digestion, lowers cholesterol and can suppress appetite for a few hours.

The essential oil, taken internally, stimulates the circulation, may promote white blood cell formation, dissolve cellulite and promote a sense of well-being. It works as an antiseptic and an antibacterial. It is used in many cosmetics and is widely used in aromatherapy. It can serve as an insect repellent and can be applied to sunburn (though see warning).

Lemon juice removes stains, cuts through grease, and is used in detergents and soaps. Both lemon and lime juice, diluted and rinsed through hair and then exposed to sunlight, act as a bleach. Too much juice can damage hair. Lemon juice, mixed with salt, is said to make a good, healthy face scrub. It can be effective against acne, boils, insect bites, warts and cold sores and has been used on freckles to bleach them. Lime juice can help calm the irritation and swelling of mosquito bites and relieve the effects of stinging corals and jellyfish. Its antiseptic properties are used for all kinds of ulcers and as a gargle for sore throats.

Warning: Large daily doses can erode tooth enamel making them more susceptible to caries. Coumarins within peel can irritate the skin, particularly if then exposed to sunlight.

How they are used

Slices of lemon and lime are served as a garnish on many dishes, added to iced or hot tea and to various cold drinks, both alcoholic and fruit. Just chilled water and lemon juice is a most refreshing drink. Lemons and limes are used in pies, tarts, as a flavouring for cakes, cookies, chocolates, etc. They can be added to jams, chutneys and preserves. Make delicious lemon curd and a delicious cheesecake mixed with sweetened condensed milk and double cream. A few drops of lemon juice added to cream before whipping gives it stability. Added to meat, it acts as a tenderiser. If added to fruits or vegetables that oxidise, lemon juice prevents them turning brown. Their outer peel can be used in all types of dishes (sweet and savoury) and adds a zingy taste as well as conferring depth of flavour to the overall dish – add just before serving to avoid being denatured by heat. Try adding peel to risotto and other rice dishes. Thinly slice the peel and add to tasty cheese and yeast extract on toast.

Limes are considered by some to be more aromatic and better flavoured. Lime juice is often used instead of lemons. It is great squeezed on fruits and desserts, but also as a juice on fish and meats. It makes a wonderful marinade (with other spices) for raw fish. The lime softens and tenderises the fish, which is then mixed with coconut cream, sliced cucumber and cherry tomatoes. In the Middle East, ripe limes are boiled in salt water and dried until their flesh darkens in colour. The resulting spice, called loomi, gives a distinctive citrus flavour to legumes, meats, rice and other dishes. Limes can be either crushed or pierced before adding them to slow-cooked dishes. In the Philippines, the chopped peel is made into a sweetmeat with milk and coconut.

Lemon balm $\circledS$

Balm, or lemon balm as it is often known, is a very common garden herb that has attractive lemon-yellow leaves with a wondrous lemon aroma when lightly crushed. Native to southern and central Europe, it has now become naturalised across Europe and elsewhere. The leaves are used for their powerful medicinal properties, including as a sedative, anti-spasmodic, antibacterial, antiviral, anti-inflammatory and antioxidant. Research has confirmed most of these uses. It also makes a great flavouring.

What it contains

The leaves contain ~0.1% **essential oil**, which is rich in **terpenes**, particularly **citronellol** and **carveol**, which give this plant much of its aroma and flavour. It also contains **flavonoids** (e.g. **rosmarinic acid**, **apigenin**) and **tannins**.

What it does

The leaves were used to treat stomach and digestive problems and to relieve stress and anxiety. The essential oil, applied as aromatherapy, is effective in relieving agitation in people with severe dementia, including those with Alzheimer's – it has been found to be clinically safe and to improve quality of life. Of the many plants tested, balm in particular enhances and restores mental functions, including memory. It has helped children with sleep problems caused by ADHD.

> Stressed and tired? Lemon balm can induce relaxation, relieve stress and rejuvenate.

It also has antibacterial and antifungal properties and is a powerful antioxidant. Leaf extracts, applied topically, have effectively controlled herpes simplex virus and are used to treat both genital and oral infections. These activities may be due to its terpenes. Other compounds seem to have potent anti-HIV-1 activity.

The plant also has anti-tumour activities, including repairing disrupted cell-cycle checkpoints, which may prevent tumours forming. Apigenin also has remarkable anti-inflammatory properties – the leaves can enhance the immune system's humoral and cellular responses. They can also reduce serum-triglyceride and total cholesterol levels, and inhibit accumulation of fat around the liver, which helps regulate weight gain and reduce the likelihood of cardiovascular disease and stroke.

Dried leaves retain their fragrance and are used in pot-pourri. Its essential oil is used in perfumes, air-fresheners, etc. Crushed leaves rubbed onto skin may help deter mosquitoes – recent research demonstrates that leaf extracts can kill the larvae of some mosquito species.

Warning: Lemon balm may inhibit the activity of some thyroid medications.

How it is used

A refreshing lemon-flavoured summer drink is prepared with chopped leaves, ice and a little honey, but it also makes a popular warming tea. A few leaves may be added to alcoholic drinks (e.g. schnapps, fruit wines). The chopped leaves can be added to fruit or green salads, though their flavour is fairly strong. They go well in Mediterranean-style dishes and in many rice dishes and their refreshing flavour cuts through oily foods. Lemon balm can be added to salad dressings, ice cream, cakes and desserts. It is used with lemons and limes to increase citrus flavour, as a lemon-peel substitute, and can be used instead of lemongrass. There is even a lemon balm wine, mixed with either white grapes or apple juice.

Lentils

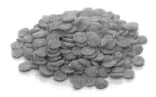

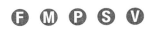

A legume crop that has been gathered as a food since Neolithic times – it was one of the first crops to be cultivated, almost 9000 years ago. Originally grown in regions around the Middle East and the Mediterranean, its tasty, highly nutritious seeds have ensured its continued cultivation by many around the world. It is a common ingredient within Asian, Indian, Middle Eastern and Mediterranean cuisine, and is popular with vegetarians for its abundant protein. India is the biggest worldwide producer. Lentils are inexpensive, easy to cook, highly nutritious, and a few go a long way.

What they contain

Cooked, they have excellent levels of **protein** (10–20%) – more than most other seeds except for soy. The protein includes **most of the essential amino acids**, including **lysine**. The seeds are rich in **fibre** (~8%) and in the **B vitamins**, particularly **folate** and **thiamine** – a serving provides 90% of the daily requirements of folate and ~25% of thiamine. They contain abundant minerals, having excellent levels of **manganese, iron, copper, zinc, magnesium** and **phosphorus**; are rich in **potassium** and also contain some **selenium**. Contain virtually no fat.

A serving of cooked lentils supplies ~35% of the RDA of protein, ~65% of the RDA of fibre, plus ~40% RDA of manganese, iron and phosphorus.

Lentils are also very rich in **phyto-oestrogens** as **isoflavones**, and contain some **saponins**. The sprouted seeds are nutrient rich and contain good amounts of vitamin C.

What they do

An excellent, nutritional food. Rich in fibre, lentils improve digestion and have long been used to ease digestive problems. B vitamin-rich lentils contribute to a healthy heart and digestive system. They reduce age-related eye disorders and seem to help fight depression, increase mental agility and verbal fluency. They may reduce the incidence of some cancers and are used to form new blood cells. They are rich in minerals too, including iron and antioxidant zinc.

Lentil's phyto-oestrogens are likely to benefit post-menopausal women and to possibly reduce the development of hormone-related cancers.

Lentils may cause flatulence in some, but much less so than beans.

> 🐾 Made with red lentils, dhal soup is inexpensive, easy to make, nutritious and filling. Fry mustard seeds, chilli, cumin, coriander, turmeric, ginger and black pepper in a pan. Add red lentils and fry for a few more minutes. Cover with coconut milk (or cream) and water, and simmer until the lentils are cooked. Add salt and serve with a generous squeeze of lemon juice and poppadoms – delicious.

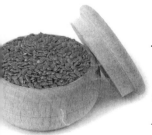

Linseed
(flax, seeds of gold)

   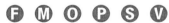

The ancient crop linseed has been cultivated for at least 5000 years, mostly for its fibre, with some estimating its usage going back 8000–10,000 years. It may be the first fibre to have been used for cloth. Linen was used by ancient Egyptians to wrap around the dead. Later, it was widely grown in the Middle East and Europe, but became less common when cotton became widely cultivated. However, the excellent oil properties of its seeds are now recognised. They are extremely rich in omega-3 fatty acids, which have significant health benefits, and its popularity within many foods has hugely increased.

What it contains

A highly nutritious food. The seeds are rich in **omega-3 fatty acids** (~55%), particularly the essential fatty acid, α-**linolenic acid**. Linseed contains much more than any other seed or fish oil. It is also rich in **omega-6** and **omega-9** essential fatty acids, and contains good amounts of the **B vitamins** – is very rich in **thiamine**. The seeds are very rich in **calcium, iron, zinc, copper, manganese, phosphates** and **selenium**. They contain **lecithin** and a fantastic 18–22% **protein**. They are also very rich in **fibre** (~25%), and in **choline**. The seeds are rich in the **phyto-oestrogens lignans**, more so, by far, than any other food (except sesame), and are also very rich in **tocopherols** (**vitamin E**).

What it does

Omega-3 fatty acids are powerful anti-inflammatories: chronic inflammation is increasingly thought to initiate several serious diseases (e.g. cardiovascular disease, arthritis, neurodegenerative disease, cancer). Omega-3 reduces high blood pressure and serum-cholesterol levels and, thus, the risk of heart disease. The crushed seeds are well known for aiding digestion and have a soothing effect on smooth-muscle contractions of the gut. They are often included in the diet of those with inflammatory bowel disease and have laxative properties. They are recommended by some for the treatment of the auto-immune disease systemic lupus erythematosus.

Increasing omega-3 in the diet is likely to reduce the incidence of depression due to the importance of this compound in nerve cell membranes. It rebalances the omega-3 to omega-6 ratio: an imbalance of omega-6 fatty acids has been shown in several studies to be related to a range of neurological and psychiatric disorders.

The seeds are very rich in the phyto-oestrogen lignans, which have protective properties against hormone-related cancers, particularly breast cancer.

Linseed not only contains abundant gamma-tocopherol, which reduces several human age-related diseases such as cancer and heart disease (a type of vitamin E), it also significantly increases the body's ability to make its own. Eating linseed seeds improves the vitamin E status of the body without the use of vitamin E supplements, which can have detrimental effects.

The oil is used to treat various skin problems, such as eczema and psoriasis, and enhances skin healing (e.g. for burns). It is often taken by those with arthritis, but also for menstrual pains and asthma.

Warning: The husk of linseed contains cyanide-like compounds, so should not be eaten in excess (i.e. >150 g), though most purchased seed is de-husked. It is advised to not apply the oil to open wounds or broken skin.

How it is used

Linseed can be used in breads, pastries, biscuits, muffins, breakfast cereals, pancakes and scones. Can be added to soups, stews, sauces, ratatouille, rice dishes, curries, salads and sprinkled on veggies or roast potatoes. Sprinkle some lightly ground linseed onto your oat-based cereal in the morning, along with a few berries and a live yoghurt topping. Are best crushed before usage as whole seeds tend to pass straight through – crushing breaks the seed coat which releases the oil, minerals and vitamins. The seeds are added to food products to raise their nutrient status. They have a pleasant, mild, nutty flavour. Its light-flavoured oil is added to dressings, stir-fries and many other foods, though is best not cooked to a high temperature as this destroys many of its health benefits and affects the flavour. The seeds can be sprouted and used in salads, and have a pleasant, spicy flavour.

> ☙ Make a salad with lightly toasted linseed, fresh watercress, raspberries and diced spring onions (scallions), sprinkled with olive oil and black pepper and served with croutons and crumbled feta.

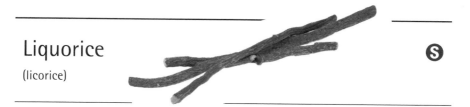

Liquorice

(licorice)

Ⓢ

Liquorice roots have been valued for at least 2300 years – within traditional Chinese and Japanese medicine it is one of the most frequently used drugs. Liquorice is derived from the plant's sweet-tasting roots. In the past, it was a popular confection. Unfortunately, much liquorice sold today does not include any 'real' liquorice, or only has a small amount, with the greater proportion being molasses, treacle and aniseed. However, liquorice is becoming re-popularised, and is now used in many dessert recipes. It has significant medicinal benefits.

What it contains

The sweetness of liquorice is derived from **glycyrrhizin**, which is reported to be 50 times sweeter than refined sugar and has many medicinal properties. Glycyrrhizin can be 2–24% of the root's dry weight. Roots also contain **saponins,** many **flavonoids** and the **phyto-oestrogen glabridin,** which is a powerful antioxidant.

What it does

Liquorice is used traditionally to treat many disorders, including to expel pulmonary phlegm, and for coughs and colds. Many of its medicinal properties are linked to glycyrrhizin. It enhances production of interferon and seems to increase the immune system's response to viruses. In research, it was the most potent inhibitor tested against SARS. Its anti-viral properties have also been used to treat HIV (though it is not fully proven or tested). It improves liver function in hepatitis C patients. Glycyrrhizin inhibits gastric secretion, significantly reduces the symptoms of gastric ulcers, has a mild laxative effect and is good for digestive problems. Liquorice also significantly reduces the ability of LDLs to form arterial plaques and helps with weight loss by inhibiting abdominal fat storage.

Glabridin's strong phyto-oestrogenic properties (more active than most phyto-oestrogens) may enable it to partially relieve menstrual cramps and adverse menopause symptoms. These compounds are also being investigated for their possible role in preventing hormone-related cancers (e.g. breast, uterine, prostate). It has been shown to inhibit growth of human breast cancer cells. With vitamin D, it may help prevent bone loss in post-menopausal women.

🐾 Liquorice makes good confectionery and has a host of significant medicinal benefits. Also, unbelievably, this sweet black root has been shown to reduce tooth decay. Compounds such as glycyrrhizin can inhibit and even kill the bacteria *Streptococcus mutans,* whose acid secretions are a major contributor to dental caries.

Warning: In moderate doses liquorice is completely safe to eat. However, at higher doses (>50 g), glycyrrhizin inhibits an enzyme responsible for inactivating the hormone cortisol. Thus, continuous high-level consumption of glycyrrhizin can result in hyper-cortisol levels, which adversely affects the body's salt–water balance to cause oedema and

Glabridin within liquorice has potential to improve cognitive functions and help improve memory, and is being researched to treat the symptoms of Alzheimer's disease. It may also stimulate the adrenal gland (which produces adrenaline), and so boost energy levels.

increased blood pressure. This can be very serious, though incidences are rare. Symptoms are reversible once consumption is stopped. Liquorice, in quantity, should be avoided by those with high blood pressure, obesity, heart problems or diabetes, and possibly pregnant women.

How it is used

The root extract can be simply eaten or a tea is made from it. Liquorice has a very sweet, distinctive flavour with aniseed or fennel overtones. It is widely used in confectionery and is popular with children and adults alike. Can be added to ice cream and to dessert puddings and pies. It is also used in alcoholic drinks (e.g. schnapps), and is sometimes added to tobacco as a flavouring. Unlike many sweets, liquorice also has the advantage of being healthy. It is also added to Chinese five-spice powder, and is used to disguise the taste of unpleasant-tasting medicines.

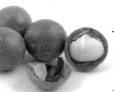

Macadamia nuts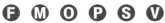

Related to the banksias and grevilleas, macadamia trees originate from subtropical Australia. Natural hybrids of these wild macadamia trees now produce one of the best-tasting nuts in the world. The nuts come within a green rounded fruit from which the husk first has to be removed. Inside, the nuts are surrounded by a very hard seed coat, which needs special crackers, or a hammer, to break open. Inside this though, is a single, creamy-white, delicious and nutritious kernel.

What they contain

The nuts contain 60–80% oils, of which >80% is **monounsaturated fatty acid** (i.e. ~80% **omega-7 palmitoleic acid** and ~20% **oleic acid**). The nuts are rich in **soluble fibre** and antioxidant **flavonoids**, which help protect against cancer and heart disease. They contain **squalene** and are rich in **phytosterols**. They are also very rich in **thiamine**, with good amounts of **niacin**.

Macadamia nuts are mineral rich, containing large amounts of **manganese**, **copper**, **magnesium**, **iron**, and phosphates, potassium, calcium. Their **protein** content (~9 g/100 g of kernel) is good, though relatively low for a nut.

A good source of fibre and protein, these nuts deliver their benefits over time, thus reducing peaks and troughs in blood-sugar levels.

What they do

Palmitoleic acid (PA) is uncommon in the plant world and there have been conflicting reports of its health effects. One study, which looked at PA in isolation, found that it increased serum LDLs and lowered HDLs in men who already had elevated cholesterol levels. In contrast, another study found that total cholesterol and LDLs were significantly decreased in a group of Japanese women who regularly ate macadamia nuts. In addition, their body weights were significantly decreased, confirming other findings that palmitoleic acid increases fat metabolism, thus reducing stored body fat. It may also have beneficial effects on joints. Oleic acid has been shown in many studies to help prevent cardiovascular disease and to improve the ratio of omega-3 to omega-6 fats in cell membranes.

Overall, macadamia nuts do reduce serum-cholesterol levels. People who eat macadamia nuts regularly (>5 times/week) have significantly lower rates of heart disease than those who eat nuts less than once a week. They also act as antioxidants, reducing thrombosis and inflammation, which are risk factors for coronary artery disease. Their phytosterol content also helps reduce serum-cholesterol levels.

Palmitoleic oil is highly beneficial to the skin – it moisturises, nourishes and conditions, does not irritate, penetrates the skin easily and can be safely used on babies. It is used in many cosmetic preparations, especially in Japan. Warning: Like all nuts, macadamias can cause allergic reactions in those susceptible.

How they are used

🐾 For a tasty, healthy appetiser try avocado slices with macadamia nuts, sprinkled with a dash of olive oil and balsamic vinegar.

The kernels are delicious, particularly roasted. To roast the nuts, place them in a shallow pan at 120°C for ~6–7 minutes, then turn them and give them a further 7 minutes. It is best to remove nuts if they start to tan. They can be dry-roasted or sprinkled with olive oil. The nuts can be added to any dish that uses nuts, but are best if their flavour can be clearly differentiated. Roasted nuts can be eaten as they are, or salted. They are excellent coated in dark chocolate, or can be honey-roasted or roasted with chilli. Chopped, they can be added to salads, rissoles, stuffing, ratatouille, couscous, rice dishes, pasta sauces and also muffins, cakes, ice cream and pancake fillings. The nuts can be stored in airtight jars in the cool and dark, or they can be frozen.

Mace   See 'Nutmeg and mace'

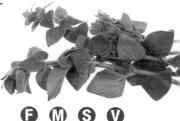

Marjoram and oregano   Ⓕ Ⓜ Ⓢ Ⓥ

Within the *Origanum* genus three species are particularly well known for their culinary, ornamental and medicinal values: sweet marjoram (*O. majorana*), pot marjoram (*O. onites*) and oregano (wild marjoram, *O. vulgare*). All are popular culinary herbs, though sweet marjoram is thought to have the finest flavour, and traditionally has symbolised youth, beauty and happiness. They all have a pleasant sweetish yet spicy flavour and are wondrously nutritional. These herbs are particularly popular in the cuisine of France, Greece and Italy, but also the Middle East.

What they contain

Marjoram leaves are enormously rich in **antioxidants**, having a higher ORAC score than most foods. Dried, the leaves of marjoram and oregano are hugely rich in **vitamin K, carotenoids** (i.e. **α-carotene** and also **lutein** and **zeaxanthin**) and contain lots of **vitamin C** (>50 mg/100 g). Dried, they have a huge amount of **calcium, iron** and **zinc**, a lot of **potassium, magnesium, copper** and **manganese**, and contain ~40% **fibre**. They are also super-rich in **B6** and **folate**, with a lot of **niacin**. These species are very rich in **terpenes** (e.g. **carvacrol, thymol, terpinene**).

What they do

These amazing herbs are packed with nutrients, with the dried herbs containing even more. Although their secondary plant compounds are the focus of most modern research, their abundant minerals, vitamins and fibre are also of great worth. Rich in calcium, which enhances bone formation, and in iron and antioxidant zinc, they also have good quantities of beneficial B vitamins, which are particularly important as we age.

Carvacrol within oregano, in particular, has antibacterial and antifungal properties, and is effective at controlling many micro-organisms. It works against *Helicobacter pylori*, which causes stomach ulcers and cancer. Its

> If you are feeling run-down with coughs, colds and infections make yourself some marjoram and cranberry cookies.

activities are enhanced when it is combined with cranberries. This treatment does not induce antibiotic resistance compared with conventional antibiotic therapies. The strange partnership of oregano with cranberries is also effective against the food pathogen *Listeria*. Oregano is effective against the yeast infection *Candida albicans*, and can reduce the growth and spread of several disease-causing protozoa. The essential oil can be effective against herpes cold sores if one drop is taken daily for 2–3 weeks, though the oil is best mixed 50:50 with olive oil or similar.

These herbs have potential to treat diabetes – they reduce blood-glucose levels in rats without affecting plasma insulin levels. Compounds strongly inhibit blood clotting, so may prevent some types of heart disease. They also have anti-cancer properties and anti-spasmodic activity. They are used to relieve flatulence and other digestive complaints. Externally, the oil is used to ease muscle aches, sprains, painful joints, sore gums and toothache. The oils are also used to perfume soaps, colognes and lotions.

Warning: A small number of people have adverse skin reactions to these herbs. Additionally, some recommend not ingesting the oil while pregnant. As with all essential oils, use in moderation and with care.

How they are used

These herbs have a spicy, peppery, almost thyme-like flavour and aroma.

> Marjoram and oregano are popular in Middle Eastern dishes, sprinkled on yoghurt, in vegetable, tahini and falafel recipes and dips, and are often mixed with other ingredients (e.g. sumac and nigella seeds, pinenuts) to form a condiment sprinkled on Mediterranean-style dishes.

Leaves harvested from plants grown in lots of sunshine have a strong flavour and can almost induce a numbing sensation to the lips. Although sweet marjoram is considered to have the finest flavour, all are used in similar recipes. A popular usage for marjoram is in stuffing for poultry; it is also popular in soups, stews, dips, herb butter, tomato sauces and in dressings. They mix well in egg dishes, such as frittatas and omelettes, and in potato or bean salads, and blend well with parsley. They are eaten in enchilada, chilli and salsa dishes and the leaves are very popular in Italian recipes, sprinkled on pizzas and pastas. Herbs such as rosemary, thyme and sage mix well with marjoram and oregano. A few sweet marjoram leaves can be added to fruit salads and desserts such as ice cream or custard. The dried leaves of sweet marjoram, in particular, are used to make a tea.

Mints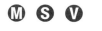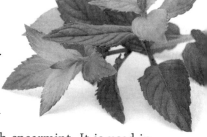

Known to all is the aroma and flavour of fresh spearmint. It is used in sauces, drinks and a wide range of cosmetic and food products. Apart from spearmint, many other *Mentha* species are utilised for their culinary, ornamental or herbal properties. The species peppermint, apple/pineapple mint, Japanese peppermint and long-leaved mint are also well known.

What they contain

Fresh spearmint leaves are very rich in **vitamin A** and contain some **vitamin C**. They also contain **folate** and are rich in **iron** and **manganese**. Spearmint, peppermint and Japanese mint are particularly rich in **menthol**, which is used in many medicinal products, and has cooling, antiseptic and analgesic properties. Spearmint is rich in **terpenes** (e.g. **linalool, limonene, caryophyllene, pinene, carvone**).

What they do

Mint has antiseptic, anti-irritant and anaesthetic properties. It is widely used in cough remedies to soothe irritation and treat minor sores. The oil, rubbed on the skin, can relieve the pain of headaches, cramps, sprains, and can reduce itching. It is inhaled or rubbed on the chest to act as a decongestant. Menthol oil, applied topically, gives a cooling sensation, which provides relief from sunburn and is soothing applied during a fever, though does not actually cause a drop in temperature.

Most mints are effective against a wide range of pathogens. They have antibacterial properties against *Staphylococcus aureus* and *Escherichia coli*, as well as yeast infections such as *Candida albicans*, and are effective against the parasite *Giardia*. Peppermint oil is topically effective against the herpes simplex virus. Research has shown that extracts from many mint species "can drastically and rapidly reduce the infectivity of HIV-1 virions at non-cytotoxic concentrations." (Geuenich at al. 2008)

Mints are rich in antioxidants and can reduce cancerous lung tumours in mice. Spearmint has

Peppermint oil has long been used and is proven to be effective in treating indigestion. It reduces smooth-muscle spasms within the gut and can give relief from irritable-bowel syndrome. It has been recommended as the best choice to alleviate the symptoms of those with non-serious or infective constipation or diarrhoea.

shown protective activity against various mutagens. The mints also protect against UV damage to the skin.

Warning: Moderate to excessive consumption of pennyroyal is not advised during pregnancy. Both pennyroyal and Corsican mint have potential adverse effects if consumed in excess. As with all essential oils, these should be diluted and used with caution.

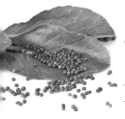

🌿 Chopped and mixed with herbs, such as lemon balm and rosemary, mint can be sprinkled on a diverse range of Mediterranean-style dishes, and added to vegetable pies and soups.

How they are used

Spearmint, finely chopped and mixed with good-quality vinegar, makes the traditional accompaniment to roast lamb. Can be added to yoghurt to make a cooling, refreshing addition to Indian curries. Is made into jellies and added to a wide range of vegetable soups, stews and pies, as well as being cooked with new potatoes. The dried or fresh leaves make a refreshing tea, and sprigs of mint can be added to iced summer drinks. A few leaves go well in fruit salads and make an attractive garnish on savoury and dessert dishes: look great with a chocolate and dark berry dessert. Is excellent with dark chocolate and added to ice cream. Mint is an ingredient in several liqueurs (e.g. Crème de Menthe, Benedictine).

Mustards

   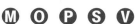

There are three main species of mustard: milder white seeds used in table mustard, with their leaves also used as salad greens; hot black mustard seeds; and medium-hot brown Indian mustard seeds, which is also grown for its edible leaves.

What they contain

Sprouted mustard seeds are super-rich in nutrients and vitamins. So too are mustard greens, which also have good amounts of **fibre** that aids digestion and helps prevent constipation. They are very rich in **carotenoids** (as α-**carotene**, **lutein** and **zeaxanthin**) and in **vitamin C** (~70 mg/100 g). Greens are also incredibly rich in **vitamin K**, with a serving providing seven times the RDA. **B vitamin** content is high, with very high quantities of **folate** present. The leaves are rich in minerals, including **calcium**, **manganese**, **iron** and **potassium**. However, prolonged cooking will reduce many of these nutrients. The seeds are very rich in **protein** (~25%) and in **fibre** (~15%). They contain large amounts of antioxidant **selenium** and are very rich in **zinc, phosphate, calcium, manganese, magnesium, sulphur** and **iron**. They also contain **omega-3 fatty acids**, are very rich in **niacin, folate, choline** and also in **vitamin E**. The hotness of the seeds and spiciness of the leaves comes from isothiocyanates (converted from **sinigrin** in black or brown seeds and **sinalbin** in white seeds).

What they do

Many of their antioxidant and isothiocyanate compounds can reduce the incidence of cancer. Ingestion of isothiocyanates is inversely correlated with the incidence of cancer. They are virtually proven to reduce the risk of developing and the spread of several cancers, including skin, lung, bladder, colon and prostate. Their abundant omega-3s and vitamin E synergistically enhance these effects.

Both seeds and greens are rich in red blood cell-enhancing iron. They are also ingested to relieve stomach and liver ailments. Mustard greens promote bone health and delay age-related visual impairment.

> Mustard seeds have blood-sugar lowering effects and have been recommended for those with diabetes mellitus.

The ground seeds have long been used in baths, as poultices, or mixed with oil and used externally to treat colds, flu, aches, sprains, headaches, toothache, etc. They can be used as an external antiseptic, but please note the following. Warning: The oil is strong – if placed undiluted on the skin (or ingested), it can cause inflammation and even skin lesions. Mustard oil also contains erucic acid (as does rape), which has been shown to induce cancers. For these reasons, although mustard oil is popular in India, its usage in foods is not advised in Europe and the United States (mustard seeds contain only very small amounts). Like other brassicas, mustard contains compounds that can interfere with thyroid function – those with thyroid problems may wish to avoid these foods

How they are used

The seeds sprout quickly in a few days and are then tasty and nutritious in salads and sandwiches. Use untreated seeds. The seed is very familiar as a ground, hot spicy condiment to accompany meats, hot dogs and chicken, and is also good with vegetable pies, in sandwiches, added to soups, stews, etc. When used at full strength it is hot enough to bring

🐾 Young mustard greens can be added to salads, or older leaves are lightly steamed as a vegetable or added to stews and soups. They have a flavoursome though fairly spicy taste and are popular in Asian and Chinese cuisine, where they are often stir-fried or added to egg dishes.

tears to the eyes; therefore, it is often mixed with flour and other ingredients. Seeds can be soaked in water, drained, macerated and then mixed with herbs, garlic and vinegar to create this condiment. However, the addition of vinegar or hot water reduces its spiciness, as it limits the conversion to isothiocyanates. The whole seeds are popular in Indian and Asian cuisine, and are usually dry-cooked (in a pan with a lid) for a few minutes over a high heat until they start to pop. Then, other ingredients such as garlic, chillies, turmeric, cumin and coriander are added to produce spicy sauces. They are also a main component in pickling spice mixes and are used with pickled onions.

Nasturtium

(Indian cress)

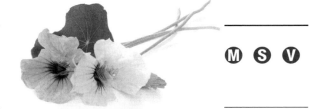

Ⓜ Ⓢ Ⓥ

This very popular and easy-to-grow ornamental originates from South America. All parts of the nasturtium plant, including its bright orange flowers, are edible – the leaves and flowers are great in salads and the seeds, caper-like in flavour, make a good addition to Italian-style dishes.

What it contains

The leaves are rich in antioxidant **carotenoids** and **vitamin C**. They also contain **calcium**, **iron** and **phosphate**. All parts of the plant, but particularly the leaves, are rich in beneficial **isothiocyanates**, which give this plant its hot, peppery flavour.

What it does

The isothiocyanates in nasturtiums, which are also found in brassicas and watercress, have natural antibiotic properties and are anticarcinogens. They can inhibit the growth of various human cancer cells.

Historically, indigenous South Americans used this plant to treat respiratory diseases; more recently, it has been used to treat coughs, flu, colds and other respiratory infections. Additionally, nasturtium, with horseradish, has been shown to effectively and safely treat people with chronic recurrent urinary tract infections, acute sinusitis and acute bronchitis, and is as effective as an antibiotic treatment but does not have the associated negatives. This combination also produces a rapid improvement in cold symptoms: for best benefits this herbal combination should be started as soon as possible after first symptoms show. Individually, but more so together, nasturtium and horseradish possess broad antibacterial activities against many bacterial pathogens.

How it is used

Nasturtium leaves have a peppery, quite hot flavour, similar to water- or landcress. They are great in salads, or can be mixed with other greens and cucumber to tone down their heat. The leaves blend well with seafoods (such as prawns, mussels and crab), fresh salmon or smoked chicken, and taste good with strawberries, apple, grapes or avocado. A nasturtium salad complements many egg recipes. The leaves make an interesting pesto, mixed with olive oil, garlic, black pepper and chopped pine or macadamia nuts. The edible flowers are delightful as a garnish, and have a

> 🌰 Feeling full of coughs and colds? Perhaps enjoy a few smoked salmon slices with either fresh nasturtium leaves or the pickled seeds, accompanied by a horseradish and live yoghurt dressing.

milder flavour than the leaves. Nasturtium seeds are spicy with a similar flavour to capers. They can be used fresh, when they are crisp and quite juicy, or are pickled. Are delicious added to Italian-style recipes such as spaghetti sauce, pizza, and ratatouille. The leaves, flowers and seeds can be steeped in good-quality vinegar to give the whole a peppery flavour. A peppery tea is made from the leaves and flowers, and is popular in Korea, China and Japan.

Nettles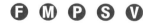

(stinging nettle)

The common stinging nettle, familiar to many as a garden weed, is infamous for its fine hairs, which, when broken, release an acid that stings the skin. However, its effects do not last too long, and it is not in the same league as plants such as poison ivy. It has long been used as a food and also medicinally in many countries worldwide. It is still gathered as a food and for its medicinal properties. In Turkey, it accounts for 93% of the herbs used for medicinal purposes.

What they contain

The leaves are very nutritious and are rich in **protein** and **minerals**, particularly **iron**, and also **calcium, magnesium, potassium** and **zinc**. They also contain good amounts of **fibre** (10–20%), and abundant **carotenoids**, and **vitamins C** and **K**. They are rich in **antioxidants**, many as **flavonoids**, including **ellagic acid**. They contain the **coumarin scopoletin**, and their 'sting' comes from **formic acid**.

What they do

Modern research has confirmed many of its traditional uses. Nettle roots and leaves can reduce the incidence of benign prostate problems, improve urine flow and improve the health of the urinary tract. It regulates and, acting as a diuretic, increases urine output. Nettles can also reduce the spread of prostate cancer, and are being researched for usage in treating HIV.

Historically, nettles were used to treat rheumatic disease and recent research has confirmed this use. Its anti-rheumatic action seems to interrupt the production of compounds that would otherwise produce inflammation. In a large study, daily consumption of a small amount of nettles resulted in 60% of patients ceasing to need non-steroidal anti-inflammatory drugs (NSAIDs) for their rheumatism. They have also been used to relieve sinusitis and other allergy-related disorders. Nettles enhance the immune system by stimulating the production of T-lymphocytes, possibly due to its lectins.

Scopoletin has antibacterial properties and helps regulate serotonin (which reduces depression and anxiety), is an analgesic and an anti-inflammatory (used to treat bronchial disease and asthma). It relaxes smooth muscle and has been used for menstrual cramps.

Nettles help prevent the formation of ulcers and act as a digestive analgesic. They are effective at treating ulcerative colitis (in mice). In addition, formic acid has antibacterial and preservative properties, and can kill *Salmonella* bacteria as well as mites.

How they are used

The younger leaves are tender and tasty; older leaves become too fibrous and bitter. Wearing gloves, harvest the younger leaves as they appear during the season and lightly steam. Much of their nutrients and flavour are lost if overcooked. Once cooked, the leaves lose all of their stinging properties, though the water they are steamed in contains the released formic acid, which some like to add to soups, gravies, etc., or it can be used as a hair wash. The leaves are used like spinach and their taste is not dissimilar. One of their most popular uses is to make a nettle soup, with chicken stock and perhaps a few oats to thicken it, a little cream or mascarpone and seasoning. Nettles are also used in stews, quiches, pies, polenta, ravioli, and served with meats such as sausages. There is a recipe for nettle, herb and chestnut risotto.

> ✿ One of the oldest recorded dishes in Britain, served about 6000 years ago, was nettle soup made with dandelion, chives, watercress, sorrel leaves, barley flour, salt and water.

They mix well with garlic or shallots, and like spinach go well with cheese and eggs. They can be added as a flavouring to white cheese to form a tasty rind. A flavoursome beer is made from the leaves and the dried leaves are used as a flavouring or to make a tea.

Nutmeg and mace

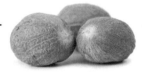 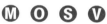

Mace and nutmeg are derived from the nuts of a tree native to the South Pacific, which is now grown in many tropical regions of the world. It was a sought-after spice during the Middle Ages in Europe, where its aromatic properties were used to disguise unpleasant smells, to flavour dull foods, and even to treat the plague. The tan-coloured fruits (~8 cm in diameter) have a thick outer skin. Within this, the large inner kernel is covered by a shiny, thin, deep-red aril, which is the source of mace. It is pleasantly aromatic and surrounds the ovoid nutmeg. Initially, the nutmeg is cream-coloured, but turns dark brown as it dries.

What they contain

Mace is rich in **protein, fibre** and **omega-6 fatty acids**, contains good amounts of **vitamins A** and **C**, and is rich in **iron, copper** and **manganese**. Nutmeg has good amounts of **protein** and **fibre**, and some **minerals** (manganese, iron). In addition, 25–40% of the nutmeg kernel consists of an orange, aromatic solid oil known as nutmeg butter or oil of mace. This is ~98% **saturated**

> It has been shown that nutmeg significantly improves the memory and learning abilities of mice, and has significant antidepressant-like effects.

fat. Nutmeg is rich in **myristicine** and **elemicin**, and also **safrole** and **eugenol**.

What they do

Nutmeg has a diverse range of medicinal uses: some good, some bad. Historically, it was used to treat diarrhoea and is still given to some cancer patients suffering from this. It has long been considered an aphrodisiac, with recent research showing that there is a significant and sustained increase in the sexual activity of normal male rats.

Nutmeg has significant antibacterial properties against many species tested, particularly against *Streptococcus mutans*, which is one of the main human oral pathogens and is also associated with carcinogenesis. Thus its compounds are included within some toothpastes. Extracts can also inhibit the growth of *Helicobacter pylori*, a bacteria that can cause gastric ulcers and cancers. These antibacterial plus its insecticidal properties are being researched to prevent food spoilage during storage.

Myristicine has been found to possess extraordinarily potent liver-protective activity and is being further researched. The essential oil is used to ease rheumatism and, like cloves, is used as an analgesic to relieve toothache. A drop or two can be taken to prevent halitosis. The essential oil is widely used in perfumery and the pharmaceutical industry, and is added to many cosmetic products including cough medicines.

Warning: Nutmeg has some serious negative effects. The compounds myristicine and elemicin, in large quantities, can cause hallucinations, transient psychosis and kidney toxicity; in very large amounts, it can even cause death. As little as 2–3 nutmegs can induce these effects and the dose needed to give hallucinogenic effects is dangerously close to the toxic dose. (Mace is considered to be much less toxic and hallucinogenic.) In large doses, safrole has been found to be a carcinogen in rats. Pregnant women should avoid ingesting nutmeg and possibly mace – it has been linked with causing birth defects and miscarriages.

How they are used

Mace and nutmeg have a similar flavour, though the taste of nutmeg is stronger and sweeter. Both are popular flavourings added to a range of desserts, particularly with milk and egg, and impart a warm, pleasant, aromatic flavour. They also mix well with

🐾 Mace and nutmeg can be added to savoury dishes – a little is added to soups and stews, and to vegetables such as spinach, chard, cauliflower and broccoli, particularly in a creamy, mascarpone or yoghurt sauce. They are a classic ingredient in pumpkin and squash recipes.

apple, pear and other autumn fruits, are added to jams and confectionery, and a little is added to fruitcakes adding lots of flavour. Small amounts are delicious in fruited breads, chocolate or coffee-flavoured cakes and desserts. It can also be used in savoury cheese, potato, chicken or egg dishes, with mace adding an attractive golden-yellow colour. Lightly cooked Brussels sprouts topped with mascarpone, sliced almonds and a little nutmeg are delicious. Can be added to milky drinks, teas and various alcoholic drinks such as mulled wine and eggnog. Both spices are popular flavourings in soft drinks. They have a strong flavour, and should be used sparingly.

Oats

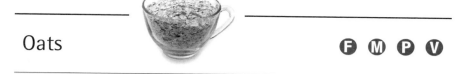

F M P V

Oats are wonderfully rich in protein, minerals and soluble fibre – its health benefits are legendary. Often only encountered as porridge or in muesli-type cereals, this food deserves to be included in more culinary dishes. Today, although most oats are grown in Canada and Russia, the country most famous for its love of oats and its use of this grain must surely be Scotland.

What they contain

Oats, and particularly the outer grain layer, are very rich in **protein**, containing 14–20%, depending on how it has been processed. It contains **soluble globulin protein** (mostly as **avenalins**), rather than glutens (as in wheat), and so those with gluten-type allergic reactions are probably safe to eat oats. Although several trials have confirmed this, there are still a few doubts – if unsure, don't take the risk. They are also rich in **soluble fibre** (~10%), particularly in the outer **bran layer**. Oats, particularly the bran and endosperm, are richer in fats (10%) than most other cereals, and most is unsaturated. Oats are rich in **B vitamins**, particularly **thiamine**. They are also rich in cholesterol-lowering **phytosterols**, and are very rich in **iron, manganese, magnesium, phosphates** and **copper**. Oat bran is considerably richer in most of the above nutrients.

What they do

The fibre occurs as β-glucan, which is soluble and fermentable, and is classed as a prebiotic – it is digested slowly, reducing peaks and troughs of blood-sugar levels (has a low GI), and provides energy at a steady rate for longer. It reduces the risk of type-2 diabetes. This fibre absorbs moisture to form a gel-like substance in the gut, which encourages development of beneficial gut bacteria. The bacteria use the fibre as a food source and produce compounds that are highly beneficial to intestinal health. These bacteria also reduce the formation of pathogenic organisms in the gut as well as colorectal cancers. In addition, this fibre directly and indirectly decreases serum-cholesterol levels. The ability of oats to reduce cholesterol is so marked that the US Food and Drug Administration allows oat-containing foods to make claims for their cholesterol-lowering properties. Soluble fibre may also reduce the risk of prostate disease. Intake of soluble fibre is best balanced with insoluble (viscous) fibre, such as that found in wheat. Note that oat products which contain their bran and have had minimum processing give the greatest health benefits.

> Oats are a wonderful convalescence food for those recovering from digestive disorders, such as gastroenteritis, and make an excellent food after antibiotic therapy.

A breakfast containing oats has been shown to enhance the spatial memory of children, and to improve short-term memory and auditory attention; these benefits are probably due to oats being a slower and more sustained energy source compared to low-fibre, high glycaemic cereals. In addition, its phytosterols effectively reduce serum-cholesterol and have anti-tumour activity.

The outer bran contains low levels of the alkaloid gramine and a saponin, which have mild relaxant properties. Oats have been used historically to treat anxiety and insomnia, as well as to reduce addictions (e.g. to nicotine). At present there is some controversy as to the usage of these alkaloids in strengthened capsule form.

Extracts from oats, which include saponins, are used in facial creams, soothing lotions and soaps to improve skin health and softness, and act as a moisturiser and anti-inflammatory. Oatmeal, made into a cream, has been used successfully to relieve the itching caused by eczema.

How they are used

The seeds can be sprouted and used in salads. A huge number of recipes, from sweet to savoury, include oats. Their mild nutty taste blends with many flavours. Oats can be prepared in several ways – as groats, oatmeal (or steel-cut or pin oats) and as rolled oats. Groats are best soaked overnight before cooking, and then need at least 30 minutes' cooking. They have a chewy, nutty taste and can be added to soups, stews or served and used in the same way as rice or bulgar wheat. Oatmeal is simply chopped seed that has undergone minimal processing – it still contains most of its nutrients. It has a pleasant chewy texture but, being more finely chopped, takes less time to cook. Rolled oats are popular in porridge, many breakfast cereals, flap-jacks, oatcakes (which can be sweet or savoury), muffins, pancakes and other biscuits, and can be added to other flours in cakes and scones. Oatmeal bread is a favourite. Mixes well with many fruits, particularly dark berries, oranges and apples, and also with chopped nuts and chocolate. There are loads of banana and oat dessert recipes – the mix of fibre and energy-boosting banana with blood-sugar stabilising oats is excellent. Oats are also added to stews and soups to thicken them, and have been used to make a beer. White fish, dipped in egg and then rolled oats and then lightly fried is delicious served with a little citrus zest and juice. Much of the oat's protein is, unusually for a cereal, soluble, which enables it to make a creamy dish. Oat flour, made from the hulls, is used commercially as an antioxidant in a variety of foods, including dairy products.

> ✿ For a super-quick crumble topping, mix rolled oats and dried fruits (e.g. raisins, cranberries, chopped apricots) with a little melted butter, light oil and a pinch of salt. Simply lay this mix on berries and apples before baking.

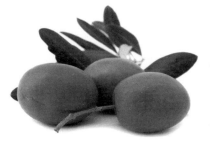

Olives

The use and cultivation of olives in Crete goes back at least as far as 4500 years. Olives then spread to Greece, Rome and other Mediterranean regions. Historically, the olive tree is associated with peace, mostly from the book of Genesis (8:11) where the dove returns to Noah's ark with an olive branch after God has made peace with man and stopped the flood. The olive tree also signifies Christ's death and resurrection. It is now very widely cultivated in Greece, Italy and Spain, with each country and its regions having their own unique cultivars. The fruits have received much publicity over the past years for their wondrous health benefits, and varieties are now being appreciated for their own individual flavours and qualities.

What they contain

The oil (~16%) is very rich in **monounsaturated oleic acid**, which promotes cardiovascular health. The fruit and oil contain many **phenolic** compounds, plus **squalene** – most of these compounds are more concentrated within extra virgin olive oil. Mediterranean people, who have always consumed lots of olives and its oil, develop far fewer heart diseases than most other Europeans and are some of the longest-lived people in the world. Olive oil promotes HDL production and reduces LDLs. The fruits are also rich in **phytosterols**, particularly **pinoresinol**, which has significant anticarcinogenic properties. They are rich in **vitamin E**, with some **carotenoids**, particularly **lutein** and **zeaxanthin**. Olives are rich in **terpenes** (e.g. **lupeol**), and in **hydroxytyrosols** (e.g. **oleuropein**). Olives can contain a lot of sodium as most have been soaked in brine.

What they do

Hydroxytyrosols have anti-inflammatory activities that have been compared to those of ibuprofen (a NSAID) in their efficacy. As antioxidants, they have been reported to be more powerful than quercetin and epicatechins. They also have antibacterial activities against several intestinal and respiratory bacteria, and are antivirals. The quantity of hydroxytyrosols is greatest in virgin olive oil, and it is better if not heated. They give the oil its peppery aroma and flavour. Long-term, regular consumption can lead to significant cardiovascular protection.

Oleic acid may inhibit a gene, particularly prevalent in breast cancer, that otherwise can increase the growth of cancer cells. It also gives up to 50-fold increase in efficacy of Herceptin, and >1000-fold sensitisation to cells that had acquired resistance to Herceptin. There is a strong synergistic interaction between oleuropein and Herceptin. Although olive oil is mostly monounsaturated, it can increase incorporation of omega-3 oils into membranes (compared to omega-6 linoleic), thus helping restore the omega-3:omega-6 balance.

The terpene, lupeol, has significant antioxidant and anticarcinogenic properties – in mice it combats testosterone-induced changes to the prostate causing the death of potential cancer cells and preventing oxidative damage to liver and skin cells. Its terpenes also help kill colon cancer cells. They also have anti-diabetic, anti-inflammatory, anti-arthritic and anti-malarial properties, which are being researched.

The oil aids digestion, is a mild laxative, soothes mucous membranes and is used externally on burns, bruises, insect bites, sprains and itching. With alcohol it makes a good hair tonic and mixed with rosemary oil is a good treatment for dandruff.

Maslinic acid, found in the skin of olives, particularly within pomace oil, inhibits an enzyme involved in releasing HIV from cells into the extracellular environment, thus preventing its further spread around the body (a 90% reduction in spread has been measured). Warning: There are concerns about the levels of polycyclic aromatic hydrocarbons (PAHs) within pomace oil, produced when it is extensively processed, which can be carcinogenic.

How they are used

The raw fruits contain an alkaloid, which makes them bitter, so need to be cured before eating. A few varieties are sweet enough to eat after sun-drying. The only difference between green and black olives is that green olives are less ripe. They are cured in oil, water, brine, lye or by drying. Green olives are soaked in a lye solution before brining; whereas ripe black olives only need brining. Black olives contain more oil than green olives. Olives make a wonderful snack, with cheese and fresh bread, and are added to pizzas, pastas, cold meat and fish dishes. They mix wonderfully with ingredients such as sun-dried tomatoes, aubergines, courgettes, onions, capers and pepperoni. Olives mix well with smoked chicken and with oily fish. Minced, with herbs, olives make a delicious tapenade dip. The oil is added to many Italian sauces and is best not overheated. Virgin oils are best used for dressings and dips. The oil can be flavoured by steeping in, for example, chilli, rosemary, sage, garlic. Dukkah, mixed with extra virgin olive oil, with freshly cooked bread makes a very simple but delicious snack. Olive oils can be sampled like wines, with their quality and taste affected by cultivar, the region and soil they were grown in. Some oils have a strong spicy taste, others are mild and nutty. Olive oil, although often kept for extended periods, is best used during the first six months of pressing.

🌰 The first cold-pressed simple oil is unheated and unchanged. This is best-quality extra virgin olive oil, and has low acidity. The second cold pressing is virgin olive oil, with slightly higher acidity. 'Regular' olive oil is a mix of refined and virgin olive oils. Pomace olive oil has been extracted with solvents and has been refined; its qualities are questionable.

Onions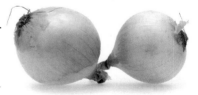

Onions were used in Middle Eastern, Bronze-Age settlements ~7000 years ago, and onion recipes written in Babylon have been unearthed. The

Egyptians may have been the first to cultivate onions. There are hundreds of onion varieties, which vary in flavour and strength from being almost sweet and mild, like shallots, to being eye-wateringly hot, even in small pieces.

What they contain

Onions have some **vitamin C** (~8 mg/100 g), **soluble fibre** (**oligofructose**), which aids digestion, and sugars (as balanced amounts of fructose and glucose). They have **sulphur-containing** compounds, which are rapidly converted to hot, eye-watering **allicin** when the plant is injured. Onions are also very rich in the antioxidant **flavonoid quercetin**, of which they contain more than most other foods. Spring onions (Welsh onions, scallions, bunching onions) are also rich in nutrients, with greater **vitamin C** (~20 mg/100 g) and **vitamin A**. They contain **folate** and have loads of **vitamin K** (~250% of RDA).

What they do

Sulphurous allicin promotes the production of powerful antioxidant enzymes that prevent the formation and multiplication of several types of cancers, including stomach, breast, prostate, colon and endometrium. Onions also have antibacterial properties, which have been utilised for thousands of years to 'cleanse the blood' and treat a wide range of infections, including colds, coughs, flu.

Onions, particularly red onions, are rich in anthocyanins and quercetin. These effectively reduce inflammation, lower serum-triglyceride levels and reduce blood pressure, so regular consumption of onions is effective at reducing cardiovascular disease. These plant compounds also promote and increase the number of white blood cells, particularly lymphocytes, thus enhancing the immune system. The onion's anti-inflammatory properties have been used to help wound healing and reduce scarring. Quercetin also increases bone formation, so could be important in the diet of post-menopausal women.

How they are used

Untreated seeds can be sprouted and are tasty and nutritious. Red and sweet onions are great sliced and used fresh in salads, whereas brown onions are usually cooked. Onions are added to sauces, salads, mayonnaise and dips; stir-fried, roasted and caramelised with other vegetables; are used to make wonderful French onion soup; and are boiled to make white onion soup (often given in convalescence), or added to burgers, hot dogs, etc. Frying makes onions sweeter and reduces their hotness, though extended heating also reduces production of beneficial allicin. Onion is a main ingredient in many spicy curry pastes and is included in numerous Asian recipes. Fresh, sliced onion mixes fabulously with matured cheddar cheese, fresh crusty

> 🐾 Quercetin within onions has antidepressive properties. Feeling low? Eat an onion!

bread and a glass of good ale – the traditional English ploughman's lunch. Onions mix well with small, sweet tomatoes and are delicious pickled. They can be mixed with vegetables, such as aubergine, courgette, tomato, herbs and garlic, to make delicious ratatouille and are added to casseroles and gravies. If onions are to be baked, roasted or steamed, do not remove their outer skins as this imparts a nutty flavour. Sweet onions can even be used in desserts. Onions are dried and ground to make a powder that is used as a flavouring. The green, tasty leaves of spring onions (scallions) are highly valued in many dishes and are usually only lightly, if at all, cooked. They are also popular in many Asian and Chinese dishes.

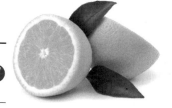

Oranges and tangerines

Oranges are hybrids between the pummelo and the mandarin. Unknown in the wild, it was probably selected in China or North-East India. Later, the orange spread to the Mediterranean, from where the Spanish took it to South America and Mexico. However, it was not until the voyages of Columbus that vitamin C's ability to stave off scurvy was discovered. Today, the orange is the most commonly grown fruit tree in the world, with Florida producing >200 million boxes of oranges a year.

What they contain

Oranges, particularly their edible pith, contain more **fibre** than most fruits. Most fibre is **soluble pectin**, which is highly beneficial to the digestive system. One orange or tangerine gives ~20% of an adult's daily **folate** needs. It has very good **vitamin C** levels (70 mg/100 g), including the peel and white pithy layer beneath. These fruits are rich in α- and β-**carotenes** (**provitamin A**), and in **lutein** and **zeaxanthin**. Their skin, in particular, is very rich in essential oils. It contains lots of **terpene** and **coumarin antioxidants**, particularly the terpene **limonene**. The skin and flesh are also rich in **flavonoids** (e.g. **apigenin** and **hesperetin**), **ferulic acid** and **anthocyanins**.

What they do

Oranges are eaten to allay colds and fevers. The flesh and particularly the skin are rich in antioxidants, which protect against oxidative damage to cells. They inhibit enzymes that might otherwise activate compounds in the body to become carcinogens. Limonene and hesperetin have been shown to reduce the risk of breast cancer. Flavonoids within tangerine peel have anti-cancer activity against leukaemia, and cancers of the head and neck (though may partially nullify the effect of Tamoxifen). In addition, these compounds, with tocotrienols (vitamin E), inhibit proliferation of cancer cells more effectively than if given individually, as each compound exerts its inhibitory effect by a different mechanism. These compounds also reduce serum-cholesterol levels and aid the digestion of fatty foods.

Their flavonoids increase flow of lymph and have been used in burns cases. They also help block the secretion of hepatitis C virus from infected liver cells, so reduce its virulence and spread. Lutein and zeaxanthin help reduce the incidence of cataracts and macular degeneration.

The roasted pulp is used as a poultice for skin diseases; the fresh peel is rubbed on acne. The essential oil from the peel, flowers and leaves is used in perfumes, soaps and household cleaners. Its high limonene content has a lethal effect on houseflies, fleas and fire ants – its potential as an insecticide is under investigation. Bergamot orange yields neroli oil, which is used in perfumery and is added to Earl Grey tea, giving it its distinctive taste and smell. Petitgrain oil, distilled from the leaves, twigs and immature fruits, is used to treat wounds, as an analgesic and an antibacterial, and to expel internal parasites. Orange oil is used in suntan lotions (it contains substances that stimulate formation of melanin) and as an anti-diarrhoeal. It helps blood clot around wounds and is an antidote to metal poisoning. Warning: Its coumarins can react adversely with skin, particularly if then exposed to sunlight.

🌿 Oranges and tangerines contain loads of flavonoids, which can reduce blood pressure by increasing the number of healthy capillaries and significantly improve the elasticity and health of blood vessels. They are used in several pharmaceutical preparations for treatment of ailments including leg ulcers, varicose veins, some diabetic complications (due to poor vascular flow) and for haemorrhoids. They improve and maintain the health of the cardiovascular system.

How they are used

Often just enjoyed fresh or added to fruit and

green leaf salads, numerous desserts. Used as a garnish, or made into juice. Reduced-sugar marmalade made with Seville oranges and rich in zest and pith is wonderfully flavourful, and is also fabulously rich in fibre, vitamins and antioxidants. Oranges can be added to cakes, muffins and biscuits. It makes an interesting wine and also a brandy. Orange slices and peel are candied; the peel is delicious in dark chocolate and it also mixes well with ginger. Oranges go well with nuts, either in rissoles, stuffing or desserts.

A spiced orange sauce, with nutmeg and cinnamon, can be poured onto crêpes. The zest is delicious scattered on top of grilled fish and seafoods, or simply mixed with mascarpone or thick yoghurt to make a very simple, yet delicious sauce for both savoury and sweet dishes. It mixes well with pumpkin and squash, and can be added to roasted vegetables to add a tangy flavour. Its essential oil is widely used commercially in many foods. The honey from orange trees is delicious.

Oregano   See 'Marjoram and oregano'

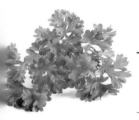

Parsley

Parsley is a very popular herbs that originates from the Mediterranean, and was popular with the Greeks and Romans. The latter served it at banquets, where its flavour was used to mask unpleasant tastes from foods probably being past what we would call their sell-by dates. It was also believed to reduce intoxication. Parsley is now probably the most commonly grown herb across Europe, North America and Australasia. It comes in two main types: Italian, with flat larger leaves, and curled (or moss-curled) parsley, which has highly crinkled leaves. In Asian countries, where parsley is less well known, it is often called Western coriander or European celery.

What it contains

Fresh parsley leaves are very nutritious. They are hugely rich in **carotenoids** (β-**carotene**, **lutein** and **zeaxanthin**) and **vitamin C**

(~160 mg/100 g). Parsley is also one of the richest sources of **vitamin K**, with two tablespoons providing ~150% of the RDA. Also contains some of the **B vitamins**, particularly **folate**. Parsley leaves are very rich in **chlorophyll**, which has anticarcinogenic and wound-healing properties. It also contains wondrous amounts of **iron** (~8 mg/100 g), greater than in most vegetables, and good amounts of other minerals. Fresh parsley leaves are wonderfully rich in **secondary plant compounds**, particularly the **flavonoid apigenin**, but also **polyacetylenes**, **coumarins** and **terpenes** (e.g. **myristicine** and **limonene**), with curly parsley being richer in myristicine. The seed oil is rich in **monounsaturated petroselinic acid**, an unusual oil, though common in this plant family. The seeds also contain myristicine and **apiole**.

What it does

Parsley's secondary plant compounds help reduce heart disease and the incidence of cancer. Apigenin has remarkable anti-inflammatory, antioxidant and anticarcinogenic properties. Apiole, from the seeds, has beneficial effects in treating kidney ailments and kidney stones, and is used by women to reduce painful menstruation. Polyacetylenes within parsley can be highly toxic towards fungi and bacteria, are anti-inflammatory and inhibit blood-clot formation. They are also responsible for allergic skin reactions. Both polyacetylenes and coumains have shown anticancer activity in several studies.

> Parsley added to a dish aids its digestion, helps you to see better in the dark and provides lots of iron.

Parsley has long been used to aid digestion and eliminate intestinal gas; recent studies have confirmed that it inhibits gastric secretion and protects the stomach lining against injury. Parsley was widely used historically as a diuretic and a laxative; recent studies have also proven these uses. It contains compounds that affect the sodium/potassium-transport pumps in cell membranes, which, in turn, stimulate electrolyte and water excretion. Parsley can also reduce some of the symptoms of memory dysfunction by inhibiting the activity of adverse enzymes.

The amounts of these nutrients are greatest within fresh leaves. Drying or cooking greatly reduces its efficacy, so it is best to eat it fresh. Parsley is often eaten to freshen the breath and may reduce the odour of garlic. Its extracts have been used as a hair tonic to prevent hair loss.

Warning: Like other members of this family, polyacetylenes and coumarins can cause contact dermatitis, particularly if then exposed to sunlight. In excess, myristicine can give feelings of euphoria, but it can also cause convulsions and other serious effects. Apiole, found within the essential oil, can induce abortions, so should not be taken during pregnancy. Parsley essential oil should be treated with caution. The fresh leaves have very low to zero risk of causing problems, though they do contain high amounts of oxalic acid, so should not be eaten in excess.

How it is used

Parsley is a popular traditional garnish, though also has many other uses. Parsley is often added to cooked dishes, including sauces, particularly those made with milk or cheese, which are made to accompany fish recipes. It goes well with all types of fish (white, oily and smoked) and with seafood. It mixes well with potatoes and is often added to salads. Try it with carrot, artichoke, garlic, asparagus, courgette, avocado, onion, green beans, tomatoes and mushrooms, and also chopped nuts, apple and ginger. May be blended with basil, dill, tarragon or mint and is excellent with citrus, especially lemon. Is one of the main ingredients, along with bulgar, in the delicious Middle Eastern salad tabbouleh. It mixes well with bean and lentil recipes. In Japan, it is dipped in a light batter to make tempura. Wonderful sauces can be made by combining garlic, parsley, lemon and orange zest. Parsley is also great added to a range of soups, and is often included in stuffing. In general, parsley leaves are best added towards the end of cooking to retain their flavour.

> 🍴 Mix fresh chopped parsley with chopped black olives and roasted almonds, chilli, black pepper and lemon zest and juice in virgin olive oil to make a delicious tapenade.

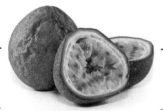

Passion fruit

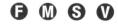

The Spanish learnt of these plants' natural sedative properties from the indigenous populations of South America and introduced the vine into warmer areas of Europe, where its leaves were popularly used as a calming herbal tea. In many countries, the passion-fruit vine has been used as a natural tranquilliser. Although there are many good-quality and fruit-producing *Passiflora* species, the most common is the passion fruit. These fruits have a tough, waxy skin, beneath which is a central cavity containing many small, dark-brown seeds surrounded by juicy sacs of wonderfully fragrant, yellow-orange, delicious, tangy-sweet pulp.

What it contains

Passion fruit have excellent amounts of **vitamin C** (30–130 mg/100 g of juice), and excellent quantities of **carotenoids** (especially yellow-fruited species), particularly **lycopene**, which has significant nutritional and medicinal benefits. The fruits are rich in **potassium** and **iron**, and in **soluble fibre** (~10%). The seeds contain ~23% oil, of which ~85% is **unsaturated** and most is **omega-6 linoleic acid**. The fruits are also rich in flavonoids (e.g. **apigenin**) and also in **alkaloids**.

Soothing, sedative, passion-fruit extracts are found in many herbal tea mixtures and medicines. Individually, its active compounds are stimulatory; it's only when they are combined that the plant has its sedative effects.

What it does

From historic to present times, passion fruit (and their leaves) have been used as a natural sedative and to relieve muscle spasms, particularly the species *P. incarnata*. It reduces spasms and acts as a pain killer by depressing the central nervous system by helping to slow down the breakdown of neurotransmitters. Passion fruit are rich in apigenin, which has remarkable anti-inflammatory and antioxidant properties, and is an anticarcinogen. Passion fruit and their leaves are used to reduce anxiety, hyperactivity, hysteria, insomnia, irritability, muscle tension, narcotic-induced hangover, nervous headache, nervous tension, anxiety related to asthma, neuralgia, pain of shingles, painful menstruation, Parkinson's disease, restlessness, anxiety during menopause, gastrointestinal complaints of nervous origin, epilepsy and as a sedative. Most importantly, it does not have the side effects that many modern pharmaceutical drugs have. Given to people before surgery, instead of a pre-med, passion fruit was found to reduce anxiety without inducing sedation. The passion fruit described here is classified by the FDA as safe to be given to both children and infants. Both the leaves and fruit can be used.

The oil from the seeds has moisturising, healing, lubricating and antibacterial properties; it is used on dry, itchy skin and in a wide range of cosmetics.

Warning: Possibly should not be eaten during pregnancy as it may stimulate the muscles of the womb. Under-ripe fruits contain cyanide-like compounds, so shouldn't be eaten.

How it is used

Passion fruits are great added to ice cream, yoghurt and to cheesecake, muffins, cakes and pies. Try them fresh on top of bananas that have been fried in a little butter and cinnamon. A spicy sauce recipe recommends blending fresh mangoes, passion fruit and chilli together. It can be added to sauces, used in sweet and savoury dishes, and is used as a glaze on red meats or chicken. It mixes well with berries and tropical fruits and particularly with banana.

Passion fruit have a fabulous aroma and a tangy, exciting flavour. They are delicious eaten fresh, scooped out from their skin, but are also fabulous added to fruit salads.

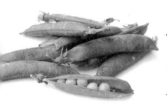

Peas

There are many varieties of peas, from small, sweet peas that can be eaten along with their pod, to common garden peas, to field peas, which are grown for forage or for drying, to sweet-smelling, delicately coloured, ornamental sweet peas. Peas are now one of the most popular vegetables in Western cuisine. Note that cowpeas, crowder peas and black-eyed peas are actually beans (see. p. 92).

What they contain

Sprouted peas are rich in **protein** and **folate** (>40% RDA), and the other **B vitamins**. They have good quantities of minerals (i.e. **iron**, **manganese**). Garden peas (without pods) also have excellent levels of protein, which includes good amounts of **lysine** and **tryptophan** that are lacking in cereal and corn crops. They have lots of **fibre**, and are rich in **vitamin C** (~40 mg/100 g) and **vitamin K**. Peas are rich in **carotenoids**, much as β-**carotene**, and even more **lutein** and **zeaxanthin**, which help improve vision and can significantly slow the progression of age-related eye disorders. They are also rich in cholesterol-lowering **phytosterols**. Because cooking and freezing reduce levels of many of the above, it is best to cook them for a minimum to enjoy their full nutritional benefits.

Research shows that out of seven major food types (which included dairy, meat, fruit, etc.), the legumes, including peas, if eaten regularly, offer the best dietary predictor for elderly people's survival.

What they do

Their fibre confers numerous benefits to the digestive tract, reduces serum LDLs, reduces blood-sugar levels and helps control insulin levels, so they are useful in reducing the development of diabetes and cardiovascular disease.

Historically, pea oil was taken as a contraceptive (it was thought to reduce progesterone levels), and was believed to reduce sperm count. There is a report that pea oil reduced pregnancy rate in women by 60% in a 2-year period and reduced sperm production by 50%. However, as peas only contain a small amount of oil, a large quantity of peas would need to be consumed.

How they are used

Peas can be used in many ways. Along with tomatoes, peas are one of the few vegetables most children enjoy. Untreated pea seeds can be sprouted and used in salads, stir-fries, etc. Edible podded peas (e.g. sugar snaps and sugar peas) are added raw to salads. They can be lightly stir-fried and added to Asian and Chinese recipes, or briefly steamed. They are often served as a speciality vegetable and are crisp, sweet and delicious. Older pods may need any stringy edges removed before use. Garden peas, without their pods, can be eaten fresh added to salads, or be lightly steamed as a vegetable to accompany many menus (e.g. meat and fish recipes) or be added to soups, stews, stir-fries, omelettes, etc. They are delicious with a dab of butter or cooked with a little mint. Marrowfat peas are a variety of pea that are picked when mature and are then dried. They are popular in the United Kingdom and the United States for making thick pea soups and in the United Kingdom, when mashed to form 'mushy peas', they are a popular accompaniment to fish and chips. Other dried peas, such as yellow split peas, can be used and cooked like lentils and have a similar flavour. They do not need soaking like many bean varieties and are much more digestible. They are excellent added to soups and stews, or used in curries and dahl. Dried peas are popular in the Middle East and Asia as a snack, where they are fried and spiced. Dried peas can also be ground to make pea flour, which may be mixed with other flour types. The young leaves and tendrils can be lightly steamed as a vegetable, particularly those from petit pois-type varieties.

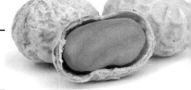

Peanuts Ⓜ Ⓞ Ⓟ Ⓢ Ⓥ

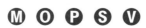

Originally from South America, peanuts were cultivated by the Incas, and were used as a currency, medicine and food. In the United States, peanuts were first grown commercially around the time of the Civil War, and were know as 'goober peas': since then, their popularity has kept increasing. Peanut seeds, although a popular snack, are mostly cultivated for their oil. Botanically, peanuts are more similar to peas and beans than to 'true' nuts.

What they contain

Peanuts are often undervalued as a nutritional food. They contain ~25% **protein**, which is higher than fish, dairy products and many meats, though are deficient in sulphur-containing methionine. They contain lots of **fermentable fibre** (8–10%). They are also very rich in the **B vitamins** – they are the richest plant-source of **biotin** – and are very rich in **thiamine**, **folate** and **niacin**. They are rich in the powerful and important antioxidant **vitamin E**. Peanuts are rich in **manganese, phosphate, copper, zinc, iron** and **magnesium**. They contain **choline**, which is intimately associated with neurotransmitters and a lack of which can cause fatty liver, neural-tube defects and neurodegenerative disease. The kernels are rich in **oils** (up to 50%) and of this 40–60% is **monounsaturated**, 20–30% is **polyunsaturated**, which virtually all is **omega-6 fatty acids**, and ~20% is **saturated**. They are rich in the powerful antioxidant **coenzyme Q10**, and in cholesterol-lowering **phytosterols**, with some **saponins**. Peanuts have very good quantities of antioxidant **resveratrol**, with levels as high as those found in red grapes.

What they do

Resveratrol inhibits tumour formation by preventing DNA damage, slowing or halting cell transformation from normal to cancerous, and slowing tumour growth (it is particularly useful in preventing colon cancer). It also inhibits the formation of arterial blockages and has anti-inflammatory properties. Its rich B vitamins content enhance neuronal and muscular transmission, including the heart and digestive system, enhance energy use, help make DNA and RNA, improve eyesight, improve how we feel (and reduce the incidence of neurodegenerative diseases), reduce the risk of cancer formation and reduce the incidence of birth defects.

Eating just a few peanuts, rich in monounsaturated fats, can reduce serum LDLs and triglycerides,

Many human studies have confirmed that eating nuts regularly can significantly reduce the likelihood of heart disease in people of all ages and socioeconomic groups who also eat a range of food types. The phytosterols in peanuts have cancer-preventive properties against colon, breast and prostate cancers.

without affecting HDL levels, and does not cause weight gain. People lost the same amount of weight on a low-fat diet as those on a diet that contained peanuts, and they enjoyed the latter more. Peanuts (and other nuts) reduce the development of cardiovascular disease – people recovering from a first heart attack, who then ate a diet that included peanuts and other nuts, decreased their risk of further heart problems by 25%. Warning: Some people are allergic to peanuts, even in small quantities.

How they are used

Peanuts are eaten fresh, or can be roasted and salted as a snack. To roast peanuts, sauté in a light oil for ~3 min, drain and sprinkle with salt or cayenne pepper. To make peanut butter, dry-roast the nuts in an oven, crush them, and add a little salt and peanut oil.

There are multitudes of peanut recipes, for both sweet and savoury dishes. Peanuts are popularly added to Asian sauces and curries and also confectionery and cookies. They are added to salads, to stir-fry mixes and go well in rice dishes. A peanut soup recipe lightly fries onions, green peppers and garlic then adds fresh tomatoes, brown rice and stock. After simmering for 45 minutes, peanut butter is added to make it creamy and the soup is served scattered with fresh peanut pieces and black pepper.

🐾 Though wonderfully nutritious, they do contain omega-6 fatty acids, so add some omega-3-rich linseed or kiwifruit to your peanut dish.

Peanuts make a great snack bar when mixed with dried fruits, rolled oats and honey. They go well with banana and chocolate. Roasted peanuts have been used as a coffee substitute. They can also be ground and added to cakes, muffins and pastry to improve flavour and raise protein levels. Peanut oil is used for frying and roasting and in dressings and spreads. It is used in cooking oils, margarine and salad oils. The germinated seeds can be eaten in salads.

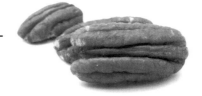

Pecans and hickory nuts

Pecans, native to the Eastern United States and Mexico, are also known as 'hickory' nuts. Native populations have long used and cultivated these trees, selecting tasty nuts with thin shells from which to propagate and thus improve quality. These nuts are still popular in North America and are used widely in confectionery and desserts.

What they contain

They have good amounts of **protein** (~10%) and are rich in **mostly soluble fibre** (10%). They are very rich in **oil** (70%), of which ~33% is **monounsaturated oleic acid**, with much of the remainder being **omega-6 linoleic acid** (they have very little saturated fats). They are wonderfully rich in **tocopherols** (**vitamin E**), and have good amounts of minerals, particularly **manganese, zinc, iron, copper, fluoride** and **magnesium**. They also contain lots of **phytosterols**.

What they do

Its quality oil can lower serum LDLs, enhance the structure of cell membranes, increase the elasticity of vessels, all of which help reduce cardiovascular disease. The oil, particularly with its very rich vitamin E content, has significant anti-inflammatory properties. Their mix of oil and fibre slows digestion and lowers peaks and troughs in blood-sugar levels – they have a low GI, and are a good food for those concerned about developing type-2 diabetes.

Pecan nut oil is used in pharmaceutical drugs, essential oils and cosmetics. Warning: Some people are allergic to pecan and hickory nuts.

How they are used

This tasty nut is eaten as a snack or can be used in pralines, cakes, desserts and the famous pecan pie. They can be covered with whipped egg white and then with sugar and spices before being toasted. In desserts, pecans go wonderfully with berries such as raspberries, blueberries and cherries; they also mix well with honey, maple syrup and chocolate. Crushed, they are delicious added to cakes, sweet pastry and muffins.

Pecans can be added to stuffing, rissoles, cheese fillings, sauces to top fish dishes and they make a good ingredient in pumpkin recipes. Pecan nut oil is used as a cooking oil, though is best not overheated or its flavours are impaired.

🐾 Enjoy pecans with vitamin A-rich apricots and vitamin-C rich guavas – perhaps on your breakfast cereal with live yoghurt.

Peppercorns
(black, green, white and red)

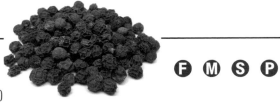

Peppercorns are the small, dried fruits from a tropical, perennial vine that, although originally from southern India, is now grown around the world. Interestingly, local varieties of peppercorn plants have developed different flavours, which are valued by connoisseurs in the same way as regional olive oils or wines – there are at least 75 varieties of peppercorns. One of the world's most popular condiments, it is particularly popular in European and New World cuisine. Peppercorns (or ground pepper) are now found in virtually every kitchen and this tasty condiment also has many nutritional benefits.

What they contain

The fruits are rich in **protein** (~10%) and **fibre** (~25%). They are also very rich in **minerals**, particularly **calcium**, **iron**, **manganese**, **fluoride**, **potassium** and **magnesium**. They contain good amounts of **vitamin C** and are very rich in **vitamin K**. Their main peppery flavour is derived from the alkaloid **piperine**. Although hot in flavour, it has only 1% the heat of capsaicin (as found in chillies). The fruits and seeds also contain a pungent resin, **chavicine**, and the outer fruits are very rich in **terpenes** (e.g. **pinene**, **limonene**, **linalool**, **caryophyllene**). It also contains **oleoresin**, a mix of oil and resin, which is used in pepper sprays, though capsicums are the main source of this.

What they do

Piperine can lower plasma LDL levels and does not affect HDLs, so it is a potential ally against cardiovascular disease. It reduces the activities of enzymes that cause oxidative stress, particularly in those on a high-fat diet. It also modulates insulin resistance in rats fed a high-fat diet. It may, therefore, protect against development of type-2 diabetes. Its compounds stimulate breakdown of fat cells and so are a good dietary addition for those worried about weight gain.

Piperine has strong antibacterial properties, including against *Staphylococcus aureus* and bacteria that cause dental disease. Historically, peppercorns were used to treat toothache and tooth decay. Peppercorns also have anticarcinogenic properties (e.g. against colon cancer). Synthetic derivatives of piperine are used to make well-known anti-diarrhoea pills: they slow down the muscular activity of the intestines.

Peppercorns, in larger amounts, can dilate capillaries in the skin which increases sweating and gives a feeling of warmth. This is followed by tightening of capillaries and a reduction in temperature. The taste of peppercorns also increases the flow of mouth saliva, stimulates secretion of stomach digestive juices and acts as an appetite enhancer.

> Piperine, when mixed with turmeric, enhances the bioavailability of its health-giving curcumin by a phenomenal 2000% in humans, with no adverse effects; so add black pepper to your curry.

Its essential oil has a warm, spicy aroma – it is strong, and should only be used in small amounts. In aromatherapy, it is used as a mind stimulant, to raise spirits and to induce warmth of emotion; it is also used on muscles to maintain suppleness and to treat deep-muscle aches and pains. It has been used, diluted, to treat chilblains, arthritis and rheumatism, neuralgia, poor circulation, sprains and stiffness. Inhaled in vapour form, it has been used to treat many pulmonary infections.

Warning: In large amounts piperine can increase the availability and slow the elimination of several pharmaceutical drugs (e.g. phenytoin, propranolol and theophylline). As with all essential oils, it should be used with caution and diluted.

How they are used

The small dried fruits are usually ground and can be used in countless savoury dishes, either added during cooking or used as a condiment along with salt. Freshly ground pepper is more aromatic, is hotter and has much more flavour than stored ground pepper. Along with being used in sauces, soups, stews, many Mediterranean and Middle Eastern recipes, cheese and egg dishes, curries and vegetable dishes, a little black pepper can be added to fresh fruits such as strawberries and pineapple, and even to chocolate recipes, to bring out their flavour. Add a little to blended raspberries and peaches and serve the mix on chilled melon slices with a sprig or two of basil. It is an ingredient in several spice mixes, including

> 🐾 Black peppercorns are fruits that are just changing from green to red, and are then steamed and dried; green peppercorns are from slightly unripe fruits, but are treated so that their greenness is maintained; white peppercorns are derived only from the inner seed, with the outer skin and flesh removed, but also much of their nutrients and flavour; pink peppercorns are derived from slightly under-ripe fruits. Most consider black peppercorns to have the fruitiest and greatest depth of flavour, and they are the most nutritious.

garam masala, and is used to coat roast meats. The generous amounts of black pepper in Cornish pasties enliven its meat, potato, carrot and swede filling. In Asian cuisine, the fresh fruits are sometimes used, and then have a fruity flavour.

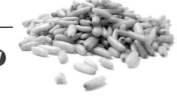

Pinenuts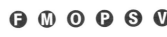

(pinyon)

There are ~20 species of *Pinus* that produce kernels large enough to be edible, but only a few are cultivated for their seeds. The stone pine from Europe and the Korean pine from China are the two most popular species. Although time-consuming to harvest (hence their cost) these delicious nuts have been especially popular within Italian cuisine, and their popularity has now spread far and wide.

What they contain

Kernels contain 12–18% **protein**, are rich in oil (50–70%), of which much is **monounsaturated oleic acid** and **omega-6 linoleic acid**. Pinenuts also contain high quantities of **pinolenic acids**. They have good amounts of **fibre** (8–10%), and are a good source of **thiamine** and **niacin**. Are rich in the minerals **manganese**, **copper**, **zinc**, **iron**, **magnesium** and **phosphates**, and contain good amounts of **lecithin**. The nuts are rich in **antioxidant compounds**.

Extracts are used to treat a condition that causes loss of vision due to blockage of fine capillaries at the back of the eye (sometimes related to diabetes), chronic venous insufficiency and several inflammatory conditions, such as asthma, eczema and arthritis.

What they do

Excellent fibre and oil content smooth out peaks and troughs in blood-sugar levels and its protein helps build muscle and promote strength. Rich in minerals, including red blood cell and muscle-enhancing iron and antioxidant zinc, which also improves sperm counts and general male well-being.

Pinenuts reduce blood pressure and blood sugar, and inhibit allergic reactions. They are being investigated for their potential in treating insulin resistance in type-2 diabetes. Their oils reduce LDLs, so decrease chances of cardiovascular disease and stroke. Lecithin also helps lower serum-cholesterol and triglycerides. Warning: Pinenuts can cause an allergic reaction.

How they are used

The kernels taste their best if very lightly roasted (they can be easily over-roasted) before eating, as this removes any slight 'turpentine' taste they may have. They can also be smoked. Pinenuts have a light, subtle, delicious flavour. They are either eaten fresh, or are added to breakfast cereals, breads, confectionery, stews, meat and vegetable dishes, curries, pastas, nut butter, as a garnish on smoked fish, in stuffing, soups, sauces, in salads or can be coated in chocolate. They are delicious in dukkah, with coriander and cumin seeds. Try them with artichokes, asparagus, watercress, aubergine, tomatoes, orange, olives, beans, capers, carrot, mushrooms, parsley or celery. Pesto made with pinenuts is a key ingredient in Italian recipes. Make your own pesto by blending together pinenuts, fresh basil, garlic, Parmesan cheese and olive oil. Add fresh lemon or lime zest and juice before use. The extracted oil is of a good quality, particularly that extracted by cold pressing. It is best added to dishes just before serving or eaten fresh – heating alters its delicate flavour. The oil is used in cosmetics and for massage.

> ✿ Pinenuts were eaten by Russians to suppress appetite and recent research verifies that the pinolenic acid within these nuts stimulates a hormone that suppresses appetite. They can significantly reduce feelings of hunger. Consequently, they are often promoted in slimming diets.

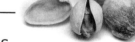

Pistachios

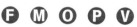 **F M O P V**

Pistachio trees used to grow wild on the hills and mountains from Lebanon to northern Iraq and Iran, and the nuts have been appreciated in Middle Eastern countries for at least 9000 years. The tree is very long-lived: ages of 700 years have been recorded, and they produce fruits throughout much of that time. The greenish kernel within the shell has a delicious flavour. It is generally considered that the deeper its shade of green, the better its flavour. The nuts are also wonderfully nutritious.

What they contain

The kernels are rich in **oil** (~45%) and have a satisfying nutty flavour. Turkish and Iranian pistachios contain ~10% **saturated fats**, ~55% **monounsaturated oils** and ~33% **polyunsaturated oils** (most as **omega-6 linoleic acid**). The oil is also rich in **vitamin E**, and contains **coenzyme Q10**, a vital compound involved in energy production and a powerful antioxidant. Pistachios are very rich in **protein** (>20%), containing a very balanced ratio of **all the essential amino acids**. They are also rich in **fibre** (~10%) and in the **B vitamins**, being an excellent source of **B6** (more than beef liver) and **thiamine**. The nuts are also a rich source of **minerals**, containing lots of **iron**, **copper**, **manganese**, **potassium** and **phosphates**. Pistachios are unusual in containing good amounts of carotenoids (i.e. **lutein** and **zeaxanthin**), which are strongly linked with reducing age-related visual degeneration. They have greater **antioxidant** activity than most fruits, vegetables and nuts, and are rich in cholesterol-lowering **phytosterols** – more so than any other nut.

Despite being rich in oil, pistachios do not cause weight gain – they reduce blood-sugar-level peaks and troughs because their energy is released slowly over time, so they are great for those worried about weight gain. As an in-shell snack, people eat them more slowly and so tend to eat less of them.

What they do

Pistachio nuts are tremendously nutritious, being an excellent source of proteins, beneficial oils, minerals, antioxidants, most vitamins and fibre. The oil can significantly reduce serum LDLs, so reduce the risk of cardiovascular disease.

Its rich vitamin B content helps build and maintain neuronal and muscular transmission, including the heart and digestive system, enhances energy use, helps make DNA and RNA, improves eyesight, helps fend off depression and reduces the incidence of neurodegenerative diseases and the risk of cancer formation. B vitamins stave off age-related health disorders, so their intake should be increased as we age.

The kernels have been used to treat sclerosis of the liver, abdominal ailments, abscesses, bruises and sores, chest ailments and circulatory problems. The Arabs consider the nuts to be an aphrodisiac.

Warning: Pistachios can cause allergic reactions in some people.

How they are used

Pistachios are used in confectionery, cakes, desserts, dressings and savoury recipes. They mix deliciously with many fruits, such as strawberries, apricots, mangoes, pears, berries, peaches, banana and citrus. Pistachios can be ground and added to stuffing, to many vegetable, fish and meat recipes. They blend well with dark chocolate in ice cream and are delicious mixed with other nuts, such as almonds, macadamias and hazelnuts. They can be combined with creamy cheeses or feta in fillings, are added to savoury rice dishes and milder curries,

> 🐾 For a delicious and healthy snack try halva made with sesame seeds, crushed pistachio nuts, honey pressed into a tasty snack bar.

as well to many pasta sauces. They are, however, usually simply enjoyed as an in-shell snack, eaten raw or roasted. They can be roasted for ~10 minutes at ~140°C and then sprinkled with salt.

Plantains

Plantain species are often overlooked and commonly considered unattractive weeds; however, several are edible and many have tremendous medicinal properties. Buckshorn plantain is often considered to be the best flavoured. It is cultivated for its leaves and seeds, which are nutritious. The seeds/seed coats have been used for thousands of years for their rich mucilage content, which is excellent in preventing and treating a wide range of intestinal and digestive problems. Its crushed seed is commonly known as psyllium.

What they contain

The leaves are rich in **carotenoids** with some **vitamin C** (~20 mg/100 g). They also contain antioxidant **flavonoids** (e.g. **apigenin**) and various **acids** (e.g. **benzoic, caffeic, chlorogenic, cinnamic, coumaric, fumaric, salicylic, ursolic, vanillic, ascorbic**). The seeds are rich in the mucilage **psyllium**. The embryo within the seeds is rich in oil, mainly as **omega-6 linoleic acid**.

What they do

Psyllium has been widely used to treat dysentery, constipation, diarrhoea, haemorrhoids and genitourinary tract infections. The mucilage is thought to also absorb toxins within the large bowel. Plantain species have been widely used in different parts of the world for these reasons.

Psyllium is being researched for its ability to lower cholesterol and control diabetes, with several studies recommending its addition to breakfast cereals. Research also indicates that psyllium, incorporated within food products, is more effective at reducing blood-glucose response than the use of soluble-fibre supplements.

🌿 Plantain seed coats contain ~30% psyllium, which expands in the gut at least 1-fold and facilitates the passage of food as well as stools. It is not actually digested and absorbed – it works in a purely mechanical way, absorbing excess water while stimulating normal bowel elimination. When eaten, it hugely benefits digestion, soothes spasms of the gut and acts as a gentle laxative.

How they are used

Young leaves have a crisp, mild, slightly salty to bitter flavour and make an interesting addition to salads. The leaves can be quickly blanched in boiling water beforehand to make them tender. They can also be lightly steamed as a vegetable, added to soups and stir-fried. The leaves are an ingredient in 'misticanze', an Italian salad composed of both wild and cultivated leaves. Try lightly roasting the seeds to give them a little more flavour and then adding them to salads, pasta dishes, breakfast cereals, breads, muffins and cakes.

Plums and prunes

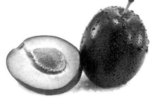

The many types of plum come in a range of sizes, colours and shapes and are mostly divided into European plums and Japanese plums, but also damsons, sloe, mirabelles (which are wilder, older cultivars) and plum cherries, which are native to North America. Their flesh is juicy and ranges from yellow to orange to rich red, depending on cultivar, is sweet, sometimes tangy, and refreshing. Their single central stone should be discarded.

What they contain

Prunes contain staggering amounts of antioxidants, higher than all other commercial fruits, and are top of the ORAC table of common fruits. Plums also have good levels of **antioxidants** with red-fleshed plums having the most, particularly lots of **anthocyanins**. Plums are nutrient rich, but prunes have most of these nutrients very concentrated. They are rich in **flavonoids** (e.g. **catechins, epicatechins**) and **chlorogenic acid**. They are a good source of **carotenoids**, with moderate levels of **vitamin C** (10 mg/100 g). Prunes are very rich in **vitamin K**. The skin contains many of their nutrients. Both prunes and plums contain fibre, mostly as **soluble fibre**, confirming the traditional usage of prunes to get the digestive system 'moving'.

What they do

Their high antioxidant content boosts the immune system, reduces inflammation, fights cancers (e.g. breast, colon), reduces cardio-vascular disease and strokes, helps repair cell damage, enhances the immune system and slows the progression of age-related disorders.

> As is popularly known, plums and particularly prunes stimulate bowel movement; these fruits can reduce and soothe many digestive problems, including irritable-bowel syndrome.

Their sugars provide energy, and prunes make a great between-meal snack. Their rich fibre content helps smooth rapid increases and decreases in blood-sugar levels. Better than a chocolate bar, they supply energy for longer and you get the benefits of their phenomenal antioxidants.

Their soluble fibre lowers blood-lipid and LDL levels in those eating a high saturated-fat diet, but also works for those with very low intakes of saturated fat.

Warning: Like all from this plant family, the stones contain cyanide-like compounds.

How they are used

Plums are wonderful eaten fresh, but can be added to many desserts, such as pies, crumbles, compote and flans. They can be bottled, made into jams, chutneys, or can be dried (to make prunes). Plums mix well with apples, ginger and cinnamon. Try them lightly poached on muesli

> ✿ Prunes, unfairly, often receive 'bad press': however, they are delicious added to fruit salads, with other soaked dried fruits, and their rich flavour goes beautifully with ice cream, mascarpone and citrus.

with live yoghurt. They make great sauces, with citrus and berries, to accompany both sweet and savoury dishes, including roasted meats and chicken. The deep red-skinned and red-fleshed plums are particularly healthy, as well as delicious. They also make a reasonable wine. Prunes make a great snack food with nuts, and deserve to be rediscovered eaten simply on their own, as a tasty pick-me-up. Soak them in tea, either green or Earl Grey, before adding to cereals or a fruit salad – the synergistic boost from the tea and prunes together is very health-giving.

Pomegranates ⓢ

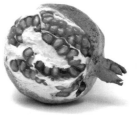

Pomegranates have been cultivated for thousands of years and have now become naturalised around the Mediterranean and North Africa. The Chinese also cultivated these fruits for more than 2000 years. Their usage has been recorded by many civilisations and only the fig is mentioned as frequently in mythical and biblical writings. Recently, the pomegranate has become highly valued for its excellent antioxidant and nutritive properties.

What they contain

A pomegranate's main nutritive value comes from its abundant anti-oxidant **polyphenols** (e.g. **anthocyanins**, **ellagitannins** and **ellagic acid**), which have greater antioxidant activity than many other fruits or vegetables. The fruits, and particularly the seeds, are rich in **phyto-oestrogens**, which may aid with menopause symptoms. The seeds are rich in oil, of which ~80% is **omega-5 punicic acid** (a type of **linolenic acid**).

What they do

Hundreds of papers have been published on the wide-ranging medicinal values of pomegranate. The fruits have significant cancer-fighting properties – particularly preventive and therapeutic activities against prostate cancer in humans, and possibly against breast, skin, colon, liver and lung cancers. The antioxidant-rich seeds, the peel and fermented juice (pomegranate wine) can cause cell death of up to 75% of human oestrogen-caused breast cancer cells, while leaving healthy breast cells mostly unaffected. Delphinidin and its ellagitannins are likely candidates for these effects, though the omega-5 oils have also shown significant anti-cancer properties. These oils can also prevent fat build-up, and its inclusion in the diet has been suggested for those who are obese.

The juice is being researched for its antiviral properties – it is hoped it could be an antiviral agent against HIV. The fruits have anti-malarial properties and are effective antimicrobials, against *Escherichia coli*, but also even methicillin-resistant *Staphylococcus aureus* (MRSA), and the yeast *Candida albicans*.

Other studies show that the juice greatly reduces levels of serum-cholesterol and LDLs while not affecting beneficial HDLs. Regular intake also prevents thickening of arteries. Therefore, pomegranates may reduce the risk of cardiovascular disease and help those with diabetes (who have hyperlipidaemia).

> Pomegranate juice is effective at reducing oral bacteria that cause dental caries and other oral disorders.

Extracts are taken for arthritis and recent animal studies have confirmed its efficacy to prevent the onset and severity of inflammatory arthritis. In addition, compounds such as ellagic acid are hypothesised to have neuroprotective activities, so are being explored for their ability to reduce diseases such as Alzheimer's.

Pomegranate, within cosmetics, has potential anti-ageing properties; it moisturises, improves skin elasticity and protects against UV damage.

How they are used

Fruits can be eaten fresh by cutting in half and the clusters of juicy sacs lifted out and enjoyed. Some people eat the seeds while others spit them out as they can be bitter in quantity. The fruits are popular made into juice, which has a sweet/tart flavour and is often mixed with apple juice. Pomegranate juice is added to a wide range of both sweet and savoury recipes – from being mixed with yoghurt on desserts and breakfast cereals, to being added to curries, chilli dishes and salads. Its tangy flavour mixes well with banana, papaya and nuts, and also with avocados in guacamole. It blends well with ginger and complements fish, seafood, chicken and lentil dishes. It is added to jellies, sorbets, makes an excellent sweet-and-sour sauce, is added to chutney, or is used to flavour cakes and desserts. Pomegranate syrup is sold commercially as grenadine and is the 'sunrise' in tequila sunrise. The juice also makes a reasonable wine. The sacs are attractive as a garnish. In India, fruits are used to make anardana –the juice sacs are dried in the sun and are then used as a spice.

Pumpkins, squash and their seeds

Pumpkin is native to Central America and the south-west of the United States, where it used to be common in the wild. Pumpkin remains have been found in settlements in Mexico dating back 10,500 years. The flesh, seeds and flowers are all edible and can be stored for long periods. The pumpkin is a popular vegetable in many regions of the world. Apart from the traditional usage of its flesh, the seeds are also popular in many recipes. Research now confirms the seeds' many nutritious properties. In the United States, pumpkins are also known as winter squash, along with varieties such as butternut, acorn, hubbard and spaghetti.

What they contain

Both the seeds and flesh are a good food source. The seeds (without shells) are very rich in **protein** (25–35%), containing **all the essential amino acids**. They are rich in oil (~45%): ~40% **omega-6 linoleic**, ~20% **omega-3** α-**linolenic**, and ~40% **monounsaturated oleic acid**. The seeds are also rich in vitamin A (as β-**carotenes**), and very rich in **tocopherols** and **tocotrienols** (**vitamin E**), and also in **chlorophyll**, giving the oil much if its green colour. They are very rich in **vitamin K**, have superb levels of **iron** and excellent quantities of **zinc, phosphates, magnesium** and **manganese. Squalene** is abundant in pumpkin seeds, as are **phytosterols**. The flesh of both pumpkin and squash is wonderfully rich in **carotenoids** – one serving providing >200% of the RDA – which includes β-**carotene**, **lutein, zeaxanthin** and **cryptoxanthin**. The low GI means pumpkin and squash are excellent for those on diets.

> Pumpkin seeds are wonderful for all, but particularly for men.

What they do

Squalene, found within the seeds (and also in shark's liver – though pumpkin seeds must surely be a preferable source), is a powerful antioxidant and is used to boost the immune system, to treat hypertension and metabolic disorders, skin problems and is a skin softener. As a food, squalene and the tocotrienols (vitamin E) significantly decrease serum-cholesterol levels. They improve the health of cell membranes, resulting in reduced blood pressure, and are therefore a good food for those with cardiovascular disease.

The seeds' high zinc and magnesium levels seem to help men with prostate problems – men in eastern Europe have long eaten the seeds and have virtually no prostate disease. In Germany, it was found that the raw seeds stimulate sex-hormone production, so eating a few raw seeds a day may help prevent impotence. The seed oil also inhibits development of testosterone-induced hyperplasia (a type of blockage) of the prostate.

Historically, in South America, the seeds were used to eradicate internal parasites. This usage has now been confirmed – the compounds responsible for this are non-toxic to humans, but toxic to parasites. They are also being investigated for their ability to inhibit certain cancer types (e.g. prostate).

The indigenous people of North America used the macerated seeds successfully on wounds and burns – their oils, vitamin E content and their high zinc levels are probable candidates for their efficacy. The oil would make a good skin moisturiser and conditioner. Their rich iron content helps build muscle and is crucial for red blood-cell formation.

Pumpkin and squash's rich vitamin A content improve night vision and their flesh helps relieve nausea and motion sickness.

How they are used

Pumpkin and squash flesh can be roasted or baked to give it a pleasant, nutty flavour and then added to soups, stews and pies. It is popular added to salads and antipasto dishes. It blends well with nuts and cheese. The cooked flesh is used in dessert and cake mixes. Spaghetti squash is used as a pasta substitute and can be added to salads; it goes well with coconut cream in sweet dessert pies.

The seeds of many pumpkin species are edible and very nutritious. However, several varieties have been selected to produce larger yields of oil-rich seeds, which have reduced or no hulls, thus making preparation easy. The seeds are used in salads, breads, cakes and trail mixes, or are eaten as a snack – raw, roasted or fried. When toasted, the seeds develop a nutty, spicy aroma and taste. Lightly toast pumpkin and sunflower seeds and add a sprinkle of tamari to make a delicious snack. The seeds are also used in confectionery and desserts. In South America, the roasted seeds are mixed with syrup to make a confection. The seeds may be ground to a flour and then added to breakfast cereals and are delicious added to bread mixes.

> Its mild flavour mixes well with many foods, such as garlic, onion, sun-dried tomato, brassicas and a range of herbs and spices (e.g. cinnamon, ginger, nutmeg, fennel, thyme, rosemary).

The oil extracted from the seeds is dark green and has a strong, distinctive flavour which is not unlike dark sesame oil. It is more usually used in dressings or where a strong flavour is required. It can be used to flavour breads, or is added to stews or soups, just before serving. A tasty salad dressing can be made by mixing pumpkin seed oil with vinegar, salt and garlic. This dressing goes well on a salad of beans, potatoes, onions, garlic and tomatoes. High-heat cooking will damage its flavour. Pumpkin flowers make a colourful, edible garnish.

Purslane

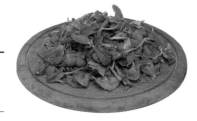

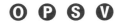

From the Middle East to eastern Asia purslane was a widely cultivated and important crop grown for food and for its medicinal properties. It was particularly popular among Arabs, who seem to have taken it to Spain, where it became naturalised. It was more popular in the United Kingdom and Europe in times past, and was used in salads and stews. Although now more usually considered a weed, the tasty succulent leaves and seeds of purslane are tremendously nutrient rich. Fortunately, it is now being rediscovered, and is often found for sale at farmers' markets or in people's home gardens.

What it contains

The leaves are rich in **carotenoids**, have some **vitamin C** (~10 mg/100 g) and are rich in **flavonoids** (e.g. **anthocyanins**) and **phytosterols**. The seeds are very rich in health-promoting **omega-3 alpha-linolenic acid**, with possibly a greater amount than any other plant. The oil is extracted and sold as a health product. The seeds also contain ~20% of good-quality protein, and **all the essential amino acids**.

What it does

Omega-3 oils are very important in reducing serum LDL cholesterol, raising HDLs and reducing the risk of various cardiovascular diseases. It has been estimated that the likelihood of cardiac death is reduced by up to an amazing 70% in those who eat diets rich in omega-3 oils. These oils also have neuroprotective properties and may reduce disorders such as depression, Alzheimer's disease, autism and schizophrenia. Omega-3 oils are also associated with reducing the incidence of some types of cancer (e.g. colon). The phytosterols significantly reduce serum LDLs and total cholesterol levels (though not HDLs), therefore reducing the development of cardiovascular disease and stroke.

The leaves' powerful antioxidants work alongside vitamin C in the body to prevent damage to cells by free radicals and the formation of some cancers. Historically, the plant was used for its soothing, mucilaginous properties. Its high mucilage content has an emollient and soothing effect on the digestive system, regulating bowel movements, reducing constipation, relieving the symptoms of irritable-bowel syndrome and healing and inhibiting gastric ulcers. Other compounds within purslane add to its benefits on the digestive system by relaxing smooth muscle.

Historically, purslane was used to reduce bladder and urinary tract problems, as an anti-inflammatory and as an eye wash. Recent research confirms its topical efficacy as an anti-inflammatory and analgesic, even when compared with some pharmaceutical drugs. It was used to relive respiratory distress and recent research has confirmed that purslane can indeed reduce the severity of asthma attacks.

> Allantoin, found within purslane, is known to heal wounds, stimulate the growth of healthy tissue and reduce skin irritations. It is used in anti-acne creams, toothpaste, mouthwash and shampoo.

Warning: Purslane leaves contain high amounts of oxalic acid, so should not be consumed in quantity by those with gout, kidney stones or rheumatism.

How it is used

The leaves are crisp, yet juicy and cooling. Young leaves and stems are added to salads and can be used instead of cucumber. When cooked the leaves become mucilaginous and are added to stews and soups. Younger leaves can be added to flans, omelettes, pies, sauces, etc., or can be lightly stir-fried with garlic and butter. In France, they are combined with sorrel to make a soup. The thick stems can be pickled in salt and vinegar for winter salads. The seeds can be ground to make flour. The oil is very nutritious and makes a good cooking and dressing oil, though should not be overheated. Its high omega-3 content means it is best used when fresh – it becomes rancid fairly quickly.

> 🐾 Charles II is believed to have enjoyed a salad prepared with purslane, lettuce, chervil, borage flowers and marigold petals, dressed with oil and lemon juice.

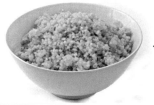

Quinoa

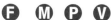

Quinoa (pronounced 'keen-wa') has recently gained popularity for its tasty and nutritional seeds, which make a good substitute for rice or bulgar wheat. Although a grain, it is not a cereal but is more closely related to spinach and buckwheat. It originates from South America and many varieties exist, though there are two main types: white-grained and red-grained quinoa.

What it contains

Quinoa has excellent **protein** content (10–18%). It contains **all the essential amino acids**, it contains more **lysine** than cereals, and is rich in **methionine** and **cysteine**, which are deficient in legumes. Quinoa protein is as digestible as other high-quality food proteins and is as or more nutritious than milk solids. The grain is rich in **fibre** (~10%), much of which is **insoluble**, which is excellent for the digestive system. It is also rich in **B vitamins**, particularly **riboflavin**, but also **niacin, thiamine, B6** and **folate**. It is very rich in the **minerals manganese** and **potassium** and also **iron** (a serving supplying ~80% RDA) and **calcium**. It also contains **magnesium, phosphorus, copper** and **zinc**. It has a variable **oil** content (2–10%), which is a balanced ratio of **omega-6, omega-3** and monounsaturated oils. It is rich in **amylose** (~20% of the starch), which makes this grain easy to digest, and contains **saponins**. It does not contain gluten, so makes a good grain substitute for those with gluten allergies. The leaves are edible, have good amounts of protein and are low in oxalic acid.

Because it is rich in protein, containing a wonderful balance of amino acids, it is a popular choice for vegetarians and is a good muscle-building and energy-producing food.

What it does

Quinoa is an excellent grain for those with cereal allergies and an interesting alternative to the usual carbohydrates. Quinoa contains more minerals than most other grains. Its B vitamins help build and maintain neuronal and muscular transmission, including in the heart and digestive system, enhance energy use, help make DNA and RNA, improve eyesight, help reduce depression and the incidence of neurodegenerative diseases, reduce the risk of cancer and of birth defects. B vitamins stave off age-related health disorders.

Historically, quinoa extracts were used as a topical antiseptic and to promote healing. The whole plant has anti-inflammatory properties and has been used to ease toothache. Saponins from quinoa are used to produce pharma-ceutical steroids, and saponins from yellow quinoa are also used in soaps, shampoos and in beer production.

Warning: The outer seed coat contains saponins – bitter quinoa is so called because of its high saponin content, whereas sweet quinoa contains much less. Although saponins can cause intestinal irritation and reduce the absorption of nutrients, virtually all can be removed by thoroughly washing de-hulled seeds in warm water before cooking.

How it is used

Quinoa's young leaves, which taste similar to beet leaves, can be lightly steamed or added fresh to salads. The cooked grain has a mild, nutty taste and can be used instead of rice. Like many grains, its flavour is enhanced by toasting in a dry pan for about 5 minutes. Cooked, the grain remains fluffy within, and enjoyably chewy and crunchy in its outer layers. It needs 10–15 minutes' cooking and is best not overcooked. Cooking in liquid triples its size and this high absorbency means it's great cooked in stock or used in risotto-type recipes.

Quinoa's mild flavour mixes well with both sweet and savoury dishes – it can be made into a sweet pudding or be added to soups, stews, pastas. It mixes well with Asian-type recipes with soy, garlic, ginger and onion. Quinoa combines readily with many vegetables (e.g. spinach, aubergine, tomatoes, peppers) and a range of herbs and spices.

🐾 Quinoa can be used to make tabbouleh with parsley, onion, olives, tomatoes and pinenuts, or can be bound with onion, herbs, smoked fish and egg to make delicious fish cakes.

The grain can be puffed and used as a breakfast food, and the flour, mixed with other flour types, can be made into tortillas, pancakes, breads, pastas, cakes, biscuits. However, gluten-containing flours need to be added to make bread rise. The grain is used to make a beverage as well as alcohol.

Raspberries

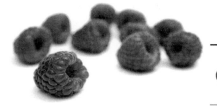

Wonderful, luscious raspberries can be grown from warmer Mediterranean regions to as far north as Iceland. Although usually a rich red colour, a few raspberry cultivars have yellow, black or light-red fruits. They have a fabulous, succulent, rich taste and a heavenly aroma – their flavours and nutritional value are hard to beat. Thimbleberries, very similar to raspberries, are native to the north-west of North America and have elongated, tasty, similarly nutritious fruits.

What they contain

Contain good quantities of **vitamin C** (25–30 mg/100 g) and are rich in secondary plant compounds – they probably have the highest amount of **ellagic acid** of any fruit. They are also rich in other **flavonoids** (e.g. **anthocyanins**, **proanthocyanins**) and **organic acids** and contain good amounts of **fibre**, much as **fermentable pectin**, and **vitamins K** and **E**.

What they do

Ellagic acid is an anticarcinogen and anti-mutagen. It has been clinically proven to cause the death of some types of cancer cells. It is readily absorbed by the body and retains its potency after heating, freezing and processing.

In rats, raspberries reduced oestrogenically produced mammary cancer volumes by 75% and their cell multiplication by 44%. Its compounds can inhibit the formation and growth of colorectal, mouth and prostate cancer cells. The anti-cancer properties of raspberries particularly apply to black fruits – the darker the berry, the better.

Raspberry's rich pectin content may be partially responsible for their effective inhibition of LDL formation, which helps reduce the risk of cardiovascular disease. Its ellagic acid also helps maintain the health and elasticity of connective tissue and vessels. Its pectins reduce blood-sugar levels and help with insulin control, so are useful in the management and prevention of type-2 diabetes. Raspberries also contain a compound that increases the breakdown of fats, so may even help with weight loss. A tea made from their leaves has long been used by pregnant women to reduce miscarriage, ease childbirth, improve lactation and alleviate heavy menstruation.

How they are used

Raspberries are wonderful just eaten fresh with cream or yoghurt and a sprinkle of brown sugar. They can be added to pies, desserts, fruit salads, sauces (for sweet and savoury dishes), made into a wonderful jam and can be added to ice cream, cheesecake and fruit fools. Imagine a mix of raspberries, chopped nuts, dark chocolate, amaretto and creamy yoghurt! Raspberries are delicious in pancakes with maple syrup and cream. As a sauce or puréed, they can enhance chicken and meat recipes. Raspberry vinegar can be made from the fruit by adding sugar and white wine, and they also make a good wine. Thimbleberries have a sweet, pleasant taste and are good for jellies, jams and preserves. They can also be dried.

> 🌿 Mix raspberries, papaya, kiwifruit and the juice and seeds from a passion fruit, sprinkle with chopped hazelnuts and a drizzle with coconut cream.

Rice

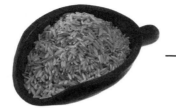

Rice is the world's second most important food crop (after wheat), and has been cultivated for thousands of years in Asia. Although there are more than 8000 varieties, there are only two main species of rice, with *Oryza sativa* being the most common. Most rice is grown in Asia, India and China, with approximately 300 million acres grown worldwide. It is also an important food in South America.

What it contains

Brown, unpolished rice (which still has its bran) is much more nutritious than white rice. Brown rice contains fibre, most as **fermentable fibre**, which has numerous nutritional benefits. It contains some **protein** (but is low in lysine), and has a low GI. Rice bran, consisting of the seed coat and embryo, is rich in **fibre** (~20%) and contains ~14% **protein**. It contains wonderful levels of the **B vitamins**, particularly **thiamine, niacin, pantothenic acid** and **B6**. Similarly, it is incredibly rich in **manganese, iron** and **magnesium**, with good amounts of **zinc, copper, potassium** and **selenium**. Brown rice, but particularly rice bran, is rich in **phytosterols, vitamin E (tocotrienols** and **tocopherols)**, and is rich in **ferulic acid**. White rice has a higher GI of 30, less fibre and protein and lower levels of B vitamins (hence the occurrence of beriberi in some Asian communities that eat predominantly white rice). White rice is often sold fortified with added minerals, etc.

What it does

Antioxidants within brown rice can reduce the formation of some cancers (e.g. mouth, colon, breast, liver), possibly due to its ferulic acid content. Rice bran can reduce bladder cancer in mice, particularly if fermented with *Aspergillus oryzae*. Research is ongoing into these fermented compounds for their use in cancer treatments.

In humans, brown rice, particularly its bran and oil, can reduce total plasma cholesterol and triglycerides and increase HDL levels; it can lower LDL levels in plasma more than most other vegetables. Rice bran also lowers blood pressure, inhibits production of blood clots and helps control glucose levels. These activities and the lower GI of brown rice, bran and brown rice flour result in reduced risk of cardiovascular disease compared with diets high in white rice.

Brown rice has been added to the FDA-approved list of whole grains that reduce the risk of heart disease and some cancers.

Rice bran is particularly rich in tocotrienols (vitamin E) – less common in foods compared to tocopherols – these lower serum-cholesterol, has neuroprotective properties, reduces the incidence of stroke-associated brain damage and has anti-cancer properties. Bran also contains oryzanol, which modulates pituitary secretion and inhibits gastric acid secretions.

Brown rice is gluten free, so can be eaten by those with allergies; however, most processed white rice has been coated with substances to refortify them. These are said not to include wheat products, but it is best to check anyway.

How it is used

There are many types of rice, including short grained (used for desserts, cakes, soups); medium grained (great for paella and risotto); long grained (popular in curries and Asian dishes); glutinous rice, which has more sugar and less starch (used in sticky desserts); aromatic Basmati (mostly from India) and Jasmine varieties. Many can be purchased as either brown or white rice.

🦐 To gain even more of brown rice's nutrients, soak it for ~20 hours in warm water (38°C) prior to cooking. This activates the germination enzymes that boost the range and amount of its nutrients, particularly ferulic acid and gamma-aminobutyric acid (GABA). This latter compound acts as an important neurotransmitter in the brain, improving neuronal communication and reducing anxiety, improving sleep and reducing blood pressure.

Rice is often the main ingredient in many people's diets, accompanied by vegetables, a few small pieces of meat or fish and various flavourings, such as soy, chilli and garlic. It is added to soups and stews, and mixes well with chicken, seafood and fish. A multitude of herbs and spices can be added to rice, as can citrus juices and peel. Rice is a part of many breakfast cereals, confectionery products and desserts. It is used to make beer and is distilled to make saki.

Rice is usually simply boiled until soft, but before it becomes mushy or sticky (except for sticky rice). In Indian cuisine, rice may be pre-fried in oil with spices before boiling to add flavour.

Like all grains and nuts, poorly stored, damp, cooked or uncooked grains can be become contaminated with toxic organisms. Quickly cooling cooked rice before putting it in the fridge significantly reduces any risk of contamination and means that it can then be stored for several days – don't let it sit around for hours before chilling.

Rocket
(arugula)

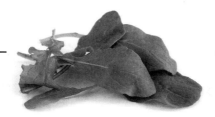

Ⓢ Ⓥ

A member of the brassica family, rocket's tasty leaves have a great flavour, which many prefer to lettuce, and are rich in nutrients. There are two main types: the more commercial *Eruca vesicaria*, and wild rocket (also called perennial wall rocket: *Diplotaxis tenuifolia*). The latter is more popular with some due its stronger flavour and greater quantity of nutrients.

What it contains

The leaves contain excellent amounts of **carotenoids** (as β-**carotene**, but mainly **lutein** and **zeaxanthin**), some **vitamin C** (~15 mg/100 g – wild rocket contains more) and **fibre**. It is also very rich in bone-enhancing **vitamin K**, with some **folate**. Rocket also contains abundant antioxidant **flavonoids** and, like all brassicas, is rich in **isothiocyanates**.

What it does

Isothiocyanates have significant anti-cancer activities and also possess anti-inflammatory and cholesterol-lowering properties. Ingestion of isothiocyanates is inversely correlated with the incidence of cancer – they are virtually proven to reduce the risk of the development and spread of several types of cancer, including skin, lung, bladder, colon and prostate. They induce enzymes that repair damaged DNA. Because these compounds are nullified by extensive cooking, eating rocket fresh in a salad promotes their full benefits.

Carotenoids also have anti-cancer properties, help reduce age-related degenerative eye disorders and are beneficial in reducing cardiovascular diseases. Rocket's rich vitamin K content encourages healthy bone formation, which benefits both young and older people.

How it is used

Rocket leaves have a fresh, peppery, mild watercress-like flavour and are popular in salads. They are also added to pasta and rice dishes just before serving, or older leaves are added to soups, stews, curries and go well with potatoes. In Italy, rocket leaves are added to a

🌿 Rocket leaves liven up a salad: some people like them on their own with a dribble of olive oil and balsamic vinegar, or perhaps also with a crumble of feta cheese or slice or two of salami.

savoury sauce with a little sugar or honey, vinegar and eaten with toasted bread. They are also used in pesto. The flower heads are edible and they make an attractive garnish. The seeds and pods can be prepared as a spicy, peppery garnish: although hot, they are less so than mustard seeds.

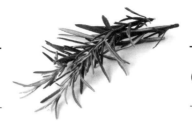

Rosemary

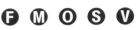

Related to sage, thyme and the mints, rosemary has been a popular herb across southern Europe for thousands of years. It has long been valued to flavour foods, but also for its many medicinal properties. Recent research has discovered new powerful benefits.

What it contains

Fresh rosemary is rich in **fibre** (~15%), and contains good amounts of **minerals** (particularly **iron**), and **vitamin C** (~22 mg/100 g), **vitamin A** and **folate**. It is rich in oil (~30%), containing lots of **omega-3** and **omega-6** oils. Rosemary is very rich in **terpenes** (e.g. **carnosol**), which are powerful antioxidants and anti-inflammatories. **Rosmarinic acid** is also abundant.

Rosemary's antiseptic properties and its oils have long made it a popular ingredient in shampoos. It has a wonderful fragrance, gives hair shine, treats dandruff, strengthens the hair and may slow hair loss and greying.

What it does

Leaf extracts significantly reduce the incidence and number of cancerous skin tumours in mice by 45–60%, reduce the incidence of colon and breast cancers in mice, and reduce cancer in human bronchial cells. Its terpenes are particularly effective. They also reduce skin damage caused by UV light and other factors.

Rosemary's terpenes (like those in its close relatives, such as sage, thyme) inhibit processes that break down bone. They lead to an increase in bone-mineral density, so are potentially useful to those concerned about osteoporosis. Rosmarinic acid has potential to treat or prevent bronchial asthma, peptic ulcers, inflammatory diseases, liver toxicity, cataracts and poor sperm motility. Rosemary is also an effective anti-thrombotic, thus reducing the risk of cardiovascular disease.

Its terpenes have strong anti-inflammatory and antimicrobial activities – they have a synergistic effect when taken with the antibiotic gentamicin. The leaves' antiseptic properties are used as a mouthwash and to clean wounds. Topical application of the oil is effective at reducing the herpes simplex virus, and is an effective antibacterial which is able to treat some drug-resistant infections. It is also an antifungal. The crushed leaves and essential oil have long been known to deter insects; research has proven it to repel at least four mosquito species. Its proven antiseptic properties have also made it a useful food preservative.

The leaves and oils are added to pot-pourri and other air-freshening products. Its scent is said to stimulate memory and to induce good dreams if a sprig is placed under the pillow. The oil is used externally to relax muscle pain and stiffness, and is inhaled to relieve chest congestion and colds.

Warning: As with all essential oils, any internal usage should be done with caution.

How it is used

The leaves can be used whole or are finely chopped and added to a wide range of dishes to impart a spicy, warm flavour. It has a peppery, eucalyptus or camphor-like aroma and taste. It mixes well with green beans and tomatoes. Unlike many herbs, cooking does not destroy its flavour, so it is used to flavour meats, particularly lamb, where sprigs (often with garlic) are inserted into the joint before it is roasted. Its flavour cuts well through greasy foods. Can be added to vinegar dressings and olive oil to add flavour. Finely chopped, a little can be added to jams, biscuits or jellies and the flowers make an attractive and unusual garnish.

> 🐾 Rosemary mixes wonderfully with other herbs, such as sage and thyme, and is great in stuffing, sauces, sprinkled on potatoes with cheese and milk (and then baked), or added to vegetable stews or ratatouille. Rosemary goes well with chicken and fish, and in pasta dishes.

Rye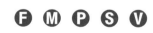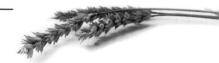

Remains of rye grains have been found in Neolithic sites in Turkey and it has been valued as a grain crop ever since. It is now often grown in cold, poorer soils where wheat struggles to survive. Though sometimes used as a whole grain or rolled, it is mostly used in bread-making and is added to other flour types. This tremendously nutritious grain is very much appreciated by the Central Europeans and Scandinavians.

What it contains

Rye grains are richer in **fibre** (~15%) than many cereals and much of this is **fermentable**. Fermentable fibre has many proven health benefits in the digestive system (dark rye flour is even richer). It has considerably greater health benefits than wheat fibre and has a low GI. Rye is also wonderfully rich in **protein** (15–20%), with good levels of **all the essential amino acids**. Is low in fat and is rich in all the **B vitamins**, including **pantothenic acid**. The grain, and particularly the dark flour, contain abundant **minerals**, particularly **manganese**, antioxidant **selenium**, **iron** (for blood and muscle health) and **zinc**, which is particularly useful to men. Rye also contains cholesterol-lowering **phytosterols**, mainly in its outer layers, and the dark flour is especially rich in **betaines**. Rye is also rich in **phyto-oestrogens** and **lignans**, and contains **choline**. All flour types retain most of the above nutrients, particularly bran-rich dark flour. Lighter rye bread, unfortunately, has lost much of its protein, fibre, minerals and vitamins.

What it does

The lignans in rye grains are more effectively converted to pre-oestrogen-like compounds in the gut than those from wheat, rice and most other cereals. These can reduce the risk of heart disease and stroke and have been shown to reduce blood cholesterol. Rye may also reduce the risk of some hormone-related cancers, such as breast cancer. Whole rye grains can reduce the risk of colon cancer, and high intake of rye bran bread has been shown to reduce human prostate cancer cells.

Its fibre significantly increases populations of 'good' gut bacteria, so prevents constipation. It is likely to reduce the development of colorectal cancers, lowers serum-cholesterol (so helping reduce the risk of cardiovascular disease) and helps reduce weight gain. Its abundant B vitamins contribute to the health and maintenance of neuronal and muscular systems, including the heart and digestive system; they also enhance energy use, help make DNA and RNA, improve eyesight, help fend off depression, reduce the development of neurodegenerative diseases and act as

Germinating and/ or fermenting (as in sour dough) rye grains increases their vitamin B levels, particularly folate, and subsequent cooking retains much of this value. This process also increases amounts of several other nutrients.

anticarcinogens. Dieticians recommend including more B vitamins in the diets of older people to stave off age-related disorders.

The grains are rich in antioxidants and these are more effective in rye breads than in most wheat breads. Rye bread also enhances early insulin secretion in people susceptible to deteriorating glucose tolerance and development of type-2 diabetes, which slows the onset of this disease.

Warning: Rye does contain some gluten, though not as much as wheat. It can cause adverse reactions in those who are sensitive or allergic.

How it is used

The seed can be sprouted and used in salads. It is then highly nutritious. It can be cooked, like rice, but does need at least 40 minutes and even then is quite chewy. Pre-soaking can reduce cooking time. The cooked grain has a pleasant nutty taste. Cooked, it can be mixed with other grains, or added to salads, soups and stews. The grain can be rolled like oats, and then added to muesli, cereal bars, cakes, muffins, bread, etc. Rye can be ground to make flour, which is very popular in some European (particularly German) breads. It gives a rich, fruity, distinctive taste, though the bread is generally heavier than wheat bread due to its lower gluten content; it is often mixed with wheat flour at a 1:3 mix. Rye flour can be made into crisp biscuits for cheese and pickles. Rye is also used to make alcohol (e.g. rye whiskey, beer and vodka). For beer, the seed is sprouted, like barley, and the sweet extract is separated out from the roasted grain.

> 🌾 Rye flour comes in three colours: dark, medium or light, depending on how much bran has been removed, with pumpernickel rye flour being the darkest, coarsest and strongest tasting, but also the most nutritious.

Safflower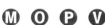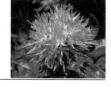

(false saffron, American saffron)

A member of the sunflower family, this plant has been utilised for thousands of years in China, India, the Middle East and Egypt. Deep yellow, to orange, to red, its dyes have long been used to colour foods and fabrics and often as a substitute for saffron. More recently, safflower seed oil has become popular – it is very rich in polyunsaturates and it has excellent culinary properties. It is most popular in Japan; in China, it is mostly grown for its medicinal properties; and a little is used in North America.

What it contains

Safflower oil is very rich in **essential unsaturated fatty acids**. Some safflower varieties are rich in **monounsaturates** (e.g. ~30% **oleic acid**), others in **polyunsaturates** (e.g. ~60% **omega-6 linoleic acid**). Has less omega-3s. Is very rich in powerful antioxidant **vitamin E**, which enhances the immune system and has cardio-protective properties; it also inhibits oils from becoming rancid. The unprocessed seeds contain good amounts of cholesterol-lowering **phytosterols** and **phyto-oestrogen lignans**. The seeds are rich in **protein**, containing 15–20%, and are wonderfully rich in all the **B vitamins**, including **B6** and **folate**. They also contain good amounts of **magnesium, copper, phosphates, zinc, iron** and **manganese**. They are also rich in serotonin-like compounds, i.e. a derivative of **ferulic acid**. The flowers are rich in **coumarins** and **flavonoids** (**apigenin** and **kaempferol**), and the leaves are rich in the flavonoids **luteolin** and **quercetin**.

What it does

Its high unsaturated oils reduce serum-cholesterol, so reduce development of cardiovascular disease. Monounsaturated oils also reduce LDLs, and raise beneficial HDLs. Compounds within the flowers significantly reduce thrombosis by extending coagulation time. Its serotonin-like compounds also have powerful atherosclerosis properties. These compounds have skin-whitening properties which work by inhibiting melanin formation.

Research shows that safflower seeds contain a phyto-oestrogen lignan that has an anti-oestrogen activity equivalent to tamoxifen. The seeds also positively affect bone formation, so are likely to be useful in treating diseases such as osteoporosis. The leaves are used as a tea in the Middle East to prevent miscarriage and to treat infertility.

Safflower seeds have antibiotic and antiviral activities – they have been traditionally used in conjunction with other herbs to treat hepatitis C and are being investigated for the treatment of HIV.

✿ Safflower oil is light in flavour and colour (is similar to sunflower oil), and its delicate flavour works well in many foods, including dressings and in general cooking. It is more heat stable than many oils, not emitting smoke or odours at high heat, and its consistency does not change at low temperatures.

The non-allergenic oil is used topically to treat rheumatism, sprains and sores, and is included in cosmetics.

How it is used

Young leaves can be eaten fresh in salads or can be lightly steamed. Safflower seeds, similar to those of sunflower, are tasty and can be gently roasted, fried or used fresh in salads, etc. The colouring extracted from its flowers may be used as a substitute for saffron and is used to colour many foods, including cheese, sausages, pickles, breads.

Sage

Sage species are closely related to mint, rosemary and thyme, and most originate from the Mediterranean and Middle East. Historically, a highly revered and widely used herb, its common name is an indicator of its traditional usage, being thought to promote long life and wisdom. Its genus name, *Salvia*, means health and salvation. The leaves have long been used as a culinary herb in Europe and, in the East, are included within traditional Chinese remedies.

What it contains

Sage leaves are rich in **essential oils** and many **phenolic** and **terpene compounds**. It is very rich in **antioxidants**. Sage species contain the following: **rosmarinic acid, cineol, camphor, borneol** and **thujone**. The leaves also contain **phyto-oestrogenic-like compounds**.

What it does

Sage has significant antiviral, antibacterial, anti-inflammatory and anti-oxidant properties. As an antiviral, applied topically, sage effectively treats the herpes virus, and a mix of sage, peppermint and lemon balm reduces the infectivity of HIV-1 virions at concentrations that are not toxic to cells. This combination is also likely to be effective against other viruses. Extracts from *S. sclarea* have shown promise in treating human cancers, especially drug-resistant cases. Its powerful antioxidant potential has been shown, in an animal model, to improve liver health – the treatment of various liver diseases has long been a medicinal use of this plant.

Sage leaves were thought to promote wisdom and health. A promising recent finding is that S. *officinalis* extracts show efficacy in relieving symptoms of mild to moderate Alzheimer's disease and help reduce agitation. It has been shown to increase the memory and concentration of both young and older human subjects. Sage tea is drunk to help relieve stress headaches.

Sage's oestrogen-like compounds can help relieve menopausal symptoms, particularly hot flushes, and help with menstrual problems. It is used as a mouthwash and to treat sore throats and mouth ulcers. The leaves are excellent in toothpaste, with their abrasive properties stimulating the gums and their antiseptic properties reducing populations of acid-forming bacteria; it is therefore effective in combating periodontal disease. The purple-leaved species are said to have the most powerful medicinal properties. Sage-leaf extracts are used in skin creams and to scent cosmetics and room fresheners. They also make a good hair conditioner. When ingested the rosmarinic acid in sage can reduce perspiration.

Warning: The leaves should not be consumed excessively during pregnancy.

How it is used

Sage mixes well with apple, pumpkin, celery, beans and lentils, Jerusalem artichokes, citrus zest, onions and garlic.

Sage leaves, particularly when fresh, have a strong, camphor-like taste and so should be used in moderation or they can overpower other flavours. Young leaves are usually chopped finely for use. They are popularly and traditionally incorporated into stuffing, often with thyme, rosemary and onion, and are a popular ingredient in sausages. Is delicious as a garnish with white cheese, sun-dried tomatoes and olives on fresh, warm bread. A tea is made from the dried leaves. The leaves can be added to vinegar or olive oil dressings to impart flavour and attractiveness. The flowers are used as a garnish.

A less common but important sage species is chia (*S. hispanica*), which has great potential as a future crop. Its oily seeds, though small, are richer in omega-3 fatty acids than virtually all other plant foods. Native to Mexico, it was important to the Aztecs, and is now being 'rediscovered'. The seed is added to a variety of dishes: it may be crushed (pinole) and added to breads, desserts and cakes, or made into porridge. The seeds are popular sprouted and used in salads and they have a spicy flavour, so are best mixed with milder-flavoured seeds (e.g. alfalfa). They can be soaked in fruit juice or water, which makes them become gelatinous. The juice is popular in Mexico. Their high affinity to absorb moisture has many digestive benefits. The seeds are also rich in protein and contain antioxidants. Research shows the seeds have no known toxic components.

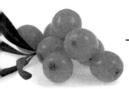

Sea buckthorn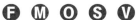

Native to China, Mongolia, Russia and northern Europe, sea buckthorn has long been valued for its juicy, orange-red berries. Recently, the berries have become of interest to many researchers around the world for their potential nutritional and medicinal benefits. The Russians started investigating substances found in the berries, leaves and bark in the 1940s. Since 1982, many hectares have been planted in China, along with 150 processing factories producing >200 products.

What it contains

The fruits are very nutritious and rich in vitamins. The flesh is rich in **organic acids** and is acidic, containing abundant **vitamin C** (200–400 mg/100 g, with some reporting 800 mg/100 g), which is much higher than most fruits. They contain good amounts of **soluble fibre**. The seeds and flesh also contain good quantities of unsaturated oil, which is an excellent balance of **omega-6 linoleic** and **omega-3 linolenic acids** (and a little **oleic acid**). The fruits are also rich in cholesterol-lowering **phytosterols** and are very rich in antioxidant **vitamin E**. The seed oil has good quantities of **carotenoids**. Sea buckthorn fruits are rich in **flavonoids** (e.g. **kaempferol**, **quercetin**), particularly **anthocyanins** and several **terpenes**. The dried berries are **rich in potassium, calcium** and **iron**.

What it does

Regular consumption of sea buckthorn berries can prevent cancer and larger quantities may even reverse the growth of some tumours. The fruits have been recommended to be added (with other highly nutritious foods) to the diets of those with serious medical conditions (e.g. breast cancer) to lower the high oxidative stress these patients experience.

The oil has anti-inflammatory, antimicrobial and analgesic properties and can promote regeneration of tissues. It has been used externally to treat mucous glands within the mouth, rectum and vagina, but also radiation damage, burns, scalds, ulcers, chilblains, to reduce scarring and other skin damage. It has significant cardiovascular-protective activity – it lowers LDLs and raises HDLs within plasma and increases the suppleness of blood vessels. In cholesterol-fed rats, it returned values to normal. The fruits are also used to treat liver problems.

More than ten different drugs have been developed from sea buckthorn in Asia and Europe and are available in different forms. The oil is used in cosmetics to soften and enhance skin quality.

Sea buckthorn fruits are highly regarded nutritionally and medicinally in Russia and China. Look out for the juice in health stores.

How it is used

Its fruits, although somewhat sour in flavour, can be eaten fresh. They are added to sauces, mixed with other sweeter fruits and are used to make jams, preserves, confectionery, salad dressing and wine. They freeze well. Blended with other fruits they make a pleasant aromatic juice. In this form it is marketed for its significant health benefits. The juice is also added to liqueurs and cocktails.

Seaweeds

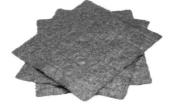

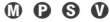

Seaweeds can be divided into three groups dependent on colour: green, brown and red. Edible seaweeds are very popular in Asia and particularly in Japanese cuisine, where they have been used as a food for at least 2500 years. About 21 seaweed species are widely utilised in Chinese, Korean and Southeast Asian cuisines. In Japan, the estimated total annual production of nori alone is >US$1 billion, making it one of the most valuable aquacrops worldwide. Seaweed accounts for ~10% of the Japanese diet. The three most popular species are nori (*Porphyra* spp., red seaweeds), kombu (*Laminaria* spp., brown seaweeds) and wakame (*Undaria* spp., brown seaweeds). Edible seaweed has also a long and traditional usage in other parts of the world: the Welsh have long eaten seaweed and it is still sold as laverbread. The Scots and Irish also appreciate seaweed. Similarly, in other countries in far-north latitudes, which have long, dark winters and a scarcity of fresh vegetables, seaweeds can be an important part of the diet.

What they contain

Seaweeds are a very important source of **iodine**, containing more than any other food. They also contain lots of **iron**, **calcium**, sometimes **magnesium** and also sodium. Kelp is very rich in **vitamin K** and most types are very rich in **folate**. Laver seaweed, in particular, is rich in **carotenoids** (as fucoxanthin). Nori is rich in **protein** (~25% dry weight) and rich in **vitamin C**, containing more than oranges. Some types (e.g. mekuba, hijiki) are rich in **phyto-oestrogens**. Seaweed has good amounts of the amino acid **taurine**. Hiziki is rich in minerals, particularly **calcium**, containing ~14 times more than cow's milk. Brown seaweeds, in particular, are rich in **fucoidan** (a compound similar to chondroitin), which has numerous health benefits. They are very low in calories.

What they do

Edible brown kelps (e.g. *Fucus* spp., bladderwrack), in particular, have been found to prolong the length of the menstrual cycle and exert anti-oestrogenic effects in pre-menopausal women. Seaweed may be an important dietary component partially responsible for the reduced risk of oestrogen-related cancers observed in Japanese women. It may also reduce the pain caused by endometriosis.

Seaweeds can inhibit intestinal tumour formation. Fucoidan reduces oxidative damage to mitochondria, which is a major cause of cancer formation and can induce cell death of some human cancer cells (e.g. leukaemia). It may prevent infection by prion diseases (e.g. scrapie). It helps protect the liver from disease and oxidative damage.

Taurine can reduce development of gallstones and helps control serum-cholesterol levels. It may also reduce liver damage caused by excess alcohol by reducing the build-up of fat around this organ and for similar reasons it helps manage obesity. In addition, brown seaweeds can enhance the breakdown of white adipose storage fats – fucoxanthin, a carotenoid, may be partially responsible for this. This carotenoid also reduces blood- glucose and plasma insulin levels, and increases levels of beneficial polyunsaturated fatty acids, so may inhibit development of type-2 diabetes and cardiovascular disease.

Seaweed extracts are added to cosmetics to rejuvenate and moisturise the skin. Through Edwardian and Victorian times seaweed baths were a popular therapy, often located in the coastal spa towns of Britain. Seaweed (bladderwrack) was heated with hot water in a bath. The heat releases gel-like alginates, as well as minerals, and these are thought to be very therapeutic, particularly for relieving arthritis, rheumatism and similar conditions. Medicinally, alginates are used in wound dressings and other products.

Warning: Some seaweeds, depending on where they are grown, accumulate high levels of heavy metals (e.g. arsenic). If possible, check where and how they have been sourced.

How they are used

No seaweeds are known to be toxic, though some may be very tough and rubbery to eat! Kombu, popular in Japan, China and Korea, is used in various fish and meat dishes, in soups, as a vegetable with rice, and is added to bean dishes to make them more flavourful and easier to digest.

Seaweeds, particularly the denser kelps (e.g. wakame), are pre-soaked before being used. Wakame soup is served with miso and is served at virtually every Japanese meal. Wakame is also toasted, added to rice dishes, is used in sunomono salads, or can be coated in sugar and then tinned. Nori sheets are typically flaked and added to sauces and soups or are used to wrap sushi. Nori may also be simply soaked and eaten as a snack and is often added to crackers and biscuits. Hiziki needs >4 hours' cooking in a pressure cooker after which it develops an astringent, but nutty, flavour.

Laverbread is made from well-cooked *Porphyra* species, which become dark green and like pâté in consistency. It is traditionally served with toast and local seafoods, such as cockles. It is now becoming re-popularised and may even be served in pastas or within a spicy batter.

Apart from its usual edible uses, seaweeds are also important for their agar, alginate and carrageen contents. These gelatinous substances are used as thickeners, emulsifiers, food additives and to retain moisture in foods. Agar is used in a range of foods as a moulding agent. Carrageen and alginates are used to thicken salad dressings and sauces and as a preservative in meat and fish products, dairy items and baked goods.

Chlorella are tiny, single-celled, simple algae that have been recently described as a 'super food'. The cells are especially rich in **protein** (i.e. ~45% dry weight), and this includes **all the essential amino acids**. It is also rich in other nutrients, though some say claims of its nutritional benefits may be exaggerated. Chlorella is rich in **chlorophyll** and contains ~20% unsaturated fats. It has good amounts of **vitamin C** and **vitamin E** and **all the B vitamins**. It may strengthen the immune response, and so reduce the incidence of several diseases. Some claim that it is a powerful anticarcinogen.

Sesame seed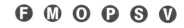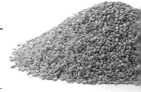

Sesame seeds are popular throughout the Near, Middle and Far East. The crushed seeds are often added to breads, made into sauces and added to desserts. The rich, distinctive oil is used in numerous dishes as well as cosmetically. There are many sesame varieties, which are often referred to in terms of their colour: white, red or black.

What it contains

The seeds have a low GI, are rich in **protein** (15–20%), with good amounts of **all the essential amino acids**. They are rich in **fibre** (~12%), and **oils** (~50%), of which most is unsaturated. They have high quantities of **monounsaturated oleic** and **omega-6 linoleic acids** and are also rich in **myristic acid**. The oil is rich in **coenzyme Q10**, a vital compound involved in energy production and a powerful antioxidant. The **B vitamins**, particularly **thiamine**, **niacin** and **B6**, are present in good quantities. The seeds boost **vitamin E**. Sesame seeds are rich in minerals, particularly **copper**, **calcium**, **iron**, **magnesium**, **manganese**, **zinc** and **phosphates**. Seeds are also very rich in **phyto-oestrogenic lignans** and quantities of these are almost as high as in linseed. They are virtually the richest food source of cholesterol-lowering **phytosterols** and contain good amounts of **lecithin** and a small amount of **saponins**.

What it does

Sesame seeds' abundant lignans are being researched for their ability to reduce hormone-related cancers. They are effectively converted to enterolactone (a pre-oestrogen). They also lower the absorption of cholesterol from the gut, as well as its production in the liver, and increase its excretion – they are effective at reducing both serum- and liver-lipid levels and thus are likely to reduce the development of cardiovascular

Human volunteers who included sesame seeds (compared to walnuts or soya beans) in their diet for a few days developed significantly increased levels of plasma gamma-tocopherol (i.e. vitamin E). This vitamin reduces ageing-related diseases such as cancer and heart disease. Eating sesame seeds boosts vitamin E status of the body, without the use of supplements, which can have detrimental side effects.

disease and stroke. These lignans are also thought to encourage fat loss, so are good for those on a diet. They also have anti-inflammatory properties that help protect the liver and reduce blood pressure. Lignans have even greater efficacy if taken with vitamin E.

Lecithin is a major source of choline, which is needed by every cell membrane in the body, particularly the brain, and is important in preventing oxidation. Choline helps reduce blood cholesterol and to digest and burn fats within the body. It is a part of a neurotransmitter that is crucial for the passage of nerve impulses, so is associated with improving mental functions.

Seeds are rich in calcium and phosphate for bone health and also in zinc, a micronutrient often deficient in the diet; and iron, which is needed for building muscles and in red blood cells.

The seeds have antibacterial and antifungal properties. The quantities of many of these active compounds (and their flavours) are greater in black than in white seeds, with red seeds being intermediate. Sesame oil and de-hulled seeds lack most vitamins (except for vitamin K) and minerals, because these are removed with the seed coat.

Sesame oil is readily absorbed by skin and is widely used in moisturisers and other skin-protection products. It is added to soaps and massage oils, and to hair conditioners to make the hair shine. It is said to reduce UV damage to hair and skin.

Warning: A few people are allergic to sesame seeds.

How it is used

The seeds can be sprouted and used in salads. More usually, the seeds are added whole, crushed or ground to breads, pastries, confectionery (including many health bars), to cereals and are sprinkled into stir-fry dishes, curries and soups. Whole seeds may be pressed into the outer layer of buns and breads. White sesame seeds are more popular than black seeds in the West, though they have a blander flavour. In Greece, the roasted seeds are mixed with honey to make a tasty snack. The seeds can be crushed and mixed with honey and pecan nuts to make delicious halva. The seeds are also used in sweets, desserts and ice cream, and are the main ingredient in tahini, which is used to make the Middle Eastern dip hummus. The oil is prepared in several ways and this affects its taste. Some oil is simply pressed (like virgin olive oil), and retains much of its nutrients; other oils are obtained from the remains of pressing, using heat. Unfortunately, this heat-treated oil has much less flavour and has lost most of its nutrients. If the seed is roasted before being pressed, it produces aromatic, dark, Oriental sesame oil, which has a rich, distinctive flavour – only a little is needed to impart a delicious flavour to marinades, sauces, curries, stir-fries, mayonnaise and dips. It has a nutty, warm flavour and a wonderful aroma when gently heated. It is also easy to digest.

> ✿ Sesame seeds can be roasted and/or toasted with vitamin E-rich pumpkin and sunflower seeds, plus a little soy sauce to bring out their nutty flavour, to make a delicious, nutritious snack.

Soya beans **F P S V**

(soybean)

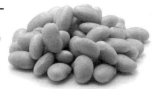

Soya beans are a major cultivated crop and this protein-rich legume is used in many foods. The Japanese, Koreans and Chinese have long used and valued soy in many preparations. The dried, mature beans are used whole, but are also used in fermented soy sauce, tempeh and miso. In addition, a few soy varieties are enjoyed as young green beans, particularly in Japan, cooked still in their pods (edamame). Much soy grown for human use is processed for its oil – and a great deal of it is now genetically modified.

What they contain

Dried soya beans are high in **protein** (up to ~35% – fresh beans have less) and are rich in **most essential amino acids**, though lack methionine. Soya beans also contain **lectins**, which can lower the uptake of amino acids, though these are largely deactivated by heat. The beans have a very low GI and contain good amounts of **fibre** (~7%), which is mostly **fermentable** and is beneficial to the digestive system. Contains the **B vitamins** and **choline**, plus **vitamin K**, and good amounts of **iron** and **phosphates**. The beans are rich in **saponins**, with tempeh containing even more. Soya beans are rich in **phyto-oestrogens** as **isoflavones**, and also cholesterol-lowering **phytosterols**. Soya beans contain good amounts of **coenzyme Q10**, a compound involved in energy production and a

Dark soy sauce is very rich in antioxidants and can decrease free-radical damage by 20%, reducing athero-sclerosis and cardiovascular disease, despite its high salt content.

powerful antioxidant. Cooked, edamame beans retain good quantities of **vitamin C** (30 mg/100 g), and are rich in **B vitamins**, particularly **folate**, with one serving supplying 50% of the RDA. They also contain **biotin**.

Only ~8% of the soya bean is fat and much of this can be **omega-3 β-linolenic acids**; however, genetically engineered soya beans (~80% of the world's soy) have much greater **omega-6 linoleic acid** than omega-3s (i.e. 40% linoleic and 4% omega-3 linolenic). Some nutrition-ists think this ratio has exacerbated inflammatory dis-ease. Biotech companies have engineered plants to produce less omega-3s as these reduce the oil's storage time: nutrition v. commerce.

What they do

Interest in soya beans has recently increased considerably, particularly because of their isoflavone content; these phyto-oestrogens occur at particularly high levels in this species (though do not occur in fermented soy sauce, miso, etc.). Isoflavones may help prevent several hormone-related diseases. Soya beans have become a popular dietary supplement, particularly with post-menopausal women as a possible replacement to pharmaceutical-based oestrogen therapies. Because these compounds are very similar in structure to oestrogen and bind to oestrogen receptors they may reduce the negative effects of high and fluctuating oestrogen levels within the body, which is sometimes associated with increased risk of breast cancer. Therefore, there is some evidence that isoflavones may inhibit the proliferation of breast cancer, but also stimulate bone form-ation and inhibit its resorption (thus, increasing bone mass and reducing post-menopausal bone density loss). It may also reduce the occurrence of prostate, colon, stomach and lung cancers. It is reported that eating isoflavone-rich foods while young and through adolescence does confer some protection, though only results in modest reductions in pre- and post-menopausal protection when only eaten later in adult life.

Soya beans can lower serum-cholesterol, particularly LDLs, thus reducing risk of cardiovascular disease and atherosclerosis. In addition, soya beans contain good quantities of lecithin and phytosterols, both of which significantly reduce cholesterol levels. Phytosterols improve fat assimilation, reduce cardiac disease and possibly reduce the formation of some cancers. They have been used in drugs to reduce blood pressure. Unfortunately, as they cause cloudiness, they are often removed in food processing, i.e. when clearing vegetable oils.

Soy sauce has antibacterial properties against several bacteria (e.g. *Staphylococcus aureus, Escherichia coli*). Soya bean saponins have been shown to prevent the formation and growth of human colon cancer cells.

Warning: Some suffer from flatulence after eating soya beans. Pre-cooking the beans and discarding the water can reduce this effect. These compunds are not present in fermented soy, tofu, etc. There are claims that a diet rich in soy can reduce thyroid function. In addition, fermented soy sauce can have quite high levels of tyramine, a compound that can increase blood pressure (and heart rate), and may also be associated with migraines. Also, it may be best to purchase genuine fermented soy products – a few brands of non-fermented soy sauce have been shown to contain dangerous levels of carcinogenic contaminants.

How they are used

Asian cultures have developed many ways to use soya beans, including fermenting them to make soy sauce, miso and tempeh, as well as the preparation of tofu. Fine-quality soy sauce is made by fermentation with a fungus that breaks down the beans' carbohydrates and proteins. The colour of a soy sauce depends on how long it has been aged. Cheap soy sauce is not fermented; instead, the beans are hydrolysed with colour added. Tamari sauce is brewed in a similar way to soy sauce, but it contains less or no wheat. Miso is made by fermenting rice, salt, cooked soya beans, lactic acid and yeast. Tofu is made by grinding the beans to make soy milk, which then may or may not be fermented. The 'milk' is then boiled and separated to make a curd, which is pressed into cakes. Tofu is often deep-fried and eaten with soy sauce and other ingredients to give it flavour. Tempeh uses whole beans that are inoculated with a fungus, and then left to incubate and form a firm block. Soya beans are also crushed to make soy milk, which is sometimes used as a replacement for dairy milk. It can also be made into soy yoghurt, ice cream and cheese. Dried soya beans are a main ingredient in many soups and stews. Soy flour can be mixed with other flour types to increase protein content and is added to many foods. Dried soya beans can be sprouted and used in salads. The extracted oil is very popular in the West; it is widely used as cooking oil, and is added to margarine and a vast number of commercial food products.

🐾 Young, green edamame soya beans are popular in stir-fries, make a tasty snack food and can be added to soups and stews. As a snack, they are steamed for a couple of minutes in their pods, rinsed, salted and then eaten like peanuts with the pods being discarded. They have a pleasant, sweet, nutty flavour.

Spinach

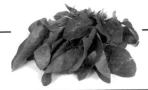

Ⓜ Ⓢ Ⓥ

Related to beets and quinoa, spinach leaves are full of vitamins and nutrients – made famous by Popeye, though perhaps misleadingly. This green vegetable is regaining popularity after going through a period of being commonly served overcooked. Now, it is prepared in many imaginative ways and its young leaves are delicious fresh in salads.

What it contains

Spinach leaves are rich in β-**carotene** and are very rich in **lutein** and **zeaxanthin**, containing more of the latter two carotenoids than any other common food. These carotenoids improve vision and significantly slow the progression of age-related macular degeneration and cataracts, while also protecting against heart disease. Spinach contains good amounts of **betaine**, which helps reduce arterial disease. It is also hugely rich in **vitamin K** (equivalent to >1000 times the RDA), contains good amounts of **vitamin C** (18 mg/100 g) and abundant **vitamin E**. The leaves are richer in **chlorophyll** (the photosynthetic molecule in plants) than other vegetables and this seems to have anticarcinogenic and wound-healing properties. Spinach contains good quantities of **folate**, with one serving providing ~65% of the RDA. The leaves are rich in **minerals**, particularly **potassium**. It contains fibre, which is beneficial to the digestive system, **saponins**, and is very rich in antioxidants **flavonoids**, particularly **quercetin**.

Spinach contains iron, though not as much as Popeye made out, as some becomes bound with oxalic acid, making it unavailable. However, vitamin C increases the absorption of iron by ~50%, so squeeze some orange juice on your spinach to get its full benefits.

What it does

Research shows that spinach protects the central nervous system and has anti-ageing activities. Its antioxidant content may retard neuronal age-related disorders and cognitive decline, thus may help prevent neurodegenerative diseases such as Alzheimer's. The leaves also contain rubiscolins, classified as opioid peptides and which seem to affect the mind. In rats, extracts of rubiscolins affected the brain: serotonin levels were increased and norepinephrine and dopamine levels were decreased.

Spinach is also unusual in being rich in lipoyllysine, a recently discovered compound containing α-lipoic acid (LA). LA is involved in the production of several vital enzymes connected with energy production, is a powerful antioxidant, stimulates activity of other antioxidants, is involved in cell signalling, and may enhance the insulin response.

Warning: Spinach contains some oxalic acids – in regular, large quantities these acids can cause kidney disorders, increased risk of gout, and interfere with calcium and iron absorption. However, recent data showing a direct relationship between oxalic acid intake and kidney stones are not conclusive; other factors (e.g. genetic, high meat diet, etc.) are now thought to be of greater importance in the growth of kidney stones. Although cooking does not significantly reduce oxalic acid content, new varieties of spinach have been selected that have lower levels of this compound.

How it is used

Older varieties of spinach (often with narrower leaves) tend to be more acidic in flavour; newer types have less oxalic acid and a milder flavour. Spinach goes wonderfully with eggs. It is also popular in soups, dips, pies, many Italian recipes, curries, meatballs, quiche and rice dishes, and mixes well with veggies such as pumpkin, artichoke, aubergine, mushrooms, potatoes and pinenuts.

Spinach only needs a brief cooking time – it can be steamed for just a minute or two. Overcooking spinach destroys its flavour and greatly reduces its vitamins and nutrient content, particularly vitamin C and folate. The water it has been cooked in can be used for stocks or gravies and this contains much of the nutrients lost from the leaves.

> 🌿 Young spinach leaves are combined with other salad greens, or can be simply enjoyed on their own. They are wonderful fresh with diced white cheese, black olives, crushed garlic, a drizzle of olive oil with black pepper, and croutons.

Spirulina

  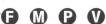

Spirulina is similar to algae and can photosynthesise and multiply rapidly. It is a highly nutritious food. A primitive life form, its cultivation takes up very little space and needs only light and a source of minerals to produce large crops of highly nutritious biomass. It is the ideal food for a world filled with so many people, though many resist spirulina as a food source due to its colour and texture. It is often added to food products to increase their nutrient and protein content, and is the base of a wonderful-tasting, nutritious drink made with bananas, mango and other fruit juices. It is commonly sold dried in powder or tablet form.

What it contains

Spirulina is packed with nutrients – when dried, it contains an amazing 55–65% **protein**, which includes **all the essential amino acids**. It has a richer and more complete protein profile than any other food. It is very rich in **iron** and **copper**; has very good amounts of **potassium**, **magnesium** and **manganese** and also quite a lot of sodium. Spirulina contains abundant quantities of the **B vitamins**, particularly **riboflavin**, **thiamine**, **pantothenic acid** and **niacin**. It contains good amounts of **choline**, **β-carotene** and **vitamin E**, and is very rich in **vitamin D** and **vitamin K**. Spirulina also contains **fermentable β-glucan fibre**.

What it does

Much research has been conducted on spirulina. It is packed with antioxidants, helps reduce triglycerides, serum LDL and total cholesterol levels, while also regulating carbohydrate metabolism, so could be good added to the diets of those at risk for type-2 diabetes. It seems also to help reduce the severity of strokes as well as improving recovery from them. It may reduce the prevalence of neurodegenerative diseases, and has been linked with reducing the symptoms of hay fever.

Its photosynthetic pigment (photocyanin) seems to stimulate the immune system. It increases production of infection-fighting compounds, the production of both red and white blood cells and T-cell counts. Spirulina has shown marked antiviral activity against influenza, herpes and HIV – it significantly inhibits HIV-1 replication. Further development of these substances could yield broad-spectrum antiviral drugs. It has even been suggested that regular consumption may help prevent HIV infection, and suppress viral load among those infected.

Spirulina's minerals, iron and B vitamins help build and maintain neuronal and muscular transmission, help make DNA and RNA, improve eyesight, help fend off depression and reduce the incidence of neurodegenerative diseases, and reduce the risk of cancer formation. The amino acid arginine, which is essential for sperm production, is also present in spirulina.

How it is used

The powder should be stored in an airtight container to avoid moisture uptake. Spirulina is used in drinks mixed with cold fruit juices, to which spices such as cinnamon or vanilla may be added. It can be added to vegetable juices, sprinkled into soups just before serving, added to stir-fries, sprinkled on salads, added to dips such as guacamole and mixed into stews or gravy at the last minute. It is best not cooked because this reduces its nutritive value. In Mexico spirulina is added to candies. In Japan, India and Singapore it is added to nutritional appetisers and is sometimes used as a colouring. In France, spirulina is incorporated into a vegetable pâté. It is also fed to poultry and is said to make the hens' eggs yellow as well as improve their health. When fed to flamingos it makes them pink, and it accelerates growth in cattle leading to earlier sexual maturation and increased fertility.

🐾 Although spirulina is super-rich in most vitamins it does not contain vitamin C, so add lemon, orange or kiwifruit juice to your spirulina to make a truly healthful and delicious drink.

Strawberries

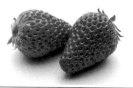

The modern strawberry is a cross between two American wild strawberry species. Because one of the main goals of modern, commercial fruit production is to select firm, large fruits with long storage times, many modern strawberry varieties lack the intensity of flavour that smaller, older-style varieties have. However, there is now a revival in these heirloom varieties, so seek them out at a farmers' market or perhaps grow your own in a pot on the window sill.

What they contain

Very rich in **vitamin C** (55–80 mg/100 g), which is highest just after harvesting on a sunny day. Are low in calories and have good amounts of **soluble, fermentable pectins**. They contain abundant **antioxidants**, much as **flavonoids** (e.g. **anthocyanins, kaempferol, quercetin, ellagitannins, ellagic acid**).

What they do

Ellagic acid is being researched as an antiviral and antibacterial and it is thought that it may reduce the activity of HIV. It also strengthens connective tissue and helps blood to clot. Together, strawberry's flavonoids have activity against human oral, colon and prostate cancer cells. Its compounds are clinically proven to rapidly bind to or cause death of cancer cells and to inhibit further division of cancer cells.

Strawberries have very high antioxidant activity, with their abundant anthocyanins significantly contributing to their healthful properties. Intake of strawberries, due to their flavonoids and pectin, is inversely correlated with serum LDLs and total cholesterol. They have the sixth greatest cholesterol-lowering effect of all berries investigated.

The antimicrobial activity of strawberries helps prevent tooth decay and mouth ulcers.

How they are used

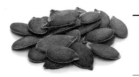

Fresh, ripe, sweet strawberries have a divine fragrance and taste delicious with a little cream or yoghurt.

Wonderful fresh, or as a dessert with a little sugar, a few drops of balsamic vinegar, and either cream, yoghurt or coconut milk. Excellent in preserves and jam – the pectins making them set wonderfully. Also great in juices, ice cream, smoothies, yoghurt, tarts, as a coulis, or as a garnish on sweet and savoury dishes. Strawberry cheesecake, amaretto or daiquiri on strawberries; strawberries with a mint-chocolate biscuit slice; or strawberries puréed and used to fill a pancake.

Strawberries are wonderful in green salads, with avocado, and really bring out the flavour of seafoods, bacon and cold chicken. They mix superbly with dark berries and banana on top of breakfast cereals, or as a simple, healthy dessert try them with kiwifruit and mango. They can be cooked with other fruit and blend well with the sharp flavours of rhubarb and gooseberry. Although cooking destroys most vitamin C and anthocyanins, some other antioxidants are more stable and are retained in jams and cooked strawberry dishes. A tea can be made from the leaves, and strawberry wine is like rosé and very pleasant.

Sunflower seeds

Sunflowers are native to North America and although original 'wild' plants were multi-stemmed with several flower heads, modern varieties usually have a single stem with a large flower head packed with seeds. Only a small proportion of these are used whole – most are used to make one of the most popular vegetable oils worldwide.

What they contain

The seeds and oil are of very good quality nutritionally and are an excellent source of **protein** (>20%), containing **all the essential amino acids**, though somewhat less tryptophan. The seeds (and oil) are very rich in **vitamin E** (300–400% of RDA). This powerful antioxidant has significant immune-improving and cardio-protective properties. The seeds are also very rich in cholesterol-lowering **phytosterols** and are rich in **betaines**. They contain good amounts of **dietary fibre** (~9%) and some **choline**. They also contain lots of the **B vitamins**, particularly **pantothenic acid, niacin, thiamine, B6** and **folate**.

Sunflower seeds are very rich in **copper, iron, phosphates, magnesium, zinc** and **manganese**. The seeds contain **terpenes**, which have anti-inflammatory properties and are rich in antioxidants (e.g. **quercetin**), as well as containing more **histidine** than most, if not all, other plants. The seeds contain ~50% of light, high-quality oil, consisting of 50:50 **omega-6 linoleic acid** to **monounsaturated oleic acid**. However, this ratio varies according to variety, with some bred to produce 80% oleic acid, while others have 65% linoleic (with the rest as saturated and oleic acids). Processed oils contain no vitamins or minerals (apart from vitamin E).

What they do

Histidine is an essential amino acid necessary for development and indirectly by the immune system (it reduces histamine production). It is used to treat arthritis and allergic disorders and is said to prolong orgasm.

Its oils are partially converted to prostaglandin E1, a dilator of smooth muscle (via gamma-linolenic acid). This may account for its effective treatment of pulmonary problems and be why it has been used to reduce premenstrual pain. In addition, its terpenes inhibit expression of many enzymes that produce harmful oxidants and inhibit the release of inflammatory cytokines. These significant inflammatory properties have been shown in animal models to reduce asthma and some forms of dermatitis.

Sunflower seeds reduce serum-triglycerides and LDLs and increase breakdown of fats around the liver, so help reduce the development of cardiovascular disease. Research is being conducted into the ability of sunflower seeds to reduce tumours in cancer patients, which may occur because of the seeds' high vitamin E content.

Rich in minerals, including iron and zinc, and also in B vitamins, which enhance heart and digestive system health, improve energy production and help in the production of DNA and RNA, increase a sense of mental well-being, reduce the incidence of neurodegenerative diseases and act as anticarcinogens. More B vitamins are recommended in the diet of older people to stave off many age-related disorders.

How they are used

The seeds can be eaten fresh or roasted which gives them a delicious nutty flavour. They can be added to cereals, breads, savoury and sweet dishes, enjoyed as a snack on their own, or can be sprouted, with the fresh shoots being tasty and nutritious. The seeds are delicious briefly dry-roasted and then sprinkled with tamari to make a delicious snack. The roasted seeds are made into a flavoursome beverage. The seed is ground to make butter or yoghurt; the latter, apparently, is best if the seed is germinated, blended with water and then left to ferment. The seed oil is used in dressings and in many recipes. It can be cooked to higher temperatures than olive oil without losing its taste or characteristics. Young flower buds can be steamed and served like globe artichokes, with sepals peeled off, dipped in yoghurt, garlic, butter or mayonnaise and then the fleshy base is eaten.

🌿 When buying sunflower oil check its ratio of oleic to linoleic acids – you may wish to choose one more rich in oleic acids because of concerns about the quantity of omega-6 fats in the diet.

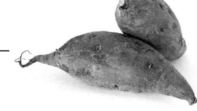

Sweet potato Ⓢ Ⓥ
(kumara, batatas)

Sweet potato is one of the world's most popular root crops, along with potato, taro and cassava. They have been cultivated in South America for at least 5000 years. They were spread to the Caribbean and Polynesia in early times and were later taken to Africa and Asia. An important crop in Asia and many South Pacific islands (e.g. Solomon and Cook Islands), they are also popular in many parts of Africa. Their good nutritional properties and ability to be stored for long periods in heat and high humidity make them particularly useful. Strangely, little is now grown in South America. In New Zealand they are known as kumara; in the United States, although sometimes known as yams, they are not related to true yams (*Dioscorea* spp.).

What it contains

The tubers are rich in **carbohydrates**, but have a fairly low GI of 44. They contain sugars as sucrose and maltose, and also starch. They are very rich in **vitamin A**, mostly as β-**carotene**, particularly those with orange flesh, with one serving providing >850% of the RDA. Sweet potatoes are also rich in **vitamin C** (~20 mg/100 g). They contain virtually no fat. The skin of red and purple sweet potatoes is particularly rich in **anthocyanins**, which can reduce the formation of colorectal cancers. The tubers are also rich in **quercetin, rutin, umbelliferone, coumarin** and **caffeic and chlorogenic acids**, and contain **phytosterols**. The leaves are rich in **vitamin A** and **vitamin K**, with some **vitamin C**. They contain good amounts of **anthocyanins**, which help prevent inflammatory disease and protect cells against oxidative damage.

What it does

Cultivation of this crop, because of its high vitamin A content, is being promoted in regions of Africa where blindness caused by vitamin A deficiency is common. Due to their coumarin compounds, the tubers have anticoagulant properties and thus reduce the development of heart diseases.

Umbelliferone strongly absorbs ultraviolet light and is often used in suncreams.

Warning: Sweet potatoes contain raffinose, which can cause flatulence. The tubers and leaves also contain some oxalates, so should not be consumed in excess by those prone to kidney stones or gout.

The tubers contain storage proteins as sporamins, which are fairly unusual antioxidant compounds that inhibit the breakdown of certain proteins and are thought to have cancer-preventive functions.

How it is used

The roots have a sweet, starchy flavour. They can be baked and served with salt and coconut cream or cheese. They can be added to soups or stews, roasted, and are delicious with other vegetables, or can be sliced or fried to make kumara chips. They can also be used in desserts.

🐾 Baked sweet potato served with asparagus and peanut sauce will easily supply your daily vitamin needs.

The mild, sweet flavour of the tubers blends well with many foods, from fruits, such as apple, apricots, citrus and even some berries, to savoury foods such as garlic, onions, chard, tomatoes and spinach. Some add them to cakes, bread and muffins. They also mix well with spices such as ginger, nutmeg and cinnamon, and herbs such as rosemary, sage and thyme.

In Japan, the sweet root is distilled to make an alcoholic spirit. The younger leaves and shoots can be lightly steamed as a vegetable.

Tamarind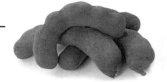

Tamarind is an attractive plant that is a popular garden and street tree in many semi-tropical and tropical regions of the world. It has delicate leaves, pretty flowers and ornamental seed pods. Tamarind is the sticky, tangy, sweet/sour pulp that surrounds the seeds within the ripe, long pods.

What it contains

Ripe pulp contains high quantities of **fruit acids** (~20%) as **citric, malic, oxalic** and **tartaric**, and **sugars** (~35%) as **fructose, glucose** and **sucrose**. It has good amounts of several **minerals**, including **magnesium, potassium** and **iron**, as well as several **B vitamins** (particularly **thiamine**). There are good amounts of soluble **pectin fibre** and the pulp is rich in **flavonoids** (e.g. **apigenin, luteolin, catechins**), and particularly **anthocyanins**.

What it does

The pulp and seeds have proven effectiveness against many and varied medical conditions. They significantly lower LDLs (by 73%), total cholesterol (by 50%) and triglycerides (by 60%), and increase HDLs (by 62%). Its flavonoids improve elasticity of blood vessels. They improve antioxidant activity by increasing the activities of important enzymes. The ripe fruits have proven ability to reduce fever, relieve wind and cure intestinal ailments, and are used as an ingredient in medicines that reduce blood-sugar levels. In the Caribbean, it is used to treat high blood pressure and diabetes and trials have partially verified these uses.

Polysaccharides from its seeds are effective at treating dry-eye syndrome; their molecular structure is similar to that produced by the cornea and conjunctiva. It has helped treat the highly damaging and serious eye disease bacterial keratitis, by increasing the efficacy of applied antibiotics. In human subjects, tamarind pulp significantly increases the bioavailability of ibuprofen and aspirin, making them considerably more efficacious. In India, seed extracts have been effective against the venom from certain snake species – it prevented oedema, haemorrhage and protected against toxic effects. The pulp is also rich in a xyloglucan, which can significantly protect human skin from UV damage, and is also used to treat skin infections, soothe sore throats, as a mild laxative, to cure nausea, for bile disorders and for alcoholic intoxication.

> 🐸 If you have sore eyes, sunburn, headaches *and* have been bitten by a snake, make sure you are not far from a tamarind tree.

How it is used

Is widely used in Asian and Indian cuisine in sauces and chutneys. The seed pulp has a sweet/sour flavour. It can be eaten fresh but is more usually added to dishes, though is also made into a flavoursome drink that is said to be similar to lemonade and is a popular drink in Latin America, Jamaica and the Middle East. It is also an ingredient of Worcestershire sauce. The pulp is often compressed and stored for later use. It is then soaked, and the juice drained from the pulp is added to savoury dishes. It makes a tasty sauce with fish, seafood, chicken and beef, but also to accompany fish and crab cakes, or with bean recipes. Try tamarind with apple, dried raisins, mango, garlic, ginger, lemongrass and baked aubergine, or combine it with coconut milk and potatoes in a curry. The seeds can be eaten, and are generally boiled or fried.

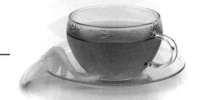

Tea ⓢ

Tea is the second most commonly drunk liquid in the world, after water. A member of the same genus as camellias and rhododendrons, the tea plant has been appreciated by the Chinese for at least 3000 years and is now grown commercially in many warmer regions of the world, with the type of tea often named after the province in which it is cultivated or the colour of its liquid. For example, Chinese teas may be described as green, red, yellow or white. Green, oolong and black teas are all made from *Camellia sinensis*; it is the 'fermentation' process that gives teas their different colours and tastes.

Green tea is made by wilting the leaves in hot air and then rapidly heating them to stop fermentation or oxidation processes. Oolong tea leaves are wilted, then bruised and allowed to partially ferment until reddening of the leaf edges occurs. Black tea leaves are produced by fermenting them in cool, humid rooms until the entire leaf has darkened, with the word 'fermentation' meaning an oxidation process and not actual fermentation, as no micro-organisms are involved.

What it contains

Both black and green teas are very rich in cholesterol-lowering **phytosterols**, with green tea containing a little more of these. Tea is especially rich in soluble polyphenolic tannins. Green tea is very rich in **catechins** (15–30% of its dry weight); whereas black tea contains **theaflavins** and **thearubigins**. Tea also contains a range of minerals, but is particularly rich in **fluoride** and **manganese** – green tea is the richest food source of manganese. Tea is also rich in the powerful antioxidant **quercetin** and contains a caffeine-like compound, **theine** (2–5%). Tannins give tea its characteristic colour and aroma.

What it does

Catechins (and theaflavins) are very potent therapeutic compounds that readily form complexes with reactive oxidative molecules, thereby rendering them harmless. There are several catechins, of which the most powerful is epigallocatechin gallate, which is 25–100 times more powerful than vitamins C and E as an antioxidant. A cup of green tea provides more antioxidant activity than a serving of broccoli or strawberries.

A study reports that people who drank hot black tea with lemon peel were 70% less likely to develop skin cancer and drinking tea alone reduced the risk by 40%. Black tea may also reduce the incidence of prostate cancer – it reacts with androgen receptors that can initiate this type of cancer. Its polyphenols can induce cell death of various tumour cells. Green tea contains more antioxidants, vitamins and minerals than other types of tea. Regular consumption of green tea can inhibit tumour development and cancer cell multiplication within skin, bladder, lung, liver, stomach, leukaemia, colon and prostate; catechins are thought to be the main active component. The Chinese consider tea to be one of the 50 fundamental herbs and have long used it as a cure for cancer, as a blood cleanser, a diuretic, to relieve phlegm, as a stimulant, for digestive problems and to treat certain heart diseases.

Tea has antibacterial, antiseptic and detoxifying properties. Regularly drinking green tea reduced the body fat of a group of Japanese men compared to those who did not drink tea. This weight loss may be due to increased calorie use promoted by greater heat loss and because green tea increases levels of norepinephrine (a form of adrenaline), which prepares the body to burn fat for the 'fight or flight' response. Elevated norepinephrine may also be linked with a reduced response to allergies and asthma, though saponins within tea can also minimise allergy-induced asthma in animals and humans. Compounds within tea also significantly reduce development of cardiovascular disease – they reduce total serum-cholesterol and LDLs, increase beneficial HDLs and reduce blood pressure.

Tea is said to give a feeling of comfort and exhilaration. It seems to enhance the immune system: as little as 3–4 cups of tea a day can lead to significant proven benefits.

> Tea has been used to protect teeth from decay due to its high fluorine content and it decreases plaque by preventing bacteria from adhering to teeth, as well as reducing their acid secretions.

Externally, tea has been used as a poultice to treat cuts, burns, bruises, insect bites, etc. Teabags can be laid on tired eyes, placed on foreheads for headaches or used to soothe sunburn. Green tea is said to have more pronounced effects used in the above ways.

In India, tea has been traditionally used as an aphrodisiac – in rats black tea is a safe aphrodisiac which prevents premature ejaculation and enhances impaired libido.

Warning: Excessive consumption can reduce the body's ability to absorb iron.

How it is used

Steam distillation of black tea yields an essential oil (theol), which is used to flavour alcoholic beverages, perfume, frozen desserts, baked goods and puddings. Soaking dried fruits in tea gives them an interesting flavour – prunes are delicious this way. Green tea ice cream is fabulous – not over-sweet and deliciously refreshing after a meal. There are several recipes where tea is gently charred, in a wok, to smoke fish, chicken, seafood or

> ❧ Adding lemon juice to your tea greatly enhances the release of beneficial compounds.

tofu that is placed above it on a wire rack. For a good cuppa, water that is slightly acidic brings out the best in your brew. Some people add milk; others add lemon or even spices such as ginger, cinnamon and cloves. It can be served hot or cold – chilled lemon tea is very refreshing. There are numerous teas to taste, such as jasmine, Earl Grey and Darjeeling; some are subtle and mild, while others are dark and astringent. A tea and raisin wine is surprisingly pleasant.

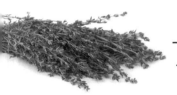

Thyme

Plants of the thyme species are related to mint, rosemary and sage. Their tiny leaves are wonderfully fragrant and have been long appreciated in the Middle East, Italy, France and Greece as a culinary herb and for their medicinal properties. The species *Thymus vulgaris* is particularly popular for its essential oil and as a culinary herb.

What it contains

The fresh leaves are rich in **fibre**, contain mega amounts of **vitamin A** (including β-**carotene**) and loads of **vitamin C** (~160 mg/100g), and are hugely rich in powerful **antioxidants**, containing more than most foods. Fresh, the leaves contain several times the RDA of **iron** and large amounts of **calcium** and **potassium**; dried, the leaves contain about 200% the RDA of calcium, an unbelievable 1600% the RDA of **iron**, a great amount of **potassium**, **manganese** and **zinc**, and lots of the other minerals. Dried thyme is also very rich in **niacin**, **folate** and **vitamin E**. Thyme is rich in **terpenes**, particularly **thymol**, which has powerful antiseptic properties, both topically and internally. It is safe to use on skin. Thyme also contains the terpene **carvacrol** and other compounds.

What it does

The antiseptic and antibacterial activities of thyme oil have been used to treat infected wounds, as a local anaesthetic, an analgesic, an effective insect repellent and an antifungal and antiviral. It can also control some disease-causing protozoa – it is more effective than most other oils at repelling mosquitoes, can control some forms of *Escherichia coli* and when applied topically has some activity against the herpes virus. Thyme is also used to reduce fevers, relieve the symptoms of coughs and sore throats and to expel phlegm.

In mice, thyme has significant activity against tumour cells resistant to chemotherapy and strongly inhibits the development of new tumours, which are actions thought to be related to its carvacrol content. When mixed with clove oil, it strongly inhibits the formation of potentially dangerous compounds within skin caused by UV damage, which may be due to its terpenes.

The oil is used in cosmetics and skin creams, and a few drops can be added to bath water. Thyme oil can be incorporated into toothpaste, where its antibacterial action helps control plaque. It is also effective against *Listeria* bacteria, and thus has potential as a food preservative.

How it is used

A versatile herb, its tiny leaves can be used whole or chopped. Thyme has a subtle spicy taste that is not too powerful. It can be added to sauces, sprinkled on meat dishes, added to stews and soups and is widely used in many Italian, Greek and Turkish recipes. It is one of the main components of bouquet garni, along with bay and parsley, and adds flavour to mustards and sauces and can be sprinkled on roast potatoes and other vegetables. A tasty pesto can be made with fresh thyme and parsley, blended with pinenuts, garlic, black pepper, Parmesan cheese and olive oil. It mixes well with rosemary, apples, apricots, citrus, onion, garlic, carrot, asparagus, artichoke, courgette, mushrooms and sweet potato.

> �_ Historically, thyme was used to reduce smooth-muscle spasms of the gut and uterus, thereby aiding digestion, reducing wind and relieving menstrual pains. Research has now confirmed this anti-spasmodic activity.

Thyme is traditionally used in stuffing, along with sage and rosemary, for poultry and various cuts of meat. It goes well in egg dishes and mixes well with oily fish, sausages and cheese. It is added to pickles and chutneys and the leaves are steeped in vinegar or olive oil to create a dressing. It is often used to flavour Creole cooking and the tiny sprigs of flowers make a pretty garnish.

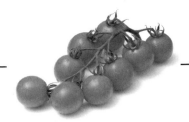

Tomatoes

Ⓜ Ⓥ

Originally from South and Central America, this fruit is well known and used extensively. It is not known whether the tomato was cultivated by the indigenous populations in South and Central America, but the Spanish took it back to Europe, the Caribbean and to Asia (via the Philippines). Its popularity rapidly spread across the Mediterranean, where it suited the climate and was soon widely adopted, particularly in Italy. There are thousands of tomato varieties – from small, sweet cherry tomatoes, to larger hot-house types with thicker skins and less flavour, to oval Italian plum tomatoes, popular canned and puréed, to large beefsteak tomatoes, ideal for grilling and barbecues.

What they contain

Tomato fruits are wonderfully rich in **carotenoids** (**vitamin A**), as β-**carotene**, and also **lycopene**, **lutein** and **zeaxanthin**. These antioxidants confer cardio-protective and anti-cancer effects. They are particularly rich in lycopene, being number one within the common vegetables and fruits (though yellow tomatoes contain less). They also contain good quantities of **vitamin C** (12–30 mg/100 g). Tomatoes have some **potassium** and **fluoride**. They have a low GI.

The antioxidant properties of tomatoes can reduce skin damage caused by UV light, particularly in those with delicate skins. It is recommended that people who work regularly in the sun include more lycopene-rich foods in their diet as studies have found reductions in UV damage ranging between 20–40%.

Unlike many vitamins, the efficacy of vitamin A actually increases with cooking and processing, as in puréed, as a sauce or as sun-dried tomatoes, where their flavours are intensified. The addition of olive oil further promotes vitamin A's absorption.

In these concentrated forms, tomatoes also have greater amounts of the **B vitamins**, particularly **niacin**, **thiamine**, **riboflavin** and **pantothenic acid**, and become much richer in **vitamin K**. They then contain ~40 mg/100 g of **vitamin C**, ~15% **protein**, 12% **fibre** (most of it **soluble**) and **choline**. Levels of **minerals** are wonderfully enriched, with much greater levels of **iron**, **potassium**, **copper**, **phosphate** and **magnesium**, but also more **sodium**.

What they do

Lycopene gives tomatoes their wonderful red colour and is a very powerful antioxidant – there is strong evidence for it preventing and reducing several forms of cancer. Several studies report that lycopene reduces the occurrence and impact of existing prostate cancers, possibly by 30–40%. It may also reduce the incidence of ovarian cancers. Smokers should include more lycopene in their diet.

Tomatoes reduce the development of several age-related diseases, reduce cardiovascular disease and have anti-inflammatory properties. They contain flavonoids that may help block the secretion of hepatitis C virus from infected cells: thus reducing its virulence and spread.

How they are used

Fresh in salads as a garnish or added to many Mediterranean-style dishes, tomatoes can be mixed with virtually any vegetable and many herbs.. They can be sun-dried, puréed, made into sauces for pastas and pizzas, are wonderful in soups, both hot and cold, are added to sandwiches, served with cheese and pickles, made into a tasty healthy juice, spicy salsas, added to pies and stews, stuffed with grains and

🌺 Serve a quick salad of watercress, sun-dried tomatoes, sliced avocado and feta cheese, sprinkled with pumpkin and sunflower seeds and topped with a drizzle of virgin olive oil.

herbs, made into ketchup and the juice is combined with vodka and spices to make a Bloody Mary. Are delicious dribbled with olive oil, black pepper and garlic, and then grilled – this way they are great for breakfast on wholemeal toast with avocado. Green and red tomatoes make wonderful chutneys. There are even a few tomato dessert recipes; they have been added to cake mixtures to make them moist and tangy, and how about tomato ice-cream?

Turmeric

(tumeric)

Related to ginger, the rhizomes of turmeric are valued for their deep-yellow spice, which is included in many dishes of Indian cuisine. It is also popular in many Asian dishes and in Chinese and Japanese recipes. Its usage in India stretches back at least 2500 years, and it is still used in ceremonies, particularly weddings, where it is associated with good luck, fertility and prosperity. Although most turmeric is grown in southern India, some is also grown in Pakistan and Bangladesh, as well other tropical regions of the world. Turmeric has recently become the focus of scientific research which studied its numerous powerful medicinal properties.

What it contains

The root contains **vitamin C**, **vitamin B6** and **niacin**. Is very rich in **iron** and **manganese** and has good amounts of **potassium, zinc** and **copper**. **Antioxidants** are abundant in turmeric. Turmeric's main compound is **curcumin**, which has diverse and very important medicinal properties. Curcumin is considered by some to be the most exciting plant compound recently researched for its potential benefits, and unlike some plant compounds, only a little is needed to offer significant effects. It also contains **oleoresin** which is a mix of oil and resin and gives turmeric a little of its aroma and flavour.

What it does

Turmeric is one of the most important foods being researched for its ability to combat or prevent serious diseases. It has exciting potential to slow the progression of the neurodegenerative disease Alzheimer's, with the frequent use of turmeric in Indian cooking being thought the reason this illness is so uncommon in India. Alzheimer's is linked to the formation of protein knots and neurofibrillary tangles in the brain. Turmeric reduces the number of these by ~50% and may also help treat people suffering from Parkinson's disease and stroke victims.

Curcumin has powerful anti-inflammatory and antioxidant properties. It inhibits enzymes that cause oxidation and inflammation, increases the activity of anticarcinogenic enzymes, prevents maturation of pre-cancerous cells and initiates cell death. It suppresses the proliferation of several types of tumour cell and may even inhibit cancer metastasis.

In humans with rheumatoid arthritis, its anti-inflammatory properties reduce morning stiffness and joint swelling and increase 'walking time' after 2

Research has shown that people who regularly eat curcumin-based spices have a much lower incidence of colon cancer. It may also have some effectiveness against cancer of the stomach, liver, mouth, pancreas, breast, ovary, prostate, rectum, as well as multiple myeloma.

weeks of curcumin supplementation. These results were comparable with those of patients taking a pharmaceutical anti-inflammatory (NSAID). In other trials it reduced inflammation caused by injury and surgery. These results confirm its traditional usage in India.

Turmeric gives some protection against the formation of cataracts, against liver injury and helps repair damage after heart attacks and strokes. There is also a little (though conflicting) evidence for it repairing genetic changes caused by cystic fibrosis.

It has antibacterial activity (e.g. *Helicobacter pylori*, which can cause stomach ulcers and cancer, and *Staphylococcus aureus*). It may even help treat some sexually transmitted diseases such as gonorrhoea and chlamydia. In trials, it shows promise in reducing cholesterol and therefore atherosclerosis, and in treating inflammatory bowel disease, ulcerative colitis, pancreatitis, psoriasis and the inherited disorder familial adenomatous polyposis. Research suggests that even in low doses curcumin enhances the immune system, which may partially explain its efficacy at relieving so many of the above medical conditions.

Curcumin is rapidly metabolised, resulting in its appearing at low serum levels soon after ingestion. However, adding black pepper enhances serum concentration and increases curcumin bioavailability by 2000% in humans.

Externally, its antiseptic properties are used for cuts and burns, including difficult-to-heal wounds. It has been used in suntan creams and to colour the skin.

Warning: Turmeric, in large amounts, should be avoided by those taking anticoagulant medications (due to its blood-thinning properties), and by women receiving chemotherapy for breast cancer.

How it is used

This deep-yellow spice is widely used in Indian curries off all types and spiciness. Its flavour is subtle compared to most spices – warm, aromatic, not hot, but slightly bitter and somewhat drying. It can be blended with many ingredients and goes wonderfully in potato and rice dishes. Turmeric mixes well with a wide range of vegetables, from aubergines and mushrooms, to cauliflower, onions and tomatoes. It imparts a strong yellow colour to food and is used commercially to colour various foodstuffs (e.g. mustards, relishes, cheese

🌿 Enjoy a turmeric-rich curry sauce with cumin and coriander seeds and black pepper on top of lightly stir-fried broccoli and Brussels sprouts. The mix of turmeric, black pepper and brassicas has a wonderful synergistic health-giving effect.

and butter) and may be used as a saffron substitute. In Japan, it is made into a popular tea. The young leaves can be used as a flavouring.

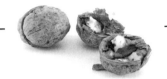

Walnuts

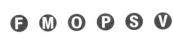

Members of the walnut family can be traced back to the Cretaceous period when dinosaurs roamed Earth. They have been used as a food source since at least Neolithic times, 8000 years ago, with remnants of roasted walnuts being found at archaeological sites in France and in caves in northern Iraq. The walnut's convoluted, deeply folded appearance is due to it being two primitive embryonic leaves, rather than the usual oily storage organ as found in most nuts. These primitive structures reflect its ancient origins. The nuts are sweet and very tasty, particularly when eaten fresh.

What they contain

Walnuts are rich in **protein** (>15%) and oils (65%), which are mostly **polyunsaturates** (50–60% **omega-6 linoleic acid**, 5–10% **omega-3 β-linolenic acid**, ~8% **monounsaturated oleic acid**). Walnuts are rich in **calcium, iron, magnesium, manganese** and **phosphates**. They are a good source of the **B vitamins** and have excellent amounts of **gamma-tocopherol (vitamin E)**. Walnuts contain **fibre** (~8%), are rich in cholesterol-lowering **phytosterols, ellagic acid** and in **cinnamic acids** (e.g. **chlorogenic, caffeic, ferulic**) and **juglone**. They are also very rich in **antioxidants**.

What they do

The good-quantity oils in walnuts reduce LDLs and total cholesterol (while maintaining HDL concentrations), reduce the risk of cancer and are effective anti-inflammatories. High levels of vitamin E offer powerful antioxidant and anti-inflammatory actions. Walnuts significantly improve the elasticity of blood vessels and reduce the adhesion of potentially damaging cells to vessel walls. These factors benefit healthy people, but also those with diabetes and cardiovascular problems. Like most nuts, although rich in fats, they do not cause an increase in weight.

Extracts, containing ellagic acid and juglone, are being investigated for their use as a cancer therapy. Ellagic acid has high anti-inflammatory activity that reduces arterial disease, but also shows some activity at repairing and retaining bone, so walnuts could be a good food for those concerned about osteoporosis.

Warning: Some people are allergic to walnuts.

How they are used

Walnuts are delicious eaten alone fresh or added to various dishes. They are included in stuffing, chocolates, pies and biscuits, go particularly well in cakes and breads along with dried fruits, apricots, apples and spices such as ginger and cinnamon. They mix well with pumpkin, asparagus, green beans, cranberries, strawberry and watercress. They are an ingredient in the famous Waldorf salad, made with celery, apple, grapes and mayonnaise. The nut yields delicate oil that can be used in both sweet and savoury dishes. Green walnuts are also made into a liqueur, nocino, in Italy.

> 🐾 Walnuts can be pickled: the nuts are harvested while still green, and marinated for 3 days in brine, which is then brought to the boil: this is repeated three times. The nuts are then drained, placed in a jar and covered with vinegar, peppercorns, allspice, cloves and crushed ginger. The sealed jars can then be matured in a cool place for several weeks, until enjoyed with freshly made bread and a mature cheese.

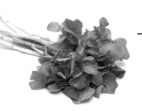

Watercress and landcress
(winter cress)

Watercress, a member of the mustard family, has dark-green, peppery, highly nutritious leaves that are great in salads and soups. It has been gathered from streams and riversides for many thousands of years. Landcress is similar in flavour, with the species *B. verna* often considered to have the finest flavour. But, unlike watercress, landcress does not need to grow in running water. This salad crop is undergoing a revival for its ease of cultivation and flavoursome leaves which can be harvested over a long period.

What they contain

Watercress contains good amounts of **calcium** and **sulphur**, and landcress also contains good amounts of **iodine, iron, potassium** and **manganese**. They are both rich in β-**carotene** (**vitamin A**), and also in **lutein** and **zeaxanthin**. They are also rich in **vitamin C** (~45 mg/100 g) and are very rich in **vitamin K**. Similar to other brassicas, their distinctive flavour is derived from **isothiocyanates**. Landcress is particularly rich in these compounds, more so than broccoli, watercress or horseradish. The sprouted seeds are also very nutritious, containing high levels of **protein** (~20%), **vitamin A** and **vitamin C**, as well as several minerals.

What they do

A herbal remedy containing watercress and horseradish root reduced acute sinusitis, bronchitis and urinary tract infections in a large group of children to the same extent as treatment with standard antibiotics.

Isothiocyanates are strongly linked with preventing cancers and heart disease – compounds from both watercress and landcress have strongly inhibited the formation of liver, breast, lung and colon cancers, and reduced the incidence of cardiovascular disease. These compounds also inhibit the formation of blood clots, much more so than aspirin, and so reduce the incidence of heart attacks and other coronary disease. They lower serum LDLs and raise HDLs and their anti-inflammatory properties are being researched to reduce the symptoms of asthma and even anaphylaxis.

Isothiocyanates are powerful antioxidants and decrease the activity of several damaging oxidising enzymes. They also have antimicrobial properties.

Watercress has been used historically to purify the blood, as a tonic and has been used to treat a wide range of ailments, including chest complaints, skin infections, kidney disorders, as well as to relieve rheumatism and as a diuretic.

Watercress, macerated, has long been valued as a hair tonic, and is said to improve the health and thickness of hair.

Warning: When gathering watercress from the wild check the pasture around it does not contain sheep. Sheep can carry parasite liver flukes and their faeces contain its eggs, which lodge on watercress. Liver fluke can infect people and may cause considerable internal damage. If gathering from the wild, thoroughly wash watercress before use, or, if in doubt, cook it.

How they are used

Both cresses make a wonderful, flavourful salad on their own, or can be mixed with other greens – a good option for people who find their flavour too hot to eat alone. The leaves can be mixed with cottage cheese and fruit to make a delightful, light snack. They are often used as a garnish, are great on potatoes with sweet cherry tomatoes and goat's cheese, and mix well with pear, asparagus, avocado, citrus, carrot, leek, pinenuts, celery, endive and ginger. A wonderful soup with Stilton cheese and/or cream can be made from watercress, or it can be puréed as an accompaniment to seafood. The cresses are also delicious in quiches and pies. Try fresh watercress leaves with a few slices of smoked salmon on rye bread accompanied by a glass of shiraz. The leaves may be lightly steamed like spinach, though note that much of their beneficial isothiocyanate content is destroyed by extended cooking. For the extremist, there are recipes that combine watercress and wasabi. The yellow flower heads of landcress make an attractive garnish.

> Watercress and landcress are rich in carotenoids (vitamin A) and isothiocyanates. It has been found that isothiocyanates increase the bioavailability of carotenoids by up to 100%, therefore the nutritional effects of the anticarcinogenic carotenoids in the cresses are hugely increased. In studies, these beneficial effects were most noticeable in smokers.

Wheat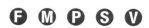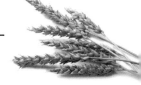

Wheat is a cereal crop with a very long history of human usage which extends back >16,000 years. Its cultivation stretches back to the very beginning of agriculture. Most species originate from the Middle East, and from there spread outwards to Europe as early as the Stone Age. Many varieties and species of wheat have been developed. It is now the most important cereal crop in temperate zones. The grain is usually ground into flour and is rich in the protein gluten. In wheat bread, gluten provides a stickiness that enables the bread to rise satisfactorily.

Some older wheat types still exist, including einkorn, which was gathered from the wild ~18,000 years ago and is still grown to a limited extent around the eastern Mediterranean and in Africa. Emmer also probably originates from the Middle East, and a little is still grown in Ethiopia and India. Spelt is a 'newer' wheat, possibly only dating back ~7000 years and also originating in the Middle East. Triticale is a fairly new (~1850 years old) wheat–rye cross, and from this many other cultivars have been developed. Kamut® is an ancient wheat, which has been recently rediscovered and given a trademark to ensure that it is always grown according to organic certification and agronomic practices. Kamut® wheat has larger grains, more protein, is said to be easier to digest and to be sweeter than other wheat types. It is often the grain used to germinate wheat grass.

What it contains

Whole-wheat grains (un-germinated) are rich in **protein**, containing 12–15%, particularly **glutamic acid**. It is rich in **fibre** (~10–20% by weight), most of which is **insoluble**, and in cholesterol-lowering **phytosterols**. Contains very little fat and is rich in the **B vitamins**, particularly **niacin**, **B6** and **thiamine**. Although some B vitamins are inactivated by heat, germinating the seeds increases vitamin B content several-fold, and even after subsequent cooking the vitamin B content remains stable.

Whole grains are wonderfully rich in antioxidant **selenium**, with one serving providing ~250% of the RDA. They are also rich in **manganese**, **phosphorus**, **magnesium**, **iron**, **zinc** and **copper**, contain antioxidant **polyphenols** such as **ferulic acid** and good amounts of **phyto-oestrogens**. The bran and germ, particularly, contain **choline**, which is intimately associated with neurotransmission and a lack of which can cause fatty liver, neural-tube defects and neurodegenerative disease.

Because selenium-rich whole wheat works synergistically with vitamin E, and is linked with reducing heart disease, as well as decreasing the symptoms of asthma and arthritis, mix crushed nuts or sunflower or pumpkin seeds in with wheat flour to get this added boost.

Whole-wheat flour still retains most of these nutrients and minerals. Old-style wheats, such as spelt, are said to contain more proteins and vitamins. Wheat germ, the embryo of the grain, is packed with protein, minerals and vitamins, particularly **folate** and **vitamin E**, and in minerals such as **manganese** and **zinc**. It is one of the richest sources of **phytosterols**.

White flour has its outer layers (the bran) and the embryo removed. With this removal, virtually all fibre, protein, vitamins and minerals are also subtracted; therefore, white flour is often sold 'enriched' with the addition of folate and niacin. However, its nutrient status is still very poor compared to whole wheat.

What it does

Whole-wheat fibre improves the formation and passage of stools by absorbing large amounts of water; this process relieves constipation, helps keep the gut flora healthy and reduces the likelihood of colon and bowel cancers. Selenium helps metabolise fats, so helps reduce the development of cardiovascular disease. Its antioxidant and enzyme-like properties also help protect and even to fight existing cancers. Selenium is essential to thyroid metabolism, so is vital for normal growth and development. It enhances the immune system and improves the health of blood vessels, thus adding to its cardio-protective properties.

Interestingly, wheat contains low levels of natural benzodiazepines, which act as sedatives, anticonvulsants, muscle relaxants, anxiety reducers and as hypnotics.

Warning: Some people are allergic to gluten and wheat is very rich in this protein. There are two main disorders. Coeliac disease (or coeliac sprue), which is usually a genetic disorder. People who have this are never able to eat gluten. In this disease, gluten reacts with the small bowel to cause an autoimmune reaction which results in damage to the delicate lining of villi. This inhibits absorption of many minerals, vitamins and compounds. This disorder can go undetected for some time and is thought to occur in about 1/300 people. Although wheat is the most problematic cereal, rye and barley can also cause this reaction. The other disorder is an allergic reaction to gluten. It can affect children (who often outgrow this condition) or people who use wheat flour a lot. After ingesting gluten, certain antibodies mistakenly become activated to cause an allergic reaction. This reaction can manifest as asthma, skin swelling, cramps and eczema, or in extreme circumstances, as anaphylaxis. Both conditions are easy to diagnose through a blood test.

How it is used

The grains (sometimes called berries) can be sprouted to form wheat grass, which is a popular additive to health juices. The whole grains can be soaked overnight and then cooked for >40 minutes and eaten as a rice substitute or can be added to a salad – they are fairly chewy and have a pleasant, nutty flavour. Wheat grain can be crushed to form small pieces, which is known as bulgar wheat. This takes much less cooking time than whole wheat and is delicious in salads, such as tabbouleh, or served as a carbohydrate source with pepper and a knob of butter. The cracked grain can be lightly toasted or roasted to add flavour. Harder durum wheat can be coarsely ground to form semolina. This is used to make milky desserts and as a thickener. It may also be rolled into small pellets to form couscous, a popular staple carbohydrate in North Africa and the Middle East. It is usually cooked by steaming until light and fluffy, though most commercially prepared couscous has been pre-steamed to reduce preparation time. Durum wheat is also popular in pasta-making. Wheat grain is used to make alcohol, including whiskey. Wheat flour is the most popular and widely used bread and pastry flour. A trip around the supermarket shows that wheat, by far, is the main cereal grain used in a huge number of both savoury and sweet foods.

🐾 Nutritious wheat germ has a pleasant flavour when very fresh, though can become bitter as it ages. It can be sprinkled on breakfast cereals or is added to pies, crumbles, as a topping for casseroles, or is added to breads, muffins and cake mixes.

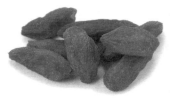

Wolfberries and Goji berries
Ⓜ Ⓞ Ⓟ Ⓢ Ⓥ

These berries, related to tomatoes and chillies, are sprawling vines that originate from Inner Mongolia and the Himalayas. Although only recently popular in the West, they have been valued in Mongolia and China for at least 3000–3400 years. Research carried out in Inner Mongolia found people who were mostly vegetarian and who ate wolfberries daily lived 20 to 40 years longer than other people in the region – they had a life expectancy of more than 100 years. They also had a lower incidence of diseases such as arthritis, cancer and diabetes. As a result, numerous clinical studies have been conducted on the benefits of these fruits. Today, in the West, they are included in many health preparations and are sold as a juice for their anti-ageing benefits.

What they contain

These berries are often described as super foods. Many of the values below probably apply to dried fruits, where their levels are concentrated. The berries contain 12–15% **protein**, which is very high for a fruit. This is rich in the **essential amino acid leucine**, and many other amino acids. The berries are rich in the **B vitamins (thiamine, riboflavin, B6)** and are reported to be exceptionally rich in **vitamin C** (up to 5000 mg/100 g of fruit). They are also very rich in **carotenoids**, particularly **zeaxanthin**, which is one of the richest food sources. The fruits contain good amounts of fatty acids, including **omega-3 linolenic acid**, and are also very rich in **flavonoids** and other **secondary plant compounds**, such as **betaine**, **phytosterols** and **p-coumaric acid**, which give them very powerful antioxidant and immune-supporting properties. They have much greater **antioxidant** levels than most fruits, including blueberries. The berries also contain good amounts of **zinc, iron, copper, calcium, selenium** and **phosphorus**. The quantities of many of the above are said to be greater within the Goji berry variety.

What they do

Many trials report that these berries significantly enhance the immune system. The juice increases the number of immune cells, enhances the transformation rate of lymphocytes within cancer patients and increases white blood cell counts. It is said to strengthen immunoglobulin A levels (an index of immune function) and because these decline with age, and from a relatively young age onwards, it is hypothesised that any increase in immunoglobulin A helps reduce tissue degeneration.

The berries also increase antioxidant levels by 40%, with many Chinese studies reporting a multitude of medicinal benefits. The berries are reported to increase red blood cell levels by 12%, to reduce LDLs, to increase HDL levels, and to activate anti-inflammatory enzymes, so are likely to reduce cardiovascular disease. In an animal study, the berries inhibited tumour growth by 50%, therefore showing a significant ability to even reverse cancer growth. They can significantly lower blood-sugar levels and can reduce insulin resistance, a symptom of type-2 diabetes.

The fruits may reduce neuronal decline in neurodegenerative diseases and have anti-ageing properties that are not only due to their antioxidant properties. Possibly due to their betaine content, they are said to improve

A recent, controlled American study found that people who took the juice for 14 days had feelings of increased energy, athletic performance, quality of sleep, ease of awakening, ability to focus on activities, mental acuity, calmness, feelings of health, contentment and happiness, and significantly reduced fatigue and stress with improved regularity of gastrointestinal function.

memory and recall, as well as act as a pick-me-up. Historically, in China, they have been used as a mild tranquilliser, to relieve insomnia, to enhance weight loss, to treat sexual dysfunction and for menopause symptoms.

Being rich in vitamin C and zinc, these berries are likely to benefit sperm production and fertility. Extracts from the berries are good for the hair and skin due to their high vitamin and antioxidant content.

Warning: These berries may reduce the effectiveness of anticoagulant drugs such as warfarin; therefore, don't eat too many if on this medication.

🐾 The abundant carotenoids within wolfberries and Goji berries enhance dark adaptation, acuity of eyesight and help protect against age-related macular degeneration. Mixing the berry juice with warm milk increases its bioavailability and therefore its effects three-fold.

How they are used

The berries are often dried and have a sweet, strong flavour which is similar to dates and raisins. The recommended dosage to get their health benefits is just 10–15 g of dried fruits a day. Goji berries are said to be sweeter and more tasty and they can be used like other dried fruits in cereals, or added to meat, vegetable or fish dishes, desserts, or muffins and cakes. The berries are made into juice – either on their own or with other fruits. They can be soaked with wine and then stored to be enjoyed later. A tea is made with the fruits, which is very popular in China.

Yeast

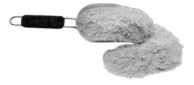

Yeast products come in several types: nutrient, brewer's, baker's and torula and yeast extract. Brewer's yeast can be referred to as nutrient yeast, though the latter is specifically produced as a nutrient additive whereas the former is usually the waste product from brewing. Yeasts are simple organisms that are closely related to fungi. Given the right conditions – warmth, moisture and the necessary nutrient media – they multiply rapidly. They partially ferment the products they are given and produce carbon dioxide but also many by-products. Yeasts have a very long history of usage, mostly for bread-making and brewing.

Yeasts are particularly valued for their **B vitamins (thiamine,**

riboflavin, niacin, pantothenic acid, B6, folate and **biotin**). These vitamins, together, are vital for neuronal and muscular transmission, are involved in conversion of carbohydrates and fats into energy for the production and repair of DNA and RNA, help delay development of several neurodegenerative diseases (such as Alzheimer's), help reduce age-related macular degeneration, are needed for production of powerful antioxidants, have cholesterol-lowering properties, are protective against cardiovascular disease (by increasing HDLs and reducing blood clotting), may reduce incidence of some cancers, help maintain steady blood-sugar levels and reduce the risk of some birth defects.

B12, produced by bacteria and not yeast cells, is often added to yeast brews. Because the B vitamins are all water-soluble and, thus, only have a short storage time within our bodies, they need to be eaten daily. There is increasing evidence that extra vitamin B in the diet is of significant benefit in reducing the progression of several age-related degenerative diseases.

> Yeast products must be the richest and best complete source of B vitamins while also being rich in many minerals. We need daily intake of B vitamins and there is significant evidence that they stave off many age-related disorders.

Brewer's yeast

This yeast is a by-product of the beer- and wine-making process. It can be *Saccharomyces cerevisiae*, though other species are sometimes used. It is grown in the presence of B12, and on a range of media, but often on grain or sugarcane sap. Compared to baker's yeast, brewer's yeast has a bitter flavour, though is often sold sweetened. It usually comes in powdered form and between 1–4 tablespoons a day are added to juice or sprinkled onto savoury foods or soups. It does have a yeasty flavour.

It is rich in **vitamin B** and also **protein** and several **minerals** (e.g. **potassium, phosphates, magnesium**), but especially **chromium** or **selenium**. Chromium is an essential trace mineral that is needed to maintain normal blood-sugar levels and to transport blood sugar into cells. Thus, it can reduce insulin intolerance, which develops in those with type-2 diabetes. Chromium may also help lower serum LDLs and raise HDLs.

Selenium aids fat metabolism and so reduces the development of cardiovascular disease. It also helps protect against the development of and even fights existing cancers. Selenium is essential to thyroid metabolism, so is vital for normal growth and development. It enhances the immune system and improves the health of blood vessels, which adds to its cardio-protective properties. This antioxidant mineral works synergistically with vitamin E and is linked with reducing heart disease, as well as decreasing the symptoms of asthma and arthritis. It should not be taken by those with existing yeast infections. This yeast also contains considerable tyramine, which can react adversely with some antidepressant medications (monoamine oxidase inhibitors) and prescribed pain killers, leading to increased blood pressure and other serious symptoms, so check with your physician if in doubt.

Baker's yeast

Their carbon dioxide production makes bread rise. This yeast contributes nutrients to bread and makes some compounds more available. *S. cerevisiae* is the yeast species used.

Nutritional yeast

This consists of yellowish flakes of yeast (*S. cerevisiae*). It, like baker's yeast, usually includes **B12**. It contains good amounts of **protein** and is particularly rich in **thiamine** and **riboflavin**. It also has lots of **niacin**, **B6** and **B12**, with some **folic acid**, **selenium** and **zinc**. It is commonly cultivated on cane or beet molasses. After ~7 days, the yeast is harvested, washed, pasteurised and then rolled to form flakes. It is deactivated, so is said to be less likely to affect any existing yeast infections. Some include it regularly in their diet as a source of nutrients and much is added to human and pet foods to boost nutritional content. It can be sprinkled on stews and soups before serving, mixed with rice or quinoa dishes and is used as a condiment. It has a surprisingly pleasant savoury, cheese-like flavour. Note, though, that heat destroys some B vitamins.

Yeast extract

This is the common name for several processed yeast products that are used as food additives and flavourings (e.g. Marmite, Vegemite). They consist of a thick, dark-coloured viscous paste that contains the contents of many yeast cells. These products can be used in the same way as monosodium glutamate (MSG) and, like MSG, they sometimes contain quite high amounts of free glutamic acids. Once a 'culture' is grown, the cells are flooded with a high-salt solution, which causes them to shrivel and die. The thicker cell walls are removed to leave the cell contents, which forms the extract. It is rich in **B vitamins**, though these may be added, and it contains lots of **sodium**.

Torula yeast

This yeast is formed on waste sugars from the spruce paper-making industry. It is then killed, pasteurised and dried with the resulting powdered yeast cells being a common additive to pet foods for their nutrition and flavour. The yeast *Candida utilis* is commonly used for this process. It is very **protein** rich, contains a lot of **glutamic acid** and also **many essential amino acids**. It is hugely rich in **niacin, pantothenic acid** and **riboflavin**, with some **B6**. Contains abundant **choline** and is rich in **zinc** and **manganese**, with some **copper** and **phosphates**.

Bibliography

The references listed below, mostly from science journals, report on some of the health research conducted on the plants described within this book. Many larger trials and recent papers are included, but by no means all (due to space limitations): thus, if wishing to follow up a specific topic, perhaps use these as a starting point. The internet site PubMed (at: www.ncbi.nlm.nih.gov/pubmed/) is also an excellent place to search for further specific information.

General references

Ackland ML, et al. Synergistic antiproliferative action of the flavonols quercitin and kaempferol in cultured human cancer cell lines. In Vivo 2005;19(1):69-76.

Aggarwal R, et al. Role of zinc administration in prevention of childhood diarrhea and respiratory illnesses: a meta-analysis. Pediatrics 2007;119(6):1120-30.

Alkhenizan A, Hafez K. The role of vitamin E in the prevention of cancer: a meta-analysis of randomized controlled trials. Ann Saudi Med 2007;27(6):409-14.

Arja T. Cereal fiber and whole-grain intake are associated with reduced progression of coronary-artery atherosclerosis in postmenopausal women with coronary artery disease. Am Heart J 2005;150(1):94-101.

Bazzano LA, et al. Dietary fiber intake and reduced risk of coronary heart disease in US men and women: the National Health and Nutrition Examination Survey I Epidemiologic Follow-up Study. Arch Intern Med 2003;163(16):1897-904.

Bijkerk CJ, et al. Systematic review: the role of different types of fibre in the treatment of irritable bowel syndrome. Aliment Pharmacol Ther 2004;19(3):245-51.

Blacklock CJ, et al. Salicylic acid in the serum of subjects not taking aspirin. Comparison of salicylic acid concentrations in the serum of vegetarians, non-vegetarians, and patients taking low dose aspirin. J Clin Pathol 2001;54(7):553-5.

Booth SL, et al. Effect of vitamin K supplementation on bone loss in elderly men and women. J Clin Endocrinol Metab 2008;93(4):1217-23.

Bradlow HL, Sepkovic DW. Diet and breast cancer. Ann NY Acad Sci 2002;963:247-67.

Brinkman M, et al. Are men with low selenium levels at increased risk of prostate cancer? Eur J Cancer 2006;42(15):2463-71.

Brown L, et al. Cholesterol-lowering effects of dietary fiber: a meta-analysis. Am J Clin Nutr 1999;69(1):30-42.

Bucher HC, et al. N-3 polyunsaturated fatty acids in coronary heart disease: a meta-analysis of randomized controlled trials. Am J Med 2002;112(4):298-304.

Chen JT, et al. Meta-analysis of natural therapies for hyperlipidemia: plant sterols and stanols versus policosanol. Pharmacotherapy 2005;25(2):171-83.

Choi SW, Mason JB. Folate and carcinogenesis: an integrated scheme. J Nutr 2000;130(2):129-32.

Cockayne S, et al. Vitamin K and the prevention of fractures: systematic review and meta-analysis of randomized controlled trials. Arch Intern Med 2006;166(12):1256-61.

Commenges D, et al. Intake of flavonoids and risk of dementia. Eur J Epidemiol 2000;16(4):357-63.

Conlin PR, et al. The effect of dietary patterns on blood pressure control in hypertensive patients: results from the Dietary Approaches to Stop Hypertension (DASH) trial. Am J Hypertens 2000;13(9):949-55.

De Jong, et al. Metabolic effects of plant sterols and stanols (review). J Nutr Biochem 2003;14:362-9.

Devine A, et al. A longitudinal study of the effect of sodium and calcium intakes on regional bone density in postmenopausal women. Am J Clin Nutr 1995;62(4):740-5.

Dragan S, et al. Role of multi-component functional foods in the complex treatment of patients with advanced breast cancer. Rev Med Chir Soc Med Nat Iasi 2007;111(4):877-84.

Erkkil C, et al. Cereal fiber and whole-grain intake are associated with reduced progression of coronary-artery atherosclerosis in postmenopausal women with coronary artery disease. Am Heart J 2005 Jul;150(1):94-101.

FDA authorizes new coronary heart disease health claim for plant sterol and plant stanol esters. FDA Talk Paper. At: http://www.fda.gov/bbs/topics/ANSWERS/ANS01033.html

Freudenheim JL, et al. Premenopausal breast cancer risk and intake of vegetables, fruits, and related nutrients. J Natl Cancer Inst 1996;88(6):340-8.

Helland IB, et al. Maternal supplementation with very-long-chain n-3 fatty acids during pregnancy and lactation augments children's IQ at 4 years of age. Pediatrics 2003;111(1):e39-44.

Hibbeln JR. From homicide to happiness – a

commentary on omega-3 fatty acids in human society. Cleave Award Lecture. Nutr Health 2007;19(1-2):9-19.

Higden J. Vitamin K. Micronutrient Information Center. Linus Pauling Institute. An excellent review on this vitamin at: http://lpi.oregonstate.edu/infocenter/vitamins/vitaminK/

Hoult JR, Payá M. Pharmacological and biochemical actions of simple coumarins: natural products with therapeutic potential. Gen Pharmacol 1996;27(4):713-22.

Hurwitz BE, et al. Suppression of human immunodeficiency virus type 1 viral load with selenium supplementation: a randomized controlled trial. Arch Intern Med 2007;167(2):148-54.

Jackson RD, et al. Calcium plus vitamin D supplementation and the risk of fractures. N Engl J Med 2006;354(7):669-83.

Jacques PF, et al. Long-term nutrient intake and 5-year change in nuclear lens opacities. Arch Ophthalmol 2005;123(4):517-26.

Joy CB, et al. Polyunsaturated fatty acid supplementation for schizophrenia. Cochrane Database Syst Rev 2003;(2):CD001257.

Katan MB, et al. Efficacy and safety of plant stanols and sterols in the management of blood cholesterol levels. Mayo Clin Proc 2003;78(8):965-78.

Knekt P, et al. Antioxidant vitamin intake and coronary mortality in a longitudinal population study. Am J Epidemiol 1994;139(12):1180-9.

Lakhan SE, Vieira KF. Nutritional therapies for mental disorders. Nutr J 2008;7:2.

Letenneur L, et al. Flavonoid intake and cognitive decline over a 10-year period. Am J Epidemiol 2007;165(12):1364-71.

Linus Pauling Institute site at: http://lpi.oregonstate.edu/infocenter/

Lippman SM, et al. Designing the Selenium and Vitamin E Cancer Prevention Trial (SELECT). J Natl Cancer Inst 2005;97(2):94-102.

Liu, Rui Hai. Health benefits of fruit and vegetables are from additive and synergistic combinations of phytochemicals. Am J Clin Nutr 2003;78(Suppl):517S-20S.

Martin JH, et al. Does an apple a day keep the doctor away because a phytoestrogen a day keeps the virus at bay? A review of the anti-viral properties of phytoestrogens. Phytochemistry 2007;68(3):266-7.

Masaki KH, et al. Association of vitamin E and C supplement use with cognitive function and dementia in elderly men. Neurology 2000;54(6):1265-72.

Mensink RP, Katan MB. Effect of dietary fatty acids on serum lipids and lipoproteins. A meta-analysis of 27 trials. Arterioscler Thromb 1992;12(8):911-9.

Meydani SN, et al. Vitamin E and respiratory tract infections in elderly nursing home residents: a randomized controlled trial.

JAMA 2004;292(7):828-36.

Morris MC, et al. Dietary folate and vitamin B12 intake and cognitive decline among community-dwelling older persons. Arch Neurol 2005;62(4):641-5.

Mozaffarian D. Does alpha-linolenic acid intake reduce the risk of coronary heart disease? A review of the evidence. Altern Ther Health Med 2005;11(3):24-30.

Negri E, et al. Selected micronutrients and oral and pharyngeal cancer. Int J Cancer 2000;86(1):122-7.

New SA, et al. Dietary influences on bone mass and bone metabolism: further evidence of a positive link between fruit and vegetable consumption and bone health? Am J Clin Nutr 2000;71(1):142-51.

Nimni ME, et al. Are we getting enough sulfur in our diet? Nutr Metab (Lond) 2007;4:24.

Niness KR. Inulin and oligofructose: what are they? J Nutr 1999;129:1402S-1406S.

Nutrient Data Laboratory and Arkansas Children's Nutrition Center. Oxygen Radical Absorbance Capacity (ORAC) of Selected Foods, 2007, at: http://www.ars.usda.gov/SP2UserFiles/Place/12354500/Data/ORAC/ORAC07.pdf

Oh K, et al. Dietary fat intake and risk of coronary heart disease in women: 20 years of follow-up of the nurses' health study. Am J Epidemiol 2005;161(7):672-9.

Paterson JR, et al. Salicylic acid content of spices and its implications. J Agric Food Chem 2006;54(8):2891-6.

Rimm EB, et al. Folate and vitamin B6 from diet and supplements in relation to risk of coronary heart disease among women. JAMA 1998;279(5):359-64.

SanGiovanni JP, Chew EY. The role of omega-3 long-chain polyunsaturated fatty acids in health and disease of the retina. Prog Retin Eye Res 2005;24(1):87-138.

Sellmeyer DE, et al. A high ratio of dietary animal to vegetable protein increases the rate of bone loss and the risk of fracture in postmenopausal women. Study of Osteoporotic Fractures Research Group. Am J Clin Nutr 2001;73(1):118-22.

Severi G, et al. Prospective studies of dairy product and calcium intakes and prostate cancer risk: a meta-analysis. J Natl Cancer Inst 2006;98(11):794-5.

Shaik YB, et al. Role of quercetin (a natural herbal compound) in allergy and inflammation. J Biol Regul Homeost Agents 2006;20(3-4):47-52.

Shapiro S, Guggenheim B. The action of thymol on oral bacteria. Oral Microbiol Immunol 1995;10(4):241-6.

Shaw GM, et al. Periconceptional dietary intake of choline and betaine and neural tube defects in offspring. Am J Epidemiol 2004;160(2):102-9.

Shearer MJ. The roles of vitamins D and K in bone health and osteoporosis prevention. Proc

Nutr Soc 1997;56(3):915-37.

Steinmetz KA, Potter JD. Vegetables, fruit, and cancer prevention: a review. J Am Diet Assoc 1996;96(10):1027-39.

Sylvester PW, Theriault A. Role of tocotrienols in the prevention of cardiovascular disease and breast cancer. Curr Topics Nutraceut Res 2003;1(1):121-35.

Traber MG, et al. Vitamin E revisited: do new data validate benefits for chronic disease prevention? Curr Opin Lipidol 2008;19(1):30-8.

Tucker KL, et al. Potassium, magnesium, and fruit and vegetable intakes are associated with greater bone mineral density in elderly men and women. Am J Clin Nutr 1999;69(4):727-36.

University of Ulster. Super sprouts could help reduce cancer risk. ScienceDaily, 2004. Retrieved from http://www.sciencedaily.com/releases/2004/06/040624094143.htm

US Library of Medicine and National Institute of Health: Medline Plus, at: http://www.nlm.nih.gov/medlineplus/print/druginfo/natural/patient-fishoil.html, information on fatty acids (omega3).

USDA National Nutrient Database for Standard Reference at http://www.nal.usda.gov/fnic/foodcomp/search/

Whanger PD. Selenium and its relationship to cancer: an update. Br J Nutr 2004;91(1):11-28.

Williams AL, et al. The role for vitamin B-6 as treatment for depression: a systematic review. Fam Pract 2005;22(5):532-7.

Williams RJ, et al. Flavonoids: antioxidants or signalling molecules? Free Radic Biol Med 2004; 36(7):838-49.

World Cancer Fund International at http://wcrf.org have produced an excellent free, downloadable book titled 'Food nutrition, physical activity, and the prevention of cancer: a global perspective', available at: http://wcrf.org/research/index.php

Youdim KA, Joseph JA. A possible emerging role of phytochemicals in improving age-related neurological dysfunctions: a multiplicity of effects. Free Radic Biol Med 2001;30(6):583-594.

Zhang S, et al. A prospective study of folate intake and the risk of breast cancer. JAMA 1999;281(17):1632-37.

Zhang S, et al. Dietary carotenoids and vitamins A, C, and E and risk of breast cancer. J Natl Cancer Inst 1999;91(6):547-56.

Fruits and Berries (blueberry, bilberry, blackberry, cherries, cranberry, currants, elderberries, juniper, raspberry, sea-buckthorn, strawberry, wolf and Goji)

Aaby K, et al. Phenolic composition and antioxidant activities in flesh and achenes of strawberries (Fragaria ananassa). J Agric Food Chem 2005;53(10):4032-40.

Amagase H, Nance DM. A randomized, double-blind, placebo-controlled, clinical study of the general effects of a standardized Lycium barbarum (Goji) juice, GoChi. J Altern Complement Med 2008;14(4):403-12.

Angioni A, et al. Chemical composition of the essential oils of Juniperus from ripe and unripe berries and leaves and their antimicrobial activity. J Agric Food Chem 2003;51(10):3073-8.

Basu M, et al. Anti-atherogenic effects of seabuckthorn (Hippophaea rhamnoides) seed oil. Phytomedicine 2007;14(11):770-7.

Benzie IF, et al. Enhanced bioavailability of zeaxanthin in a milk-based formulation of wolfberry (Gou Qi Zi; Fructus barbarum L.). Br J Nutr 2006;96(1):154-60.

Burdulis D, et al. Study of diversity of anthocyanin composition in bilberry (Vaccinium myrtillus L.) fruits. Medicina (Kaunas) 2007;43(12):971-7.

Canel C, et al. Molecules of interest: podophyllotoxin. Phytochemistry 2000;54(2):115-120.

Chang RC, So KF. Use of anti-aging herbal medicine, Lycium barbarum, against aging-associated diseases. What do we know so far? Cell Mol Neurobiol 2008;28(5):643-52.

Chao JC, et al. Hot water-extracted Lycium barbarum and Rehmannia glutinosa inhibit proliferation and induce apoptosis of hepatocellular carcinoma cells. World J Gastroenterol 2006;12(28):4478-84.

Chaudhury RR. The quest for a herbal contraceptive. Natl Med J India 1993;6(5):199-201.

Chauhan AS, et al. Antioxidant and antibacterial activities of aqueous extract of seabuckthorn (Hippophae rhamnoides) seeds. Fitoterapia 2007;78(7-8):590-2.

Chrubasik C, et al. An observational study and quantification of the actives in a supplement with Sambucus nigra and Asparagus officinalis used for weight reduction. Phytother Res 2008;22(7):913-8.

Connolly DA, et al. Efficacy of a tart cherry juice blend in preventing the symptoms of muscle damage. Br J Sports Med 2006;40(8):679-83.

Drăgan S, et al. Role of multi-component functional foods in the complex treatment of patients with advanced breast cancer. Rev Med Chir Soc Med Nat Iasi 2007;111(4):877-84.

Erlund I, et al. Bioavailability of quercetin from berries and the diet. Nutr Cancer 2006;54(1):13-7.

Filipowicz N, et al. Antibacterial and antifungal activity of juniper berry oil and its selected components. Phytother Res 2003;17(3):227-31.

Gan L, et al. Immunomodulation and antitumor activity by a polysaccharide-protein complex from Lycium barbarum. Int

Immunopharmacol 2004;4(4):563-9.

Geetha S, et al. Anti-oxidant and immunomodulatory properties of seabuckthorn (Hippophae rhamnoides): an in vitro study. J Ethnopharmacol 2002;79(3):373-8.

Hannum SM. Potential impact of strawberries on human health: a review of the science. Crit Rev Food Sci Nutr 2004;44(1):1-17.

Harokopakis E, et al. Inhibition of proinflammatory activities of major periodontal pathogens by aqueous extracts from elder flower (Sambucus nigra). J Periodontal 2006;77(2):271-9.

Kim DO, et al. Sweet and sour cherry phenolics and their protective effects on neuronal cells. J Agric Food Chem 2005;53(26):9921-7.

Knox YM, et al. Anti-influenza virus activity of crude extract of Ribes nigrum L. Phytother Res 2003;17(2):120-2.

Kresty LA, et al. Cranberry proanthocyanidins induce apoptosis and inhibit acid-induced proliferation of human esophageal adenocarcinoma cells. J Agric Food Chem 2008;56(3):676-80.

Lengsfeld C, et al. High molecular weight polysaccharides from blackcurrant seeds inhibit adhesion of Helicobacter pylori to human gastric mucosa. Planta Med 2004;70(7):620-6.

Li XM, et al. Effect of the Lycium barbarum polysaccharides on age-related oxidative stress in aged mice. J Ethnopharmacol 2007;111(3):504-11.

Luo Q, et al. Hypoglycemic and hypolipidemic effects and antioxidant activity of fruit extracts from Lycium barbarum. Life Sci 2004;76(2):137-49.

McDougall GJ, et al. Berry extracts exert different antiproliferative effects against cervical and colon cancer cells grown in vitro. J Agric Food Chem 2008;56(9):3016-23.

Morimoto C, et al. Anti-obese action of raspberry ketone. Life Sci 2005;77(2):194-204.

Neto CC. Cranberry and blueberry: evidence for protective effects against cancer and vascular diseases. Mol Nutr Food Res 2007;51(6):652-64.

Nohynek LJ, et al. Berry phenolics: antimicrobial properties and mechanisms of action against severe human pathogens. Nutr Cancer 2006;54(1):18-32.

Pepeljnjak S, et al. Antimicrobial activity of juniper berry essential oil (Juniperus communis L., Cupressaceae). Acta Pharm 2005;55(4):417-22.

Piccolella S, et al. Antioxidant properties of sour cherries (Prunus cerasus L.): role of colorless phytochemicals from the methanolic extract of ripe fruits. J Agric Food Chem 2008;56(6):1928-35.

Puupponen-Pimia R, et al. Bioactive berry compounds – novel tools against human pathogens. Appl Microbiol Biotechnol 2005;67(1):8-18.

Ramassamy C. Emerging role of polyphenolic compounds in the treatment of neurodegenerative diseases: a review of their intracellular targets. Eur J Pharmacol 2006;545(1):51-64.

Ruel G, Couillard C. Evidences of the cardioprotective potential of fruits: the case of cranberries. Mol Nutr Food Res 2007;51(6):692-701.

Seeram NP, et al. Blackberry, black raspberry, blueberry, cranberry, red raspberry, and strawberry extracts inhibit growth and stimulate apoptosis of human cancer cells in vitro. J Agric Food Chem 2006;54(25):9329-39.

Seeram NP. Berry fruits: compositional elements, biochemical activities, and the impact of their intake on human health, performance, and disease. J Agric Food Chem 2008;56(3):627-9.

Suzutani T, et al. Anti-herpes virus activity of an extract of Ribes nigrum L. Phytother Res 2003;17(6):609-13.

Torri E, et al. Anti-inflammatory and antinociceptive properties of blueberry extract (Vaccinium corymbosum). J Pharm Pharmacol 2007;59(4):591-6.

Van Slambrouck S, et al. Effects of crude aqueous medicinal plant extracts on growth and invasion of breast cancer cells. Oncol Rep 2007;17(6):1487-92.

Wilson T, et al. Human glycemic response and phenolic content of unsweetened cranberry juice. J Med Food 2008;11(1):46-54.

Wu X, et al. Characterization of anthocyanins and proanthocyanidins in some cultivars of Ribes, Aronia, and Sambucus and their antioxidant capacity. J Agric Food Chem 2004;52(26):7846-56.

Zafra-Stone S, et al. Berry anthocyanins as novel antioxidants in human health and disease prevention. Mol Nutr Food Res 2007;51(6):675-83.

Zakay-Rones Z, et al. Randomized study of the efficacy and safety of oral elderberry extract in the treatment of influenza A and B virus infections. J Int Med Res 2004;32(2):132-40.

Other fruits (apples, bananas, citrus, dates, figs, grapes, kiwifruits, passion fruits, plums and prunes, pomegranates)

Akazome Y. Characteristics and physiological functions of polyphenols from apples. Biofactors 2004;22(1-4):311-4.

Al-Shahib W, Marshall RJ. The fruit of the date palm: its possible use as the best food for the future? Int J Food Sci Nutr 2003;54(4):247-59.

Ataka S, et al. Effects of Applephenon and ascorbic acid on physical fatigue. Nutrition 2007;23(5):419-23.

Aviram M, et al. Pomegranate juice consumption

for 3 years by patients with carotid artery stenosis reduces common carotid intima-media thickness, blood pressure and LDL oxidation. Clin Nutr 2004;23(3):423-33.

Bae JM, et al. Citrus fruit intake and stomach cancer risk: a quantitative systematic review. Gastric Cancer 2008;11(1):23-32.

Benavente-García O, Castillo J. Update on uses and properties of citrus flavonoids: New findings in anti-cancer, cardiovascular, and anti-inflammatory activity. J Agric Food Chem 2008;56(15):6185-205.

Bradamante S, et al. Cardiovascular protective effects of resveratrol. Cardiovasc Drug Rev 2004;22(3):169-88.

Chan AO, et al. Increasing dietary fiber intake in terms of kiwifruit improves constipation in Chinese patients. World J Gastroenterol 2007;13(35):4771-5.

Chaturvedi PK, et al. Lupeol: connotations for chemoprevention. Cancer Lett 2008;263(1):1-13.

Collins BH, et al. Kiwifruit protects against oxidative DNA damage in human cells and in vitro. Nutr Cancer 2001;39(1):148-53.

Dani C, et al. Intake of purple grape juice as a hepatoprotective agent in Wistar rats. J Med Food 2008;11(1):127-32.

Delmas D, et al. Resveratrol: preventing properties against vascular alterations and ageing. Mol Nutr Food Res 2005;49(5):377-95.

Dhawan K, et al. Passiflora: a review update. J Ethnopharmacol 2004;94(1):1-23.

Duttaroy AK, Jørgensen A. Effects of kiwi fruit consumption on platelet aggregation and plasma lipids in healthy human volunteers. Platelets 2004;15(5):287-92.

Englberger L, et al. Carotenoid-rich bananas: a potential food source for alleviating vitamin A deficiency. Food Nutr Bull 2003;24(4):303-18.

Esmaillzadeh A, et al. Cholesterol-lowering effect of concentrated pomegranate juice consumption in type II diabetic patients with hyperlipidemia. Int J Vitam Nutr Res. 2006;76(3):147-51.

Folts JD. Potential health benefits from the flavonoids in grape products on vascular disease. Adv Exp Med Biol 2002;505:95-111.

German JB, Walzem RL. The health benefits of wine. Annu Rev Nutr 2000;20:561-93.

Green RJ, et al. Common tea formulations modulate in vitro digestive recovery of green tea catechins. Mol Nutr Food Res 2007;51(9):1152-62.

Hakim IA, Harris RB. Joint effects of citrus peel use and black tea intake on the risk of squamous cell carcinoma of the skin. BMC Dermatol 2001;1:3.

Heber D. Multitargeted therapy of cancer by ellagitannins. Cancer Lett 2008;269(2):262-8.

Hong YJ, et al. The flavonoid glycosides and procyanidin composition of Deglet Noor dates (Phoenix dactylifera). J Agric Food Chem 2006;54(6):2405-11.

Jung KA, et al. Cardiovascular protective properties of kiwifruit extracts in vitro. Biol Pharm Bul 2005;28(9):1782-5.

Kar P, et al. Flavonoid-rich grapeseed extracts: a new approach in high cardiovascular risk patients? Int J Clin Pract 2006;60(11):1484-92.

Khan N, et al. Cancer chemoprevention through dietary antioxidants: progress and promise. Antioxid Redox Signal 2008;10(3):475-510.

Kiani J, Imam SZ. Medicinal importance of grapefruit juice and its interaction with various drugs. Nutr J 2007;6:33.

Ko SH, et al. Comparison of the antioxidant activities of nine different fruits in human plasma. J Med Food 2005;8(1):41-6.

Lansky EP, Newman RA. Punica granatum (pomegranate) and its potential for prevention and treatment of inflammation and cancer. J Ethnopharmacol 2007;109(2):177-206.

Lekakis J, et al. Polyphenolic compounds from red grapes acutely improve endothelial function in patients with coronary heart disease. Eur J Cardiovasc Prev Rehabil 2005;12(6):596-600.

Malik A, et al. Pomegranate fruit juice for chemoprevention and chemotherapy of prostate cancer. Proc Natl Acad Sci USA 2005;102(41):14813-8.

Manthey JA, et al. Biological properties of citrus flavonoids pertaining to cancer and inflammation. Curr Med Chem 2001;8(2):135-53.

Menezes SM, et al. Punica granatum (pomegranate) extract is active against dental plaque. J Herb Pharmacother 2006;6(2):79-92.

Miller EG, et al. Inhibition of oral carcinogenesis by citrus flavonoids. Nutr Cancer 2008;60(1):69-74.

Motohashi N, et al. Cancer prevention and therapy with kiwifruit in Chinese folklore medicine: a study of kiwifruit extracts. J Ethnopharmacol 2002;81(3):357-64.

Movafegh A, et al. Preoperative oral Passiflora incarnata reduces anxiety in ambulatory surgery patients: a double-blind, placebo-controlled study. Anesth Analg 2008;106(6):1728-32.

Nahmias Y, et al. Apolipoprotein B dependent hepatitis C virus secretion is inhibited by the grapefruit flavonoid naringenin. Hepatology 2008;47(5):1437-44.

Neurath AR, et al. Punica granatum (pomegranate) juice provides an HIV-1 entry inhibitor and candidate topical microbicide. BMC Infect Dis 2004;4:41.

Reddy MK, et al. Antioxidant, antimalarial and antimicrobial activities of tannin-rich fractions, ellagitannins and phenolic acids from Punica granatum L. Planta Med 2007;73(5):461-7.

Saiko P, et al. Resveratrol and its analogs: defense against cancer, coronary disease and neurodegenerative maladies or just a fad? Mutat Res 2008;658(1-2):68-94.

Sarris J. Herbal medicines in the treatment of psychiatric disorders: a systematic review. Phytother Res 2007;21(8):703-16.

Shukla M, et al. Consumption of hydrolyzable tannins-rich pomegranate extract suppresses inflammation and joint damage in rheumatoid arthritis. Nutrition 2008;24(7-8):733-43.

Silalahi J. Anti-cancer and health protective properties of citrus fruit components. Asia Pac J Clin Nutr 2002;11(1):79-84.

Solomon A, et al. Antioxidant activities and anthocyanin content of fresh fruits of common fig (Ficus carica L.). J Agric Food Chem 2006;54(20):7717-23.

Stacewicz-Sapuntzakis M, et al. Chemical composition and potential health effects of prunes: a functional food? Crit Rev Food Sci Nutr 2001;41(4):251-86.

Sun J. D-Limonene: safety and clinical applications. Altern Med Rev 2007;12(3):259-64.

Tinker LF, et al. Consumption of prunes as a source of dietary fiber in men with mild hypercholesterolemia. Am J Clin Nutr 1991;53(5):1259-65.

Vinson JA, et al. Dried fruits: excellent in vitro and in vivo antioxidants. J Am Coll Nutr 2005;24(1):44-50.

Willers SM, et al. Maternal food consumption during pregnancy and asthma, respiratory and atopic symptoms in 5-year-old children. Thorax 2007;62(9):773-9.

Yi LT, et al. Antidepressant-like behavioral and neurochemical effects of the citrus-associated chemical apigenin. Life Sci 2008;82(13-14):741-51.

Zern TL, Fernandez ML. Cardioprotective effects of dietary polyphenols. J Nutr 2005;135(10):2291-4.

Grains and cereals including barley, oats, rice, wheat

Adom KK, et al. Phytochemical profiles and antioxidant activity of wheat varieties. J Agric Food Chem 2003;51(26):7825-34.

Amano Y, et al. Correlation between dietary glycemic index and cardiovascular disease risk factors among Japanese women. Eur J Clin Nutr 2004;58(11):1472-8.

Ardiansyah, Shirakawa H, et al. Rice bran fractions improve blood pressure, lipid profile, and glucose metabolism in stroke-prone spontaneously hypertensive rats. J Agric Food Chem 2006;54(5):1914-20.

Bird AR, et al. Wholegrain foods made from a novel high-amylose barley variety (Himalaya 292) improve indices of bowel health in human subjects. Br J Nutr 2008;99(5):1032-40.

Bylund A, et al. Randomised controlled short-term intervention pilot study on rye bran bread in prostate cancer. Eur J Cancer Prev 2003;12(5):407-15.

Food and Drug Administration. Food labeling: health claims; soluble fiber from certain foods and risk of coronary heart disease. Interim final rule. Fed Regist 2008 Feb 25;73(37):9938-47.

Hallmans G, et al. Rye, lignans and human health. Proc Nutr Soc 2003;62(1):193-9.

Ito S, Ishikawa Y. Marketing of value-added rice products in Japan: germinated brown rice and rice bread. FAO International Rice Year, 2004 Symposium Rome, Italy February 12, 2004.

Kariluoto S, et al. Effect of germination and thermal treatments on folates in rye. J Agric Food Chem 2006;54(25):9522-8.

Katina K, et al. Bran fermentation as a means to enhance technological properties and bioactivity of rye. Food Microbiol 2007;24(2):175-86.

Kemppainen T, et al. No observed local immunological response at cell level after five years of oats in adult coeliac disease. Scand J Gastroenterol 2007;42(1):54-9.

Kurtz ES, Wallo W. Colloidal oatmeal: history, chemistry and clinical properties. J Drugs Dermatol 2007;6(2):167-70.

Larsson SC, et al. Whole grain consumption and risk of colorectal cancer: a population-based cohort of 60,000 women. Br J Cancer 2005;92(9):1803-7.

Leinonen KS, et al. Rye bread decreases serum total and LDL cholesterol in men with moderately elevated serum-cholesterol. J Nutr 2000;130(2):164-70.

Mahoney CR, et al. Effect of breakfast composition on cognitive processes in elementary school children. Physiol Behav 2005;85(5):635-45.

Michalska A, et al. Antioxidant contents and antioxidative properties of traditional rye breads. J Agric Food Chem 2007;55(3):734-40.

Mori H, et al. Chemopreventive effects of ferulic acid on oral and rice germ on large bowel carcinogenesis. Anti-cancer Res 1999;19(5A):3775-8.

Osawa T. Protective role of rice polyphenols in oxidative stress. Anti-cancer Res 1999;19(5A):3645-50.

Ripsin CM, et al. Oat products and lipid lowering. A meta-analysis. JAMA 1992;267(24):3317-25.

Stallknecht GF, et al. Alternative wheat cereals as food grains: Einkorn, emmer, spelt, kamut, and triticale. In: Janick J (ed.), Progress in new crops. ASHS Press, Alexandria, VA, pp. 156-70, 1996.

Starr Moake, W. Make your own malt. In: Brew (homebrew magazine) Aug, 1997, pp 32–36.

Storsrud S, et al. Beneficial effects of oats in the gluten-free diet of adults with special reference to nutrient status, symptoms and subjective experiences. Br J Nutr

2003;90(1):101-7.

Wildmann J, et al. Occurrence of pharmacologically active benzodiazepines in trace amounts in wheat and potato. Biochem Pharmacol 1988;37(19):3549-59.

Other grains (amaranth, buckwheat, quinoa)

Li SQ, Zhang QH. Advances in the development of functional foods from buckwheat. Crit Rev Food Sci Nutr 2001;41(6):451-64.

Martirosyan DM, et al. Amaranth oil application for coronary heart disease and hypertension. Lipids Health Dis 2007;5;6:1.

Ogungbenle HN. Nutritional evaluation and functional properties of quinoa (Chenopodium quinoa) flour. Int J Food Sci Nutr 2003;54(2):153-8.

Ruales J, Nair BM. Nutritional quality of the protein in quinoa (Chenopodium quinoa, Willd) seeds. Plant Foods Hum Nutr 1992;42(1):1-11.

Herbs (borage, chamomile, dill, fennel, lemon balm, basil, parsley, rosemary, thyme, sage, mint)

Ait M'barek L, et al. Cytotoxic effect of essential oil of thyme (Thymus broussonettii) on the IGR-OV1 tumor cells resistant to chemotherapy. Braz J Med Biol Res 2007;40(11):1537-44.

Akhondzadeh S, et al. Melissa officinalis extract in the treatment of patients with mild to moderate Alzheimer's disease: a double blind, randomised, placebo controlled trial. J Neurol Neurosurg Psychiatry 2003;74(7):863-6.

Akhondzadeh S, et al. Salvia officinalis extract in the treatment of patients with mild to moderate Alzheimer's disease: a double blind, randomized and placebo-controlled trial. J Clin Pharm Ther 2003;28(1):53-9.

Alexandrovich I, et al. The effect of fennel (Foeniculum vulgare) seed oil emulsion in infantile colic: a randomized, placebo-controlled study. Altern Ther Health Med 2003;9(4):58-61.

Allahverdiyev A, et al. Antiviral activity of the volatile oils of Melissa officinalis L. against Herpes simplex virus type-2. Phytomedicine 2004;11(7-8):657-61.

Alma MH, et al. Screening chemical composition and in vitro antioxidant and antimicrobial activities of the essential oils from Origanum syriacum L. growing in Turkey. Biol Pharm Bull 2003;26(12):1725-9.

Amzazi S, et al. Human immunodeficiency virus type 1 inhibitory activity of Mentha longifolia. Therapie 2003;58(6):531-4.

Ballard CG, et al. Aromatherapy as a safe and effective treatment for the management of agitation in severe dementia: the results of a double-blind, placebo-controlled trial with Melissa. J Clin Psychiatry 2002;63(7):553-8.

Belch JJ, Hill A. Evening primrose oil and borage oil in rheumatologic conditions. Am J Clin Nutr 2000;71(1 Suppl):352S-6S.

Beric T, et al. Protective effect of basil (Ocimum basilicum L.) against oxidative DNA damage and mutagenesis. Food Chem Toxicol 2008;46(2):724-32.

Betoni JE, et al. Synergism between plant extract and antimicrobial drugs used on Staphylococcus aureus diseases. Mem Inst Oswaldo Cruz 2006;101(4):387-90.

Bozin B, et al. Characterization of the volatile composition of essential oils of some Lamiaceae spices and the antimicrobial and antioxidant activities of the entire oils. J Agric Food Chem 2006;54(5):1822-8.

Burt SA, Reinders RD. Antibacterial activity of selected plant essential oils against Escherichia coli O157:H7. Lett Appl Microbiol 2003;36(3):162-7.

Dadalioglu I, Evrendilek GA. Chemical compositions and antibacterial effects of essential oils of Turkish oregano (Origanum minutiflorum), bay laurel (Laurus nobilis), Spanish lavender (Lavandula stoechas L.), and fennel (Foeniculum vulgare) on common foodborne pathogens. J Agric Food Chem 2004;52(26):8255-60.

de Sousa AC, et al. Melissa officinalis L. essential oil: antitumoral and antioxidant activities. J Pharm Pharmacol 2004;56(5):677-81.

Dimpfel W, et al. Effects of lozenge containing lavender oil, extracts from hops, lemon balm and oat on electrical brain activity of volunteers. Eur J Med Res 2004;9(9):423-31.

Dragon S, et al. Role of multi-component functional foods in the complex treatment of patients with advanced breast cancer. Rev Med Chir Soc Med Nat Iasi 2007;111(4):877-84.

El SN, Karakaya S. Radical scavenging and iron-chelating activities of some greens used as traditional dishes in Mediterranean diet. Int J Food Sci Nutr 2004;55(1):67-74.

Feres M, et al. In vitro antimicrobial activity of plant extracts and propolis in saliva samples of healthy and periodontally-involved subjects. J Int Acad Periodontol 2005;7(3):90-6.

Geuenich S, et al. Aqueous extracts from peppermint, sage and lemon balm leaves display potent anti-HIV-1 activity by increasing the virion density. Retrovirology 2008;5:27.

Gilani AH, et al. Pharmacological basis for the use of Borago officinalis in gastrointestinal, respiratory and cardiovascular disorders. J Ethnopharmacol 2007;114(3):393-9.

Goun E, et al. Antithrombin activity of some constituents from Origanum vulgare. Fitoterapia 2002;73(7-8):692-4.

Grigoleit HG, Grigoleit P. Gastrointestinal clinical pharmacology of peppermint oil. Phytomedicine 2005;12(8):607-11.

Gülçin I, et al. Determination of antioxidant and radical scavenging activity of basil (Ocimum basilicum L. Family Lamiaceae) assayed by different methodologies. Phytother Res 2007;21(4);354-61.

Hazzit M, et al. Composition of the essential oils of Thymus and Origanum species from Algeria and their antioxidant and antimicrobial activities. J Agric Food Chem 2006;54(17):6314-21.

Henz BM, et al. Double-blind, multicentre analysis of the efficacy of borage oil in patients with atopic eczema. Br J Dermatol 1999;140(4):685-8.

Hohmann J, et al. Protective effects of the aerial parts of Salvia officinalis, Melissa officinalis and Lavandula angustifolia and their constituents against enzyme-dependent and enzyme-independent lipid peroxidation. Planta Med 1999;65(6):576-8.

Huang MT, et al. Inhibition of skin tumorigenesis by rosemary and its constituents carnosol and ursolic acid. Cancer Res 1994;54(3):701-8.

Imanshahidi M, Hosseinzadeh H. The pharmacological effects of Salvia species on the central nervous system. Phytother Res 2006;20(6):427-37.

Jagetia G. Radioprotective potential of plants and herbs against the effects of ionizing radiation. J Clin Biochem Nutr 2007;40(2):74-81.

Javidnia K, et al. Antihirsutism activity of Fennel (fruits of Foeniculum vulgare) extract. A double-blind placebo controlled study. Phytomedicine 2003;10(6-7):455-8.

Joshi H, Parle M. Cholinergic basis of memory-strengthening effect of Foeniculum vulgare Linn. J Med Food 2006;9(3):413-7.

Kreydiyyeh SI, Usta J. Diuretic effect and mechanism of action of parsley. J Ethnopharmacol 2002;79(3):353-7.

Kristinsson KG, et al. Effective treatment of experimental acute otitis media by application of volatile fluids into the ear canal. J Infect Dis 2005;191:1876-80.

Kulisic T, et al. Antioxidant properties of thyme (Thymus vulgaris L.) and wild thyme (Thymus serpyllum L.) essential oils. It J Food Sci 2005;17(3):315-24.

Lachowicz, et al. The synergistic preservative effects of the essential oils of sweet basil (Ocimum basilicum L.) against acid-tolerant food microflora. Letts Appl Microbiol 1998;26(3):209-14.

Lin YT, et al. Inhibition of Helicobacter pylori and associated urease by oregano and cranberry phytochemical synergies. Appl Environ Microbiol 2005;71(12):8558-64.

Luqman S, et al. Potential of rosemary oil to be used in drug-resistant infections. Altern Ther Health Med 2007;13(5):54-9.

Matern U. Coumarins and other phenylpropanoid compounds in the defense response of plant cells. Planta Med 1991;57(7 Suppl):S15-20.

Meeran SM. Cell cycle control as a basis for cancer chemoprevention through dietary agents. Front Biosci 2008;13:2191-202.

Mimica D, et al. Antimicrobial and antioxidant activities of Melissa officinalis L. (Lamiaceae) essential oil. J Agric Food Chem 2004; 52(9):2485-9.

Mimica D, et al. Antimicrobial and antioxidant activities of three Mentha species essential oils. Planta Med 2003;69(5):413-9.

Monsefi M, et al. The effects of Anethum graveolens L. on female reproductive system. Phytother Res 2006;20(10):865-8.

Mühlbauer RC, et al. Common herbs, essential oils, and monoterpenes potently modulate bone metabolism. Bone 2003;32(4):372-80.

Namavar Jahromi B, et al. Comparison of fennel and mefenamic acid for the treatment of primary dysmenorrhea. Int J Gynaecol Obstet 2003;80(2):153-7.

Nascimento GGF, et al. Antibacterial activity of plant extracts and phytochemicals on antibiotic-resistant bacteria. Brazil J Microbiol 2002;31(4).

Nolkemper S, et al. Antiviral effect of aqueous extracts from species of the Lamiaceae family against Herpes simplex virus Type 1 and Type 2 in vitro. Planta Med 2006;72(15):1378-82.

Ozbek H, et al. Hepatoprotective effect of Foeniculum vulgare essential oil. Fitoterapia 2003;74(3):317-9.

Patel D, et al. Apigenin and cancer chemoprevention: progress, potential and promise (review). Int J Oncol 2007;30(1):233-45.

Petersen M, Simmonds MS. Rosmarinic acid. Phytochemistry 2003;62(2):121-5.

Putnam SE, et al. Natural products as alternative treatments for metabolic bone disorders and for maintenance of bone health. Phytother Res 2007;21(2):99-112.

Rasooli I, et al. Ultrastructural studies on antimicrobial efficacy of thyme essential oils on Listeria monocytogenes. Int J Infect Dis 2006;10(3):236-41.

Ruberto G, et al. Antioxidant and antimicrobial activity of Foeniculum vulgare and Crithmum maritimum essential oils. Planta Med 2000;66(8):687-93.

Satyanarayana S, et al. Antioxidant activity of the aqueous extracts of spicy food additives – evaluation and comparison with ascorbic acid in in-vitro systems. J Herb Pharmacother 2004;4(2):1-10.

Schirmer MA, Phinney SD. Gamma-linolenate reduces weight regain in formerly obese humans. J Nutr 2007;137(6):1430-5.

Scholey AB, et al. An extract of Salvia (sage) with anticholinesterase properties improves memory and attention in healthy older volunteers. Psychopharmacology (Berl) 2008;198(1):127-39.

Schuhmacher A, et al. Virucidal effect of peppermint oil on the enveloped viruses herpes simplex virus type 1 and type 2 in vitro. Phytomedicine 2003;10(6-7):504-10.

Singh G, et al. Studies on essential oils: part 10; antibacterial activity of volatile oils of some spices. Phytother Res 2002;16(7):680-2.

Srivastava JK, Gupta S. Antiproliferative and apoptotic effects of chamomile extract in various human cancer cells. J Agric Food Chem 2007;55(23):9470-8.

Stavri M, Gibbons S. The antimycobacterial constituents of dill (Anethum graveolens). Phytother Res 2005;19(11):938-41.

Tampieri MP, et al. The inhibition of Candida albicans by selected essential oils and their major components. Mycopathologia 2005;159(3):339-45.

Tildesley NT, et al. Positive modulation of mood and cognitive performance following administration of acute doses of Salvia lavandulaefolia essential oil to healthy young volunteers. Physiol Behav 2005;83(5):699-709.

Van Den Broucke CO, Lemli JA. Spasmolytic activity of the flavonoids from Thymus vulgaris. Pharm Weekbl Sci 1983;25;5(1):9-14.

Wake G, et al. CNS acetylcholine receptor activity in European medicinal plants traditionally used to improve failing memory. J Ethnopharmacol 2000;69(2):105-14.

Wei A, Shibamoto T. Antioxidant activities of essential oil mixtures toward skin lipid squalene oxidized by UV irradiation. Cutan Ocul Toxicol 2007;26(3):227-33.

Wu CC, et al. Metabolism of omega-6 polyunsaturated fatty acids in women with dysmenorrhea. Asia Pac J Clin Nutr 2008;17(Suppl 1):216-9.

Yamamoto J, et al. Testing various herbs for antithrombotic effect. Nutrition 2005;21(5):580-7.

Yu TW, et al. Antimutagenic activity of spearmint. Environ Mol Mutagen 2004;44(5):387-93.

Zheng GQ, et al. Anethofuran, carvone, and limonene: potential cancer chemopreventive agents from dill weed oil and caraway oil. Planta Med 1992;58(4):338-41.

Zhu J, et al. Adult repellency and larvicidal activity of five plant essential oils against mosquitoes. J Am Mosq Control Assoc 2006;22(3):515-22.

Zidorn C, et al. Polyacetylenes from the Apiaceae vegetables carrot, celery, fennel, parsley, and parsnip and their cytotoxic activities. J Agric Food Chem 2005;53(7):2518-23.

Nuts (Brazils, cashews, hazelnuts, macadamias, peanuts, pistachios, walnuts)

Alexander J. Selenium. Novartis Found Symp 2007;282:143-9; discussion 149-53, 212-8.

Blomhoff R, et al. Health benefits of nuts: potential role of antioxidants. Br J Nutr 2006;96(Suppl 2):S52-60.

Burk RF. Selenium, an antioxidant nutrient. Nutr Clin Care 2002;5(2):75-9.

Cortés B, et al. Acute effects of high-fat meals enriched with walnuts or olive oil on postprandial endothelial function. J Am Coll Cardiol 2006;48(8):1666-71.

Curb JD, et al. Serum lipid effects of a high-monounsaturated fat diet based on macadamia nuts. Arch Intern Med 2000;160(8):1154-8.

Garg ML, et al. Macadamia nut consumption modulates favourably risk factors for coronary artery disease in hypercholesterolemic subjects. Lipids 2007;42(6):583-7.

Hiraoka-Yamamoto J, et al. Serum lipid effects of a monounsaturated (palmitoleic) fatty acid-rich diet based on macadamia nuts in healthy, young Japanese women. Clin Exp Pharmacol Physiol 2004;31(Suppl 2):S37-8.

Hughes GM, et al. The effect of Korean pine nut oil (PinnoThin) on food intake, feeding behaviour and appetite: a double-blind placebo-controlled trial. Lipids Health Dis 2008;7:6.

Klein EA, et al. SELECT: the next prostate cancer prevention trial. Selenium and Vitamin E Cancer Prevention Trial. J Urol 2001;166(4):1311-5.

Kocyigit A, et al. Effects of pistachio nuts consumption on plasma lipid profile and oxidative status in healthy volunteers. Nutr Metab Cardiovasc Dis 2006;16(3):202-9.

Li L, et al. Polyphenolic profiles and antioxidant activities of heartnut (Juglans ailanthifolia Var. cordiformis) and Persian walnut (Juglans regia L.). J Agric Food Chem 2006;54(21):8033-40.

Maguire LS, et al. Fatty acid profile, tocopherol, squalene and phytosterol content of walnuts, almonds, peanuts, hazelnuts and the macadamia nut. Int J Food Sci Nutr 2004;55(3):171-8.

Nestel P, et al. Effects of increasing dietary palmitoleic acid compared with palmitic and oleic acids on plasma lipids of hypercholesterolemic men. J Lipid Res 1994;35(4):656-62.

Papoutsi Z, et al. Walnut extract (Juglans regia L.) and its component ellagic acid exhibit anti-inflammatory activity in human aorta endothelial cells and osteoblastic activity in the cell line KS483. Br J Nutr 2008;99(4):715-22.

Rayman MP. The argument for increasing selenium intake. Proc Nutr Soc 2002;61(2):203-15.

Ros E, et al. A walnut diet improves endothelial function in hypercholesterolemic subjects: a randomized crossover trial. Circulation 2004;109(13):1609-14.

Ryan E, et al. Fatty acid profile, tocopherol, squalene and phytosterol content of brazil, pecan, pine, pistachio and cashew nuts. Intl J

Food Sci Nutr 2006;57(3-4):219-28.

Sabaté J, et al. Does regular walnut consumption lead to weight gain? Br J Nutr 2005;94(5):859-64.

Shahidi F, et al. Antioxidant phytochemicals in hazelnut kernel (Corylus avellana L.) and hazelnut byproducts. J Agric Food Chem. 2007;55(4):1212-20.

Trevisan MT, et al. Characterization of alkyl phenols in cashew (Anacardium occidentale) products and assay of their antioxidant capacity. Food Chem Toxicol 2006;44(2):188-97.

Seeds (alfalfa, linseed, plantain, pumpkin, safflower, sesame, sunflower)

Abraham ZD, Mehta T. Three-week psyllium husk supplementation: Effect on plasma cholesterol concentrations, fecal steroid excretion, and carbohydrate absorption in men. Am J Clin Nutr 1988;47(1):67-74.

Anderson JW, et al. Cholesterol-lowering effects of psyllium intake adjunctive to diet therapy in men and women with hypercholesterolemia: meta-analysis of 8 controlled trials. Am J Clin Nutr 2000;71(2):472-9.

Baumgaertel A. Alternative and controversial treatments for attention-deficit/hyperactivity disorder. Pediatr Clin of North Am 1999;46(5):977-92.

Belluzzi A, et al. Polyunsaturated fatty acids and inflammatory bowel disease. Am J Clin Nutr 2000;71(Suppl):339S-42S.

Boelsma E, et al. Nutritional skin care: health effects of micronutrients and fatty acids. Am J Clin Nutr 2001;73(5):853-64.

Bruinsma KA, Taren DL. Dieting, essential fatty acid intake, and depression. Nutr Rev 2000;58(4):98-108.

Cooney RV, et al. Effects of dietary sesame seeds on plasma tocopherol levels. Nutr Cancer 2001;39(1):66-71.

Coulman KD, et al. Whole sesame seed is as rich a source of mammalian lignan precursors as whole flaxseed. Nutr Cancer 2005;52(2):156-65.

Danao-Camara TC, Shintani TT. The dietary treatment of inflammatory arthritis: case reports and review of the literature. Hawaii Med J 1999;58(5):126-31.

Deutch B. Menstrual pain in Danish women correlated with low n-3 polyunsaturated fatty acid intake. Eur J Clin Nutr 1995;49(7):508-16.

Fernandez D, et al. Randomized clinical trial of Plantago ovata seeds (dietary fiber) as compared with mesalamine in maintaining remission in ulcerative colitis. Am J Gastroenterol 1999;94(2):427-33.

Frank J. Beyond vitamin E supplementation: an alternative strategy to improve vitamin E status. J Plant Physiol 2005;162(7):834-43.

Galvez M, et al. Cytotoxic effect of Plantago spp. on cancer cell lines. J Ethnopharmacol 2003;88(2-3):125-30.

Hannan JM, et al. Aqueous extracts of husks of Plantago ovata reduce hyperglycaemia in type 1 and type 2 diabetes by inhibition of intestinal glucose absorption. Br J Nutr 2006;96(1):131-7.

Harper CR, Jacobson TA. The fats of life: the role of omega-3 fatty acids in the prevention of coronary heart disease. Arch Intern Med 2001;161(18):2185-92.

Heo JC, et al. Aqueous extract of the Helianthus annuus seed alleviates asthmatic symptoms in vivo. Int J Mol Med 2008;21(1):57-61.

Horrobin DF, Bennett CN. Depression and bipolar disorder: relationships to impaired fatty acid and phospholipid metabolism and to diabetes, cardiovascular disease, immunological abnormalities, cancer, ageing and osteoporosis. Prostaglandins Leukot Essent Fatty Acids 1999;60(4):217-34.

Kremer JM. N-3 fatty acid supplements in rheumatoid arthritis. Am J Clin Nutr 2000;(Suppl 1):349S-51S.

Kusum M, et al. Preliminary efficacy and safety of oral suspension SH, combination of five chinese medicinal herbs, in people living with HIV/AIDS; the phase I/II study. J Med Assoc Thai 2004;87(9):1065-70.

Lim JS, et al. Comparative analysis of sesame lignans (sesamin and sesamolin) in affecting hepatic fatty acid metabolism in rats. Br J Nutr 2007;97(1):85-95.

Lockwood K, et al. Apparent partial remission of breast cancer in 'high risk' patients supplemented with nutritional antioxidants, essential fatty acids, and coenzyme Q10. Mol Aspects Med 1994;15(Suppl):s231-s40.

Prasad K. Dietary flaxseed in prevention of hypercholesterolemic atherosclerosis. Atherosclerosis 1997;132(1):69-76.

Ryan E, et al. Phytosterol, squalene, tocopherol content and fatty acid profile of selected seeds, grains, and legumes. Plants Food Hum Nutr 2007;62(3):85-91.

Salas-Salvadó J, et al. Effect of two doses of a mixture of soluble fibres on body weight and metabolic variables in overweight or obese patients: a randomised trial. Br J Nutr 2008;99(6):1380-7.

Samuelsen AB. The traditional uses, chemical constituents and biological activities of Plantago major L. A review. J Ethnopharmacol 2000;71(1-2):1-21.

Simopoulos AP. Essential fatty acids in health and chronic disease. Am J Clin Nutr 1999;70(2 Suppl):560S-9S.

Solà R, et al. Effects of soluble fiber (Plantago ovata husk) on plasma lipids, lipoproteins, and apolipoproteins in men with ischemic heart disease. Am J Clin Nutr 2007;85(4):1157-63.

Stampfer MJ, et al. Primary prevention of coronary heart disease in women through diet and lifestyle. N Eng J Med 2000;343(1):16-22.

Stoll BA. Breast cancer and the Western diet: role of fatty acids and antioxidant vitamins. Eur J Cancer 1998;34(12):1852-6.

Visavadiya NP, Narasimhacharya AV. Sesame as a hypocholesteraemic and antioxidant dietary component. Food Chem Toxicol 2008;46(6):1889-95.

Wu CC, et al. Metabolism of omega-6 polyunsaturated fatty acids in women with dysmenorrhea. Asia Pac J Clin Nutr 2008;17(Suppl 1):216-9.

Wu WH, et al. Sesame ingestion affects sex hormones, antioxidant status, and blood lipids in postmenopausal women. J Nutr 2006;136(5):1270-5.

Yamashita K, et al. Comparative effects of flaxseed and sesame seed on vitamin E and cholesterol levels in rats. Lipids 2003;38(12):1249-55.

Yoo HH, et al. An anti-estrogenic lignan glycoside, tracheloside, from seeds of Carthamus tinctorius. Biosci Biotechnol Biochem 2006;70(11):2783-5.

Zhang HL, et al. Antioxidative compounds isolated from safflower (Carthamus tinctorius L.) oil cake. Chem Pharm Bull (Tokyo) 1997;45(12):1910-4.

Spices (anise, cardamom, chilli (and sweet capsicums), cinnamon, coriander, cumin, ginger, nutmeg and cloves, peppercorns, tamarind, turmeric)

Aggarwal BB, et al. Curcumin: the Indian solid gold. Adv Exp Med Biol 2007;595:1-75.

Ali BH, et al. Some phytochemical, pharmacological and toxicological properties of ginger (Zingiber officinale Roscoe): a review of recent research. Food Chem Toxicol 2008;46(2):409-2.

American Chemical Society. Ginger may combat deadly infant diarrhea in developing world. ScienceDaily 2007. Retrieved May 2008, from http://www.sciencedaily.com/releases/2007/10/071001092216.htm.

Anand P, et al. Bioavailability of curcumin: problems and promises. Mol Pharm 2007;4(6):807-18.

Baker WL, et al. Effect of cinnamon on glucose control and lipid parameters. Diabetes Care 2008;31(1):41-3.

Banerjee S, et al. Clove (Syzygium aromaticum L.), a potential chemopreventive agent for lung cancer. Carcinogenesis 2006;27(8):1645-54.

Bano G, et al. Effect of piperine on bioavailability and pharmacokinetics of propranolol and theophylline in healthy volunteers. Eur J Clin Pharmacol 1991;41(6):615-7.

Betoni JE, et al. Synergism between plant extract and antimicrobial drugs used on Staphylococcus aureus diseases. Mem Inst Oswaldo Cruz 2006;101(4):387-90.

Chaudhry NM, Tariq P. Bactericidal activity of black pepper, bay leaf, aniseed and coriander against oral isolates. Pak J Pharm Sci 2006;19(3):214-8.

Chile-man website provides a wealth of information about chillis, including providing a database of nearly 3600 varieties, at: http://www.thechileman.org/search.php

Chithra V, Leelamma S. Hypolipidemic effect of coriander seeds (Coriandrum sativum): mechanism of action. Plant Foods Hum Nutr 1997;51(2):167-72.

Cole GM, et al. Neuroprotective effects of curcumin. Adv Exp Med Biol 2007;595:197-212.

Davis PB, Drumm ML. Some like it hot: curcumin and CFTR. Trends Mol Med 2004;10(10):473-5.

Delaquis PJ, et al. Antimicrobial activity of individual and mixed fractions of dill, cilantro, coriander and eucalyptus essential oils. Int J Food Microbiol 2002;74(1-2):101-9.

Deodhar SD, et al. Preliminary study on antirheumatic activity of curcumin (diferuloyl methane). Indian J Med Res 1980;71:632-4.

Dorman HJD, Deans SG. Antimicrobial agents from plants: antibacterial activity of plant volatile oils. J Appl Microbiol 2000;88(2):308.

Egan ME, et al. Curcumin, a major constituent of turmeric, corrects cystic fibrosis defects. Science 2004;304(5670):600-2

Garba M, et al. Effect of Tamarindus indica L on the bioavailability of ibuprofen in healthy human volunteers. Eur J Drug Metab Pharmacokinet 2003;28(3):179-84.

Ghayur MN, Gilani AH. Pharmacological basis for the medicinal use of ginger in gastrointestinal disorders. Dig Dis Sci 2005;50(10):1889-97.

Gilani AH, et al. Gut modulatory, blood pressure lowering, diuretic and sedative activities of cardamom. J Ethnopharmacol 2008;115(3):463-72.

Goel A, et al. Curcumin as 'Curecumin': from kitchen to clinic. Biochem Pharmacol 2008;75(4):787-809.

Golembiewski J, et al. Prevention and treatment of postoperative nausea and vomiting. Am J Health-Syst Pharm 2005;62(12):1247-60.

Gulcin I, et al. Screening of antioxidant and antimicrobial activities of anise (Pimpinella anisum L.) seed extracts. Food Chem 2003;83(3):371-82.

Iacobellis NS, et al. Antibacterial activity of Cuminum cyminum L. and Carum carvi L. essential oils. J Agric Food Chem 2005;53(1):57-61.

Iftekhar AS, et al. Effect of Tamarindus indica fruits on blood pressure and lipid-profile in human model: an in vivo approach. Pak J Pharm Sci 2006;19(2):125-9.

Jagetia GC, Aggarwal BB. 'Spicing up' of the immune system by curcumin. J Clin Immunol 2007;27(1):19-35.

Kalemba D, Kunicka A. Antibacterial and antifungal properties of essential oils. Curr Med Chem 2003;10(10):813-29.

Khan A, et al. Cinnamon improves glucose and lipids of people with type 2 diabetes. Diabetes Care 2003;26(12):3215-8.

Kosalec I, et al. Antifungal activity of fluid extract and essential oil from anise fruits (Pimpinella anisum L., Apiaceae). Acta Pharm 2005;55(4):377-85.

Lans CA. Ethnomedicines used in Trinidad and Tobago for urinary problems and diabetes mellitus. J Ethnobiol Ethnomed 2006;2:45.

Lim GP, et al. The curry spice curcumin reduces oxidative damage and amyloid pathology in an Alzheimer transgenic mouse. J Neurosci 2001;21(21):8370-7.

Lim K, et al. Dietary red pepper ingestion increases carbohydrate oxidation at rest and during exercise in runners. Med Sci Sports Exerc 1997;29(3):355-61.

Lopez P, et al. Solid- and vapor-phase antimicrobial activities of six essential oils: susceptibility of selected foodborne bacterial and fungal strains. J Agric Food Chem 2005;53(17):6939-46.

López-Lázaro M. Anti-cancer and carcinogenic properties of curcumin: Considerations for its clinical development as a cancer chemopreventive and chemotherapeutic agent. Mol Nutr Food Res 2008;52(S1):103-27.

Macho A, et al. Non-pungent capsaicinoids from sweet pepper synthesis and evaluation of the chemopreventive and anti-cancer potential. Eur J Nutr 2003;42(1):2-9.

Mahady GB, et al. In vitro susceptibility of Helicobacter pylori to botanical extracts used traditionally for the treatment of gastrointestinal disorders. Phytother Res 2005;19(11):988-91.

Maheshwari RK, et al. Multiple biological activities of curcumin: a short review. Life Sci 2006;78(18):2081-7.

Mau J, et al. Antimicrobial effect of extracts from Chinese chive, cinnamon, and corni fructus. J Agric Food Chem 2001;49(1):183-8.

Mujumdar AM, et al. Anti-inflammatory activity of piperine. Jpn J Med Sci Biol 1990;43(3):95-100.

Narasimhan B, Dhake AS. Antibacterial principles from Myristica fragrans seeds. J Med Food 2006;9(3):395-9.

Norajit K, et al. Antibacterial effect of five Zingiberaceae essential oils. Molecules. 2007;12(8):2047-60.

Ono K, et al. Curcumin has potent anti-amyloidogenic effects for Alzheimer's beta-amyloid fibrils in vitro. J Neurosci Res 2004;75(6):742-50.

Perez C, Anesini C. Antibacterial activity of alimentary plants against Staphylococcus aureus growth. Am J Chin Med 1994;22(2):169-74.

Portnoi G, et al. Prospective comparative study of the safety and effectiveness of ginger for the treatment of nausea and vomiting in pregnancy. Am J Obstet Gynecol 2003;189(5):1374-7.

Prajapati V, et al. Insecticidal, repellent and oviposition-deterrent activity of selected essential oils against Anopheles stephensi, Aedes aegypti and Culex quinquefasciatus. Bioresour Technol 2005;96(16):1749-57.

Preuss HG, et al. Whole cinnamon and aqueous extracts ameliorate sucrose-induced blood pressure elevations in spontaneously hypertensive rats. J Am Coll Nutr 2006;25(2):144-50.

Rolando M, Valente C. Establishing the tolerability and performance of tamarind seed polysaccharide (TSP) in treating dry eye syndrome: results of a clinical study. BMC Ophthalmol 2007;7:5.

Sharma RA, et al. Pharmacokinetics and pharmacodynamics of curcumin. Adv Exp Med Biol 2007;595:453-70.

Shishodia S, et al. Curcumin: getting back to the roots. Ann N Y Acad Sci 2005;1056:206-17.

Shoba G, et al. Influence of piperine on the pharmacokinetics of curcumin in animals and human volunteers. Planta Med 1998;64(4):353-6.

Shukla Y, Singh M. Cancer preventive properties of ginger: a brief review. Food Chem Toxicol 2007;45(5):683-90.

Strickland FM, et al. Natural products as aids for protecting the skin's immune system against UV damage. Cutis 2004;74(5 Suppl):24-8.

Strimpakos AS, Sharma RA. Curcumin: preventive and therapeutic properties in laboratory studies and clinical trials. Antioxid Redox Signal 2008;10(3):511-45.

Suneetha, WJ, Krishnakantha TP. Cardamom extract as inhibitor of human platelet aggregation. Phytother Res 2005;19(5):437-40.

Surh YJ, Lee SS. Capsaicin in hot chili pepper: carcinogen, co-carcinogen or anticarcinogen? Food Chem Toxicol 1996;34(3):313-6.

Tajuddin, Ahmad S, et al. An experimental study of sexual function improving effect of Myristica fragrans Houtt. (nutmeg). BMC Complement Altern Med 2005;5:16.

Thangapazham RL, et al. Multiple molecular targets in cancer chemoprevention by curcumin. AAPS J 2006;8(3):E443-9.

Trongtokit Y, et al. Comparative repellency of 38 essential oils against mosquito bites. Phytother Res 2005;19(4):303-9.

Ushanandini S, et al. The anti-snake venom properties of Tamarindus indica (leguminosae) seed extract. Phytother Res 2006;20(10):851-8.

Yoshioka M, et al. Effects of red pepper on appetite and energy intake. Br J Nutr 1999;82(2):115-23.

Vegetables: General (avocado, beans, beetroots, capers, carrots, celery, celeriac, chard, chicory, dandelion, endive, globe artichoke and cardoon, Jerusalem artichoke, nettles, olives, purslane, seaweeds, spinach, sweet potatoes, tomatoes)

Ahmed B, et al. Antihepatotoxic activity of seeds of Cichorium intybus. J Ethnopharmacol 2003;87(2-3):237-40.

Araya H, et al. Digestion rate of legume carbohydrates and glycemic index of legume-based meals. Int J Food Sci Nutr 2003;54(2):119-26.

Arena A, et al. Antiviral and immunomodulatory effect of a lyophilized extract of Capparis spinosa L. buds. Phytother Res 2008;22(3):313-7.

Aust O, et al. Supplementation with tomato-based products increases lycopene, phytofluene, and phytoene levels in human serum and protects against UV-light-induced erythema. Int J Vitam Nutr Res 2005;75(1):54-60.

Bhuvaneswari V, Nagini S. Lycopene: a review of its potential as an anti-cancer agent. Curr Med Chem Anti-cancer Agents 2005;5(6):627-35.

Blackberry I, et al. Legumes: the most important dietary predictor of survival in older people of different ethnicities. Asia Pac J Clin Nutr 2004;13(Suppl):S126.

Bond, RE, The caper bush. The Herbalist 1990;56:77-85.

Bonina F, et al. In vitro antioxidant and in vivo photoprotective effects of a lyophilized extract of Capparis spinosa L buds. J Cosmet Sci 2002;53(6):321-35.

Branca F, Lorenzetti S. Health effects of phytoestrogens. Forum Nutr 2005;57:100-1.

Brat P, et al. Daily polyphenol intake in France from fruit and vegetables. J Nutr 2006;136(9):2368-73.

Bundy R, et al. Artichoke leaf extract reduces symptoms of irritable bowel syndrome and improves quality of life in otherwise healthy volunteers suffering from concomitant dyspepsia: a subset analysis. J Altern Complement Med 2004;10(4):667-9.

Cardador-Martínez A, et al. Relationship among antimutagenic, antioxidant and enzymatic activities of methanolic extract from common beans (Phaseolus vulgaris L). Plants Food Hum Nutr 2006;61(4):161-8.

Cassidy A. Potential risks and benefits of phytoestrogen-rich diets. Int J Vitam Nutr Res 2003;73(2):120-6.

Celleno L, et al. A dietary supplement containing standardized Phaseolus vulgaris extract influences body composition of overweight men and women. Int J Med Sci 2007;4(1):45-52.

Chan K, et al. The analgesic and anti-inflammatory effects of Portulaca oleracea L.

subsp. sativa (Haw.) Celak. J Ethnopharmacol 2000;73(3):445-51.

Chaturvedi PK, et al. Lupeol: connotations for chemoprevention. Cancer Lett 2008;263(1):1-13.

Choi MS, Rhee KC. Production and processing of soybeans and nutrition and safety of isoflavone and other soy products for human health. J Med Food 2006;9(1):1-10.

Christensen LP, Brandt K. Bioactive polyacetylenes in food plants of the Apiaceae family: occurrence, bioactivity and analysis. J Pharm Biomed Anal 2006;41(3):683-93.

Chu YF, et al. Antioxidant and antiproliferative activities of common vegetables. J Agric Food Chem 2002;50(23):6910-6.

Clair RS, Anthony M. Soy, isoflavones and atherosclerosis. Handb Exp 2005;170:301-23.

Das S, et al. Lycopene, tomatoes, and coronary heart disease. Free Radic Res 2005;39(4):449-55.

de Mejía EG, et al. Antimutagenic effects of natural phenolic compounds in beans. Mutat Res 1999;441(1):1-9.

Ding H, et al. Chemopreventive characteristics of avocado fruit. Semin Cancer Biol 2007;17(5):386-94.

Doh-Ura K, et al. Prophylactic effect of dietary seaweed Fucoidan against enteral prion infection. Antimicrob Agents Chemother 2007;51(6):2274-7.

Durak I, et al. Aqueous extract of Urtica dioica makes significant inhibition on adenosine deaminase activity in prostate tissue from patients with prostate cancer. Cancer Biol Ther 2004;3(9):855-7.

Dweck AC. Puslane (Portulaca oleracea): the global panacea. Personal Care Mag 2001;2(4):7-15.

El SN, Karakaya S. Radical scavenging and iron-chelating activities of some greens used as traditional dishes in Mediterranean diet. Int J Food Sci Nutr 2004;55(1):67-74.

Frestedt JL, et al. A natural mineral supplement provides relief from knee osteoarthritis symptoms: a randomized controlled pilot trial. Nutr J 2008;7:9.

Germano MP, et al. Evaluation of extracts and isolated fraction from Capparis spinosa L. buds as an antioxidant source. J Agric Food Chem 2002;50(5):1168-71.

Giovannucci E. A review of epidemiologic studies of tomatoes, lycopene, and prostate cancer. Exp Biol Med (Maywood) 2002;227(10):852-9.

Gozum S, et al. Complementary alternative treatments used by patients with cancer in eastern Turkey. Cancer Nurs 2003;26(3):230-6.

Gulcin I, et al. Antioxidant, antimicrobial, antiulcer and analgesic activities of nettle (Urtica dioica L.). J Ethnopharmacol 2004;90(2-3):205-15.

Guns ES, Cowell SP. Drug insight: lycopene in the prevention and treatment of prostate cancer.

Nat Clin Pract Urol 2005;2(1):38-43.

Habtemariam S, et al. The muscle relaxant properties of Portulaca oleracea are associated with high concentrations of potassium ions. J Ethnopharmacol 1993;40(3):195-200.

Hornykiewicz O. L-DOPA: from a biologically inactive amino acid to a successful therapeutic agent. Amino Acids 2002;23(1-3):65-70.

Huseini HF, et al. The efficacy of Liv-52 on liver cirrhotic patients: a randomized, double-blind, placebo-controlled first approach. Phytomedicine 2005;12(9):619-24.

Islam MS, et al. Anthocyanin compositions in sweetpotato (Ipomoea batatas L.) leaves. Biosci Biotechnol Biochem 2002;66(11):2483-6.

Jeon HJ, et al. Anti-inflammatory activity of Taraxacum officinale. J Ethnopharmacol 2008;115(1):82-8.

Joseph JA, et al. Long-term dietary strawberry, spinach, or vitamin E supplementation retards the onset of age-related neuronal signal-transduction and cognitive behavioral deficits. J Neurosci 1998;18(19):8047-55.

Juan ME, et al. Erythrodiol, a natural triterpenoid from olives, has antiproliferative and apoptotic activity in HT-29 human adenocarcinoma cells. Mol Nutr Food Res 2008;52(5):595-9.

Karimi G, et al. Evaluation of the gastric antiulcerogenic effects of Portulaca oleracea L. extracts in mice. Phytother Res 2004;18(6):484-7.

Kataoka S. Functional effects of Japanese style fermented soy sauce (shoyu) and its components. J Biosci Bioeng 2005;100(3):227-34.

Kataria A, Chauhan BM. Contents and digestibility of carbohydrates of mung beans (Vigna radiata L.) as affected by domestic processing and cooking. Plant Foods Hum Nutr 1988;38(1):51-9.

Kiani F, et al. Dietary risk factors for ovarian cancer: the Adventist Health Study (United States). Cancer Causes Control 2006;17(2):137-46.

Kim MH, Joo HG. Immunostimulatory effects of fucoidan on bone marrow-derived dendritic cells. Immunol Lett 2008;115(2):138-43.

Konrad A, et al. Ameliorative effect of IDS 30, a stinging nettle leaf extract, on chronic colitis. Int J Colorectal Dis 2005;20(1):9-17.

Kucharz EJ. Application of avocado/soybean unsaponifiable mixtures (piascledine) in treatment of patients with osteoarthritis. Ortop Traumatol Rehabil 2003;5(2):248-51.

Kurata R, et al. Growth suppression of human cancer cells by polyphenolics from sweet potato (Ipomoea batatas L.) leaves. J Agric Food Chem 2007;55(1):185-90.

Lomnitski L, et al. Composition, efficacy, and safety of spinach extracts. Nutr Cancer 2003;46(2):222-31.

Long LH, et al. The antioxidant activities of seasonings used in Asian cooking. Powerful antioxidant activity of dark soy sauce revealed using the ABTS assay. Free Radic Res 2000;32(2):181-6.

López-Molina D, et al. Molecular properties and prebiotic effect of inulin obtained from artichoke (Cynara scolymus L.). Phytochemistry 2005;66(12):1476-84.

Maeda H, et al. Seaweed carotenoid, fucoxanthin, as a multi-functional nutrient. Asia Pac J Clin Nutr 2008;17(Suppl 1):196-9.

Malek F, et al. Bronchodilatory effect of Portulaca oleracea in airways of asthmatic patients. Phytother Res 2004;18(6):484-7.

Maruyama H, Yamamoto I. An antitumor fucoidan fraction from an edible brown seaweed, Laminaria religiosa. Hydrobiologia 2002;116/117(1):534-6.

Menendez JA, et al. Olive oil's bitter principle reverses acquired autoresistance to trastuzumab (Herceptin) in HER2-overexpressing breast cancer cells. BMC Cancer 2007;7:80.

Momin RA, Nair MG. Antioxidant, cyclooxygenase and topoisomerase inhibitory compounds from Apium graveolens Linn. seeds. Phytomedicine 2002;9(4):312-8.

Nottingham, S. Beetroot. http://ourworld. compuserve.com/homepages/Stephen_ Nottingham/beetroot.htm

Owen RW, et al. Olive-oil consumption and health: the possible role of antioxidants. Lancet Oncol 2000;1:107-12.

Parmenter, G. Taraxacum officinale: Common dandelion, lion's tooth. New Zealand Institute for Food and Crop Research Ltd at: file http://www.crop.cri.nz/home/products-services/publications/broadsheets/058dandelion.pdf

Petri Nahas E, et al. Benefits of soy germ isoflavones in postmenopausal women with contraindication for conventional hormone replacement therapy. Maturitas 2004;48(4):372-80.

Philpott M, et al. In situ and in vitro antioxidant activity of sweetpotato anthocyanins. J Agric Food Chem 2004;52(6):1511-3.

Pool-Zobel BL. Inulin-type fructans and reduction in colon cancer risk: review of experimental and human data. Br J Nutr 2005;93(Suppl 1):S73-90.

Sacks FM, et al. Soy protein, isoflavones, and cardiovascular health: an American Heart Association Science Advisory for professionals from the Nutrition Committee. Circulation 2006;113(7):1034-44.

Safarinejad MR. Urtica dioica for treatment of benign prostatic hyperplasia: a prospective, randomized, double-blind, placebo-controlled, crossover study. J Herb Pharmacother 2005;5(4):1-11.

Schutz K, et al. Taraxacum: a review on its phytochemical and pharmacological profile. J Ethnopharmacol 2006;107(3):313-23.

Seaweeds website at http://www.innvista.com/HEALTH/foods/vegetables/seaveg.htm

Sigstedt SC, et al. Evaluation of aqueous extracts of Taraxacum officinale on growth and invasion of breast and prostate cancer cells. Int J Oncol 2008;32(5):1085-90.

Simopoulos AP, et al. Common purslane: a source of omega-3 fatty acids and antioxidants. J Am Coll Nutr 1992;11(4):374-82.

Skibola CF. The effect of Fucus vesiculosus, an edible brown seaweed, upon menstrual cycle length and hormonal status in three pre-menopausal women: a case report. BMC Complement Altern Med 2004;4:10.

Stahl W, et al. Dietary tomato paste protects against ultraviolet light-induced erythema in humans. J Nutr 2001;131:1449-51.

Truong VD, et al. Phenolic acid content and composition in leaves and roots of common commercial sweetpotato (Ipomea batatas L.) cultivars in the United States. J Food Sci 2007;72(6):C343-9.

Tuetun B, et al. Repellent properties of celery, Apium graveolens L., compared with commercial repellents, against mosquitoes under laboratory and field conditions. Trop Med Int Health 2005;10(11):1190-8.

University of Granada. Compound from olive-pomace oil inhibits HIV spread. ScienceDaily 2007;at: http://www.sciencedaily.com/releases/2007/07/070709111536.htm

Visioli F, et al. Mediterranean food and health: building human evidence. J Physiol Pharmacol 2005;56(Suppl 1):37-49.

Visioli F, et al. Antioxidant and other biological activities of phenols from olives and olive oil. Med Res Rev 2002;22(1):65-75.

Warri A, et al. The role of early life genistein exposures in modifying breast cancer risk. Br J Cancer 2008;98(9):1485-93.

Waterman E, Lockwood B. Active components and clinical applications of olive oil. Altern Med Rev 2007;12(4):331-42.

Wegener T, Fintelmann V. Pharmacological properties and therapeutic profile of artichoke (Cynara scolymus L.). Wien Med Wochenschr 1999;149(8-10):241-7.

World carrot museum: A website full of information on all aspects of the carrot at: http://www.carrotmuseum.co.uk/index.html

Xiao CW . Health effects of soy protein and isoflavones in humans. J Nutr 2008;138(6):1244S-9S.

Yuan YV, Walsh NA. Antioxidant and antiproliferative activities of extracts from a variety of edible seaweeds. Food Chem Toxicol 2006;44(7):1144-50.

Zhu X, et al. Phenolic compounds from the leaf extract of artichoke (Cynara scolymus L.) and their antimicrobial activities. J Agric Food Chem 2004;52(24):7272-8.

Zidorn C, et al. Polyacetylenes from the Apiaceae vegetables carrot, celery, fennel, parsley, and parsnip and their cytotoxic activities. J Agric Food Chem 2005;53(7):2518-23.

Brassicas (broccili, nasturtium, watercress), garlic and onions

Albrecht U, et al. A randomised, double-blind, placebo-controlled trial of a herbal medicinal product containing Tropaeoli majoris herba (nasturtium) and Armoraciae rusticanae radix (horseradish) for the prophylactic treatment of patients with chronically recurrent lower urinary tract infections. Curr Med Res Opin 2007;23(10):2415-22.

Avcı A, et al. Effects of garlic consumption on plasma and erythrocyte antioxidant parameters in elderly subjects. Gerontology 2008;54(3):173-6.

Barillari J, et al. Direct antioxidant activity of purified glucoerucin, the dietary secondary metabolite contained in rocket (Eruca sativa Mill.) seeds and sprouts. J Agric Food Chem 2005;53(7):2475-82.

Beecher CW. Cancer preventive properties of varieties of Brassica oleracea: a review. Am J Clin Nutr 1994;(Suppl 5):1166S-70S.

Borek C. Garlic reduces dementia and heart-disease risk. J Nutr 2006;136(3 suppl):810S-2S.

Boyd LA, et al. Assessment of the anti-genotoxic, anti-proliferative, and anti-metastatic potential of crude watercress extract in human colon cancer cells. Nutr Cancer 2006;55(2):232-41.

Brandi G, et al. Mechanisms of action and antiproliferative properties of Brassica oleracea juice in human breast cancer cell lines. J Nutr 2005;135(6):1503-9.

Challier B, et al. Garlic, onion and cereal fibre as protective factors for breast cancer: a French case-control study. Eur J Epidemiol 1998;14(8):737-47.

Draelos ZD. The ability of onion extract gel to improve the cosmetic appearance of postsurgical scars. J Cosmet Dermatol 2008;7(2):101-4.

El D, et al. Cancer chemoprevention by garlic and garlic-containing sulfur and selenium compounds. J Nutr 2006;136(Suppl 3):864S-9S.

Fahey JW, et al. Broccoli sprouts: an exceptionally rich source of inducers of enzymes that protect against chemical carcinogens. Proc Natl Acad Sci USA 1997;94:10367-72.

Finley JW, Davis CD. High-selenium broccoli vs. colon cancer. Agric Res, New Zealand, July, 2000.

Fleischauer AT, et al. Garlic consumption and cancer prevention: meta-analyses of colorectal and stomach cancers. Am J Clin Nutr 2000;72(4):1047-52.

Fowke JH, et al. Brassica vegetable consumption shifts estrogen metabolism in healthy postmenopausal women. Cancer Epidemiol Biomarkers Prev 2000;9(8):773-9.

Galeone C, et al. Onion and garlic use and human

cancer. Am J Clin Nutr 2006;84(5):1027-32.

Gill CI, et al. Watercress supplementation in diet reduces lymphocyte DNA damage and alters blood antioxidant status in healthy adults. Am J Clin Nutr 2007;85(2):504-10.

Goos KH, et al. On-going investigations on efficacy and safety profile of a herbal drug containing nasturtium herb and horseradish root in acute sinusitis, acute bronchitis and acute urinary tract infection in children in comparison with other antibiotic treatments. Arzneimittelforschung 2007;57(4):238-46.

Henneicke-von Zepelin H, et al. Efficacy and safety of a fixed combination phytomedicine in the treatment of the common cold (acute viral respiratory tract infection): results of a randomised, double blind, placebo controlled, multicentre study. Curr Med Res Opin 1999;15(3):214-27.

Ishikawa H, et al. Aged garlic extract prevents a decline of NK cell number and activity in patients with advanced cancer. J Nutr 2006;136(Suppl 3):816S-20S.

Keum YS, et al. Chemopreventive functions of isothiocyanates. Drug News Perspect 2005;18(7):445-51.

Martínez-Sánchez A, et al. A comparative study of flavonoid compounds, vitamin C, and antioxidant properties of baby leaf Brassicaceae species. J Agric Food Chem 2008;56(7):2330-40.

Mayer B, et al. Effects of an onion-olive oil maceration product containing essential ingredients of the Mediterranean diet on blood pressure and blood fluidity. Arzneimittelforschung 2001;51(2):104-11.

Mennen LI, et al. Consumption of foods rich in flavonoids is related to a decreased cardiovascular risk in apparently healthy French women. J Nutr 2004;134(4):923-6.

Milner JA. Preclinical perspectives on garlic and cancer. J Nutr 2006;136(Suppl 3):827S-31S.

Morihara N, et al. Garlic as an anti-fatigue agent. Mol Nutr Food Res 2007;51(11):1329-34.

Nagini S. Cancer chemoprevention by garlic and its organosulfur compounds-panacea or promise? Anti-cancer Agents Med Chem 2008;8(3):313-21.

Rahman K, Lowe GM. Garlic and cardiovascular disease: a critical review. J Nutr 2006;136(Suppl 3):736S-40S.

Ribnicky DM, et al. Seed of Barbarea verna as a rich source of phenyl isothiocyanate to provide natural protection from environmental and dietary toxins. J Nutraceut Funct Med Foods 2001;3(3):43-65.

Song K, Milner JA. The influence of heating on the anti-cancer properties of garlic. J Nutr 2001;131(3s):1054S-7S.

Srinivasan K. Plant foods in the management of diabetes mellitus: spices as beneficial anti-diabetic food adjuncts. Int J Food Sci Nutr 2005;56(6):399-414.

Thomson M, et al. Including garlic in the diet may help lower blood glucose, cholesterol, and triglycerides. J Nutr 2006;136(Suppl 3):800S-2S.

van Poppel G, et al. Brassica vegetables and cancer prevention. Epidemiology and mechanisms. Adv Exp Med Biol 1999;472:159-68.

Verhagen H, et al. Reduction of oxidative DNA-damage in humans by Brussels sprouts. Carcinogenesis 1995;16(4):969-70.

Verhoeven DT, et al. A review of mechanisms underlying anticarcinogenicity by brassica vegetables. Chem Biol Interact 1997;103(2):79-129.

Weil MJ, et al. Tumor cell proliferation and cyclooxygenase inhibitory constituents in horseradish (Armoracia rusticana) and wasabi (Wasabia japonica). J Agric Food Chem 2005;53(5):1440-4.

Wong RW, Rabie AB. Effect of quercetin on bone formation. J Orthop Res 2008;26(8):1061-6.

Others (cocoa, hops, liquorice, spirulina, tea, yeast)

Allen RR, et al. Daily consumption of a dark chocolate containing flavanols and added sterol esters affects cardiovascular risk factors in a normotensive population with elevated cholesterol. J Nutr 2008;138(4):725-31.

Anderson RA. Chromium in the prevention and control of diabetes. Diabet Metab 2000;26:22-7.

Antonello M, et al. Prevention of hypertension, cardiovascular damage and endothelial dysfunction with green tea extracts. Am J Hypertens 2007;20(12):1321-8.

Asl MN, Hosseinzadeh H. Review of pharmacological effects of Glycyrrhiza sp. and its bioactive compounds. Phytother Res 2008;22(6):709-24.

Barclay L. Eating chocolate may decrease risk for preeclampsia. Medscape Medical News. May 2008.

Bertipaglia de Santana M, et al. Association between soy and green tea (Camellia sinensis) diminishes hypercholesterolemia and increases total plasma antioxidant potential in dyslipidemic subjects. Nutrition 2008;24(6):562-8.

Cabrera C, et al. Beneficial effects of green tea – a review. J Am Coll Nutr 2006;25(2):79-99.

Chen D, et al. Green tea and tea polyphenols in cancer prevention. Front Biosci 2004;9:2618-31.

Chen D, et al. Tea polyphenols, their biological effects and potential molecular targets. Histol Histopathol 2008;23(4):487-96.

Cui YM, et al. Effect of Glabridin from Glycyrrhiza glabra on learning and memory in mice. Planta Med 2008;74(4):377-80.

Dallard I, et al. Is cacao a psychotropic drug? Psychopathologic study of a population of subjects self-identified as chocolate addicts. Encephale 2001;27(2):181-6.

Delmulle L, et al. Anti-proliferative properties of prenylated flavonoids from hops (Humulus lupulus L.) in human prostate cancer cell lines. Phytomedicine 2006;13(9-10):732-4.

Ding EL, et al. Chocolate and prevention of cardiovascular disease: A systematic review. Nutr Metab (Lond) 2006;3(1):2.

Gerhäuser C. Beer constituents as potential cancer chemopreventive agents. Eur J Cancer 2005;41(13):1941-54.

Grassi D, et al. Cocoa reduces blood pressure and insulin resistance and improves endothelium-dependent vasodilation in hypertensives. Hypertension 2005;46(2):398-405.

Hayashi K, et al. A natural sulfated polysaccharide, calcium spirulan, isolated from Spirulina platensis: in vitro and ex vivo evaluation of anti-herpes simplex virus and anti-human immunodeficiency virus activities. AIDS Res Hum Retroviruses 1996;12(15):1463-71.

Hegoczki J, et al. Preparation of chromium enriched yeasts. Acta Aliment 1997;26:345–58.

Hertog M, et al. Dietary antioxidant flavonoids and risk of coronary heart disease: the Zutphen Elderly Study. Lancet 1993;342:1007-11.

Hodgson JM, et al. Chocolate consumption and bone density in older women. Am J Clin Nutr 2008;87(1):175-80.

Hollenberg KN. Vascular action of cocoa flavanols in humans: the roots of the story. J Cardiovasc Pharmacol 2006;47(Suppl 2):S99-102; discussion S119-21.

Inaba H, et al. Identification of hop polyphenolic components which inhibit prostaglandin E2 production by gingival epithelial cells stimulated with periodontal pathogen. Biol Pharm Bull 2008;31(3):527-30.

Isbrucker RA, Burdock GA. Risk and safety assessment on the consumption of licorice root (Glycyrrhiza sp.), its extract and powder as a food ingredient, with emphasis on the pharmacology and toxicology of glycyrrhizin. Regul Toxicol Pharmacol 2006;46(3):167-92.

Khan Z, et al. Nutritional and therapeutic potential of Spirulina. Curr Pharm Biotechnol 2005;6(5):373-9.

Kurahashi N, et al. Green tea consumption and prostate cancer risk in Japanese men: a prospective study. Am J Epidemiol 2008;167(1):71-7.

Lee KW, et al. Cocoa has more phenolic phytochemicals and a higher antioxidant capacity than teas and red wine. J Agric Food Chem 2003;51(25):7292-5.

Mani UV, et al. Studies on the long-term effect of spirulina supplementation on serum lipid profile and glycated proteins in NIDDM patients. J Nutraceut Funct Med Foods 2000;2(3):25-32.

Marcus DA, et al. A double-blind provocative study of chocolate as a trigger of headache. Cephalalgia 1997;17(8):855-62; discussion 800.

Maron DJ, et al. Cholesterol-lowering effect of a theaflavin-enriched green tea extract: a randomized controlled trial. Arch Intern Med 2003;163(12):1448-53.

Monteiro R, et al. Modulation of breast cancer cell survival by aromatase inhibiting hop (Humulus lupulus L.) flavonoids. J Steroid Biochem Mol Biol 2007;105(1-5):124-30.

Morin CM, et al. Valerian-hops combination and diphenhydramine for treating insomnia: A randomized placebo-controlled clinical trial. Sleep 2005;28(11):1465-71.

Nagao T, et al. A green tea extract high in catechins reduces body fat and cardiovascular risks in humans. Obesity (Silver Spring) 2007;15(6):1473-83.

Natarajan P, et al. Positive antibacterial co-action between hop (Humulus lupulus) constituents and selected antibiotics. Phytomedicine 2008;15(3):194-201.

Overk CR, et al. Comparison of the in vitro estrogenic activities of compounds from hops (Humulus lupulus) and red clover (Trifolium pratense). J Agric Food Chem 2005;53(16):6246-53.

Porter D, et al. Chromium: friend or foe? Arch Fam Med 1999;8:386-90.

Ratnasooriya WD, Fernando TS. Effect of black tea brew of Camellia sinensis on sexual competence of male rats. J Ethnopharmacol 2008;118(3):373-7.

Rechter S, et al. Antiviral activity of Arthrospira-derived spirulan-like substances. Antiviral Res 2006;72(3):197-206.

Sarma DN, et al. Safety of green tea extracts: a systematic review by the US Pharmacopeia. Drug Saf 2008;31(6):469-84.

Shibata S. A drug over the millennia: pharmacognosy, chemistry, and pharmacology of licorice. Yakugaku Zasshi 2000;120(10):849-62.

Shukla Y. Tea and cancer chemoprevention: a comprehensive review. Asian Pac J Cancer Prev 2007;8(2):155-66.

Singh S, et al. Bioactive compounds from cyanobacteria and microalgae: an overview. Crit Rev Biotechnol 2005;25(3):73-95.

Teas J, et al. Algae – a poor man's HAART? Med Hypotheses 2004;62(4):507-10.

Usmani O, et al. Theobromine inhibits sensory nerve activation and cough. FASEB J 2005;19(2):231-3.

Vlachopoulos C, et al. Effect of dark chocolate on arterial function in healthy individuals. Am J Hypertens 2005;18(6):785-91.

Wang Y, et al. Dietary supplementation with blueberries, spinach, or spirulina reduces ischemic brain damage. Exp Neurol 2005;193(1):75-84.

Index